Cognitive and Behavioral Dysfunction in Schizophrenia

Cognitive and Behavioral Dysfunction in Schizophrenia

Ahmed A. Moustafa

ELSEVIER

ACADEMIC PRESS
An imprint of Elsevier

Academic Press
125 London Wall, London EC2Y 5AS, United Kingdom
525 B Street, Suite 1650, San Diego, CA 92101, United States
50 Hampshire Street, 5th Floor, Cambridge, MA 02139, United States
The Boulevard, Langford Lane, Kidlington, Oxford OX5 1GB, United Kingdom

Library of Congress Cataloging-in-Publication Data
A catalog record for this book is available from the Library of Congress

British Library Cataloguing-in-Publication Data
A catalogue record for this book is available from the British Library

ISBN: 978-0-12-820005-6

For information on all Academic Press publications
visit our website at https://www.elsevier.com/books-and-journals

Publisher: Nikki Levy
Acquisitions Editor: Joslyn Chaiprasert-Paguio
Editorial Project Manager: Devlin Person
Production Project Manager: Kiruthika Govindaraju
Cover Designer: Greg Harris

Typeset by SPi Global, India

Contents

Contributors

Ahmed A. Moustafa School of Psychology & Marcs Institute for Brain and Behaviour, Western Sydney University, Sydney, NSW, Australia; Department of Human Anatomy and Physiology, the Faculty of Health Sciences, University of Johannesburg, South Africa

Alaa Eldin A. Ayoub College of Graduate Studies, Arabian Gulf University, Bahrain

Noémi Báthori Budapest University of Technology and Economics, Budapest, Hungary

Victor Counted School of Psychology & Marcs Institute for Brain and Behaviour, Western Sydney University, Sydney, NSW, Australia

Abeer M. Eissa Faculty of Medicine, Ain Shams University, Cairo, Egypt

Nagla N. El Mahallawy Institute of Psychiatry, Faculty of Medicine, Ain Shams University, Cairo, Egypt

Mahmoud H.I. El-Essawy Faculty of Medicine, Ain Shams University, Cairo, Egypt

Hossam ElKhatib Misr International University, Cairo, Egypt

Belinda Favaloro School of Psychology, University of Western Sydney, Sydney, NSW, Australia

Dorota Frydecka Department of Psychiatry, Wroclaw Medical University, Wroclaw, Poland

Pronab Ganguly Flourish, Australia

Anchal Garg School of Psychology, Western Sydney University, Sydney, NSW, Australia

Shadi Gray School of Psychology, Western Sydney University, Sydney, NSW, Australia

Eid Abo Hamza Faculty of Education, Department of Mental Health, Tanta University, Egypt; College of Graduate Studies, Arabian Gulf University, Bahrain

Ahmed A. Helal Faculty of Education, Department of Mental Health, Tanta University, Egypt

Doaa H. Hewedi Institute of Psychiatry, Faculty of Medicine, Ain Shams University, Cairo, Egypt

Pedja Ilic. School of Psychology, Western Sydney University, Sydney, NSW, Australia

Glessia Matar School of Psychology, Western Sydney University, Sydney, NSW, Australia

Daniel Miezah School of Psychology, Western Sydney University, Sydney, NSW, Australia

Błażej Misiak Department of Genetics, Wroclaw Medical University, Wroclaw, Poland

Alejandro Morris School of Psychology & Marcs Institute for Brain and Behaviour, Western Sydney University, Sydney, NSW, Australia

Patryk Piotrowski Department of Psychiatry, Wroclaw Medical University, Wroclaw, Poland

Bertalan Polner Budapest University of Technology and Economics, Budapest, Hungary

Alaa M.A. Soliman Faculty of Medicine, Ain Shams University, Cairo, Egypt

Kristina Ulm Faculty of Built Environment, University of New South Wales, Sydney, NSW, Australia

Ahmad Valikhani Department of Clinical Psychology, School of Education and Psychology, Shiraz University, Shiraz, Iran

Part One

Behavioral impairment in schizophrenia and related disorders

Masking impairments in schizophrenia and schizotypal personality disorder

1

Glessia Matar[a], Anchal Garg[a], Alejandro Morris[b], Shadi Gray[a], Pedja Ilic.[a], Daniel Miezah[a], and Ahmed A. Moustafa[b,c]
[a]School of Psychology, Western Sydney University, Sydney, NSW, Australia [b]School of Psychology & Marcs Institute for Brain and Behaviour, Western Sydney University, Sydney, NSW, Australia [c]Department of Human Anatomy and Physiology, the Faculty of Health Sciences, University of Johannesburg, South Africa

Chapter outline

Schizophrenia

Schizophrenia is a debilitating psychotic disorder characterized by a breakdown in thinking and poor emotional functioning with an onset typically occurring during late adolescence or early adulthood (Cicero, Martin, Becker, Docherty, & Kerns, 2014; Mikanmaa et al., 2019). Schizophrenia spectrum and other psychotic disorders are characterized by abnormalities in one or more of the following five domains: delusions, hallucinations, disorganized thinking (i.e., speech), grossly disorganized or abnormal motor behavior (including catatonia), and negative symptoms (American Psychiatric Association, 2013). Moreover, individuals with schizophrenia often show distractibility, disassociation, and neural impairments in the mesolimbic cortical structures, namely over-activation of dopaminergic pathways from the ventral segmental area (VTA) to the nucleus accumbens, amygdala, and hippocampus. In addition, there is an under-activation of the frontal cortex (hypofrontality) (Braver, Barch, & Cohen, 1999; Fernandes et al., 2019; Ganguly, Soliman, & Moustafa, 2018; Langdon, Connors, & Connaughton, 2014; Lauffs et al., 2016; Meehl, 1962; Moustafa et al., 2016; Pariyadath, Gowin, & Stein, 2016; Tamminga & Medoff, 2002; Veit, Hakim, Jadi, Sejnowski, & Adesnik, 2017).

Cognitive and Behavioral Dysfunction in Schizophrenia. https://doi.org/10.1016/B978-0-12-820005-6.00009-8

The pathogenesis of schizophrenia is considered to be multifactorial as it has been linked to gene–environment interactions (Nimgaonkar, Prasad, Chowdari, Severance, & Yolken, 2017; Tarbox, Almasy, Gur, Nimgaonkar, & Pogue-Geile, 2012). For instance, *COMT*, *BDNF*, and *FKBP5* genes have been found to interact with cannabis use and childhood trauma (Misiak et al., 2018). Interestingly, schizophrenia also shares a genetic predisposition with other disorders including schizoaffective disorder, affective psychoses, and schizotypal personality disorder as they share considerable overlap by implicating similar polymorphisms in their phenotypes (Butler, McGuire, Masoud, & Manzardo, 2016; Ettinger, Meyhöfer, Steffens, Wagner, & Koutsouleris, 2014; Flückiger et al., 2019; Kendler et al., 1993; Loh et al., 2015). However, the relationships among cognitive and neural impairments and the effect they have on individual symptoms in schizophrenia (positive, negative, and cognitive symptoms) remains to be elucidated in future studies (Mikanmaa et al., 2019; Thoenes & Oberfeld, 2017; Veit et al., 2017).

Schizotypal personality disorder

Schizotypal personality disorder (SPD) is characterized by both positive and negative symptoms (Lenzenweger, 2018; McClure, Harvey, Bowie, Iacoviello, & Siever, 2013; Racioppi et al., 2018). The diagnosis of schizotypal personality disorder follows a categorical approach as prescribed by the Diagnostic and Statistical Manual Of Mental Disorders-5th Edition (DSM-5; American Psychiatric Association, 2013). Further, individuals must demonstrate that the disorder affects different areas of their life (e.g. family, work, social environments), with a minimum of five out of the nine criteria that broadly include areas of unusual thoughts, behavior, speech, or limited social interest and contact (American Psychiatric Association, 2013). In other words, a schizotypal personality disorder is a pervasive pattern of social and interpersonal deficits marked by acute discomfort, reduced capacity for a close relationship as well as by cognitive or perceptual distortions and eccentricities of behavior (American Psychiatric Association, 2013).

Schizotypal personality disorder involves a subthreshold presentation of some schizophrenia symptoms (Callaway, Cohen, Matthews, & Dinzeo, 2014). Individuals who are high in schizotypal personality disorder personality traits usually exhibit a presence of attenuated psychotic, emotional, and cognitive symptoms often observed in schizophrenia (Callaway et al., 2014). As a result, individuals who exhibit high schizotypal personality disorder traits have greater liability for the future development of schizophrenia (Cicero et al., 2014). Schizotypal personality disorder's symptoms (e.g., hallucinations and delusions) are also prevalent in undiagnosed relatives of patients with schizophrenia (Nuechterlein et al., 2002; Takayanagi et al., 2018). Further, magnetic resonance imaging (MRI) studies have reported that persons with schizotypal personality disorder show similar abnormalities in gray-matter volume (a major component of the central nervous system) as in individuals with chronic schizophrenia (Lenzenweger, 2018; Modinos et al., 2010; Nishikawa et al., 2016; Takayanagi et al., 2018). Thus, early identification and treatment for individuals who are at risk of developing schizophrenia can provide multiple benefits, including a delay in the onset of the psychotic disorder, a reduced period of untreated psychosis, or even the prevention of such disorders (Cohen, Callaway, Najolia, Larsen, & Strauss, 2012).

Perceptual deficits in schizophrenia and schizotypal personality disorder

Patients with schizophrenia exhibit cognitive deficits in various domains such as attention, memory, and executive functioning (Crouse, Moustafa, Bogaty, Hickie, & Hermens, 2018; Hazlett et al., 2014; Olivier et al., 2017; Stramecki et al., 2018; Tadin et al., 2006; Yang et al., 2013). They display difficulties producing speech, maintaining and manipulating informative stimuli, as well as performing executive functions such as goal-directed behavior and flexible thinking (Fan et al., 2019; Tripathi, Kar, & Shukla, 2018). However, less is known regarding the role perceptual functions can play in maintaining and exacerbating schizophrenia symptomology (Lauffs et al., 2016). Some studies reaffirm that deficits in perceptual processes are key factors that relate to the state, severity, and treatment of schizophrenia, which may even last post-treatment (Kim & Park, 2011; Kogata & Iidaka, 2018; Olivier et al., 2017). Furthermore, perceptual deficits may influence cognitive functioning or occur on their own, but perceptual deficits are usually not associated with clinical symptoms (Kim & Park, 2011; Olivier et al., 2017). One study did find the poor perceptive ability to be negatively correlated with positive clinical symptoms in patients with first-episode schizophrenia (Olivier et al., 2017).

Schizophrenia patients display deficits in perceptual processes including visual, auditory, or somatosensory modalities (Ettinger et al., 2015; Kogata & Iidaka, 2018). These patients exhibit visual perceptual deficits as a result of a disconnection between the occipital and parietal lobe in the dorsal pathway, which hinders their ability to motion and spatial information processing (Demmin, Fradkin, & Silverstein, 2019; Deng et al., 2019; Grzeczkowski et al., 2018; Herzog, Roinishvili, Chkonia, & Brand, 2013; Thormodsen et al., 2011). In addition, a recent study found that neuroanatomical deficits in the visual cortex (reduced V1/V2 area and overall volume) were associated with an increased severity of schizophrenia symptomology on the Clinical Global Impression scale (CGI scale), as well as greater propensity to express negative symptoms that resulted in decreased velocity discrimination (Adhan et al., 2020). Moreover, studies have also found distorted visual experience involving the perception of color, size, facial expressions, and motion in samples of schizophrenia patients (Fernandes et al., 2019; Hazlett et al., 2014;Kim & Park, 2011 ; Lauffs et al., 2016). Deficits in visual perception are also related to poor performance on discrimination tasks (Cadenhead, Dobkins, McGovern, & Shafer, 2013; Fernandes et al., 2019), altered visual backward masking effect (Favrod et al., 2017; Myamlin, Kirenskaya, & Novototsky-Vlasov, 2016; Slaghuis & Bakker, 1995), impaired motion perception (Elshaikh, Sponheim, Chafee, & MacDonald, 2015), decrease in contrast sensitivity (Dakin, Carlin, & Hemsley, 2005), and poor discrimination of biological motion (Kim & Park, 2011; Lauffs et al., 2016).

Studies of the visual systems have proven to be a useful method for ascertaining the neural mechanisms that underlie perceptual deficits in schizophrenia patients (Bedwell, Rassovsky, Orem, & Kamath, 2011; Butler, Silverstein, & Dakin, 2008; Ettinger et al., 2015). The human subcortical visual system can be divided into magnocellular and parvocellular pathways. These pathways begin in the retina via the lateral geniculate nucleus and project to various layers of the primary visual cortex (Butler et al., 2008;

Ettinger et al., 2015; Marosi, Fodor, & Csukly, 2019). Generally, the neurons in the magnocellular system are more sensitive to low spatial frequencies, have momentary responses, and faster transmission (Bedwell et al., 2011; Kim & Park, 2011). The magnocellular system orients information to the space (where system) and projects to the dorsal visual system, which is involved in eye-movement control, motion perception and location, and action guidance (Kim & Park, 2011). Meanwhile, neurons in the parvocellular system are selected for high spatial frequencies with low sustained responses. This system is critical for object identification ("what" system) and color processing, and it projects to the ventral visual system (Butler & Javitt, 2005; Lima, Gracitellia, Junior, & Bressan, 2013; Marosi et al., 2019). As a result of neuroanatomical and neurophysiological studies highlighting altered activation of motion perception in the dorsal pathways, individuals with schizophrenia show dysfunctional magnocellular visual pathways (Chieffi, 2019; Jahshan, Wolf, Karbi, Shamir, & Rassovsky, 2017; Jurišic, Ćavar, Sesar, Vukojević, & Ćurković, 2020; Kim & Park, 2011; Martínez et al., 2008).

Research of the visual system in schizophrenia patients has focused on experimental designs such as backward masking, contrast sensitivity, contour detection, and perceptual closure to determine the extent to which magnocellular and parvocellular pathways influence the visual perceptual deficits found in this patient group (Chieffi, 2019). Findings employing these methodological designs suggest schizophrenia patients exhibit disturbances at early processing of visual information due to the magnocellular visual pathway being hypoactive, while the parvocellular remains relatively intact (Bedwell et al., 2011; Jahshan et al., 2017). Moreover, studies on contrast sensitivity, which measures the ability to detect luminance changes within a unit of space, have found that magnocellular-biased stimuli are decreased in patients with schizophrenia (Ansorge, Francis, Herzog, & Ögmen, 2007; Butler & Javitt, 2005). At the same time, they exhibit poor perceptual closure in object recognition tasks as a result of impaired magnocellular dorsal stream crossover input which produces processing alterations at the lateral occipital complex level (Chieffi, 2019). Considering these findings, early visual processing deficits may serve as an endophenotypic marker for individuals with schizophrenia (Fan et al., 2019).

The nature of time perception is linked to attention and arousal as research has suggested hypervigilance to be a contributing factor in the dysregulation of time perception in individuals with schizophrenia (Peterburs, Nitsch, Miltner, & Straube, 2013; Thoenes & Oberfeld, 2017; Ueda, Maruo, & Sumiyoshi, 2018). More specifically, integrated time perception processes such as interval timing (Snowden & Buhusi, 2019) and time perception impairment are associated with general functioning difficulties in everyday life situations in schizophrenia (Roy, Grondin, & Roy, 2012). Moreover, extensive research suggests time processing impairment in individuals with schizophrenia (Peterburs et al., 2013; Thoenes & Oberfeld, 2017). For instance, schizophrenia patients are less accurate and underestimate movement times compared to controls (Peterburs et al., 2013). Additionally, higher positive symptoms scores have been shown to correlate with stronger underestimation of movement time (Peterburs et al., 2013). Recently, it has been proposed individuals with schizophrenia exhibit interval timing deficits as a result of the malfunction in the neurotransmission of dopamine and gamma-amino butyric acid (GABA) through the cortico-striatal-thalamo-cortical loop that leads to a misrepresentation in the sequence of actions, and can result in a misattribution of the causes of consequences (e.g., false beliefs) (Snowden & Buhusi, 2019). In addition, there is abnormal functioning of the supplementary motor area (SMA), which in turn results in a failure in early time processing (Snowden & Buhusi, 2019; Tucci, Buhusi, Gallistel, & Meck, 2014).

Individuals with schizotypal personality disorder show abnormalities in perceptual processes including visual, auditory, and somatosensory modalities (Ettinger et al., 2015). For instance, visual abnormalities in schizotypal personality disorder are marked at early stages of processing, commencing with irregular dorsal stream (Bedwell, Chan, Trachik, & Rassovsky, 2013; Koychev, El-Deredy, Haenschel, & Deakin, 2010), backward masking (Cappe, Herzog, Herzig, Brand, & Mohr, 2012), depth perception, localization (Gruzelier, 1994), organization (Ettinger et al., 2015; Uhlhaas & Silverstein, 2005), and overall rigidity marked by systemic fixation patterns and ordered visual scanning (Gross, Araujo, Zedelius, & Schooler, 2019). The neural mechanism underlying visual abnormalities in schizotypal personality disorder has also been associated with magnocellular dysfunction as well as the precision and degree to which neurons are recruited to complete particular visual and higher cognitive tasks (Ettinger et al., 2015; Gruzelier, 1994; Koychev, Deakin, Haenschel, & El-Deredy, 2011). In the context of schizotypal personality disorder traits, visual processes impairment has been associated with disorganization and positive schizotypal personality disorder traits (Koychev et al., 2011). Despite evidence of abnormalities in visual processes, individuals with high schizotypal personality disorder show intact performance throughout a wide range of visual–spatial tasks that may be due to their ability to access compensatory mechanisms.

Visual masking deficits in schizophrenia

Studies often employ visual masking procedures to assess the earliest components of visual information processing in schizophrenia as they have been proven to be a reliable method of measuring visual processing deficits (Bakanidze et al., 2013; Chkonia et al., 2010; Green, Lee, Wynn, & Mathis, 2011; Herzog & Brand, 2015; Luber, Stanford, Malaspina, & Lisanby, 2007; Silverstein, 2016). According to the visual masking model, individuals' ability to process the target stimulus is reduced by another stimulus that is presented shortly before or after the target, which acts as a mask stimulus (Bakanidze et al., 2013; Herzog & Brand, 2015; Luber et al., 2007). In the masking paradigm, the individual's ability to process one stimulus (e.g., target) is reduced by the presentation of another stimulus shortly before or after (e.g., mask; Rassovsky, Horan, Lee, Sergi, & Green, 2011). There are two types of visual masking procedures that is, forward masking and backward masking. A forward masking procedure is a process whereby a "mask" is presented shortly before the visual target (Green et al., 2011). A backward visual masking procedure is a process whereby a "mask" is presented shortly after the visual target (Green et al., 2011). The "mask" can either overlap or surround the target but never touches the target (Green et al., 2011). Most often, masking appears at stimulus onset asynchronies (SOAs) of approximately 0–100 ms in both backward and forward masking. Visual masking has key advantages such as control over timing up to a millisecond (Green et al., 2011).

Visual masking performance has been indicated to be an interaction between two visual channels that form the basis for complex visual processing, which are the sustained channels and the transient channels (Thormodsen, Juuhl-Langseth, Holmèn, & Rishovd Rund, 2012). The sustained channels convey detailed information for the identification as well as a detailed analysis of visual stimuli, whereas the transient channels convey information about the onset, offset, and location of a visual stimulus (Rund, Oie, & Sundet, 1996). Disrupted performance in visual masking tasks has been identified as a characteristic of individuals with schizophrenia which is likely to be the result of dysfunction within or between the transient or sustained visual channels (da Cruz et al., 2020; Enns & di Lollo, 2000; Herzog et al., 2013; Thormodsen et al., 2011). Alternatively, visual masking is also considered to be a possible indicator of vulnerability in schizophrenia (Thormodsen et al., 2012; Türkörzer et al., 2018).

In the visual backward masking, as the intervals between the target and mask increase in a healthy person, the visual backward masking effect is weakened and disappears (Kim & Park, 2011). The neural basis of the visual backward masking is that the visual stimulus initiates activity in the magnocellular visual channel before it activates the parvocellular visual channel (Kim & Park, 2011). The visual backward masking is closely related to the activities of the two visual channels and their interactions; proposing that different display patterns of the visual backward masking depend on the duration and intensity of the mask (Green et al., 2011; Green, Nuechterlein, & Mintz, 1994; Kim & Park, 2011). When the mask has high duration and intensity, masking by the fusion of two images occurs and is dominated by the parvocellular channel (Kim & Park, 2011). Interruption by the magnocellular activity of the mask to the parvocellular activity of the target is effective but obscured by integration (Butler et al., 2003; Kim & Park, 2011). On the other hand, when the mask has low duration and intensity, masking by the fusion of two images does not occur, as the parvocellular activity of the target is interrupted by magnocellular activity that the onset of the mask triggers (Kim & Park, 2011).

It has been proposed that individuals with schizophrenia have deficits in the very early stages of visual information processes, therefore, requiring a longer stimulus time than others to identify a target stimulus (McClure, 2001). Further, studies have consistently found impairments in individuals with schizophrenia performance during backward masking tasks compared to healthy controls (Butler et al., 2003; Cadenhead, Perry, & Braff, 1996; Green, Nuechterlein, Breitmeyer, & Mintz, 1999; Rund et al., 1996, 2004). Specifically, individuals with schizophrenia have consistently demonstrated poorer performance, a significantly prolonged masking effect, and required longer SOAs to accurately detect the target in comparison to healthy controls (Butler et al., 2003; Green, Hugdahl, & Mitchell, 1994; Kim & Park, 2011). Moreover, masking performance in these paradigms has yielded a nonmonotonic U-shaped function congruent with the proposition that visual perception deficits in schizophrenia exist even when masking is limited to interruption (Rassovsky, Green, Nuechterlein, Breitmeyer, & Mintz, 2004). On the other hand, Green et al. (1999) found that siblings of patients with schizophrenia performed poorly on masking performance as compared to the normal controls which supports the evidence that masking is an indicator of vulnerability in schizophrenia. It has been suggested that such visual backward masking deficits in schizophrenia are due to the dysfunction in the magnocellular visual channels (Green et al., 2011; Kim & Park, 2011). Further, it has been suggested that a hyperactive magnocellular activity mask can interrupt the parvocellular activity for the target and, thus, increasing the masking effect in schizophrenia (Butler et al., 2003; Kim & Park, 2011). It is thought that perception during backward masking is a consequence of frequent communication between lower and higher levels of the various neural pathways within the visual cortex that is needed to resolve ambiguity in perception (Dux, Visser, Goodhew, & Lipp, 2010). During visual processing, information is initially processed by lower-level sensory units in a fast "feed-forward" sweep (Green, Nuechterlein, & Breitmeyer, 1997). However, it was found that "re-entrant" cortical feedback sweeps from higher to lower visual processing areas which are crucial in order to refine the visual percept into visual conscious perception (Dux et al., 2010).

Early disturbances of visual processing in individuals with schizophrenia have also been assessed using the visual masking paradigms (Cadenhead, Serper, & Braff, 1998; Cappe et al., 2012). Moreover, results have consistently demonstrated that deficits on these tasks in patients with schizophrenia, as they required longer time intervals between target and mask to be able to identify the target (Cadenhead et al., 1998; Rassovsky et al., 2011). It is also important to focus on early visual processing deficits in schizophrenia because they are related to poor real-world functioning experiences, including educational, employment, socialization, self-care, and home-care activities (Bakanidze et al., 2013; Chkonia et al., 2010; Granholm et al., 2020; Rassovsky et al., 2011). This visual processing deficit was also found in early-onset schizophrenia (Rund et al., 1996), remission cases of schizophrenia (Green et al., 1999), and their unaffected siblings and first-degree relatives (Chkonia et al., 2010; Green, Nuechterlein, Breitmeyer, & Mintz, 2006) indicating that this effect may be a possible trait marker which reflects the vulnerability to schizophrenia. Therefore, visual masking can be a potential endophenotype for schizophrenia.

The masking deficits are also found in at-risk individuals, with remitted symptoms of psychosis or prone to psychosis without exhibiting symptoms (Green et al., 2006; Keri, Kelemen, Benedek, & Janka, 2001). Furthermore, backward visual masking studies on nonclinical college-age students and community samples have indicated that high levels of schizotypal symptoms are also associated with diminished masking performance (Bedwell & Donnelly, 2005; Bedwell & Orem, 2008; Cadenhead et al., 1996; Cappe et al., 2012). Lastly, Bakanidze et al. (2013) assessed five genes in the nicotinic system and their association with individuals with schizophrenia using a visual backward masking task and shine through paradigm, which employs a sensitive backward masking technique that overcomes floor and ceiling effects by determining an interstimulus interval (ISI) with an adaptive technique that yields a good signal to noise ratio (Chkonia et al., 2010). The results demonstrated that performance deficits within the visual backward masking were more distinct in individuals with schizophrenia and their unaffected relatives compared to the healthy controls. Visual backward masking also correlated with the genes investigated (Bakanidze et al., 2013). Thus, highlighting the importance of focusing on visual backward masking deficits in both clinical and nonclinical samples.

The contrast-contrast illusion is a spatial task where the stimuli are presented together; it is selective for texture spatial frequency as well as for texture contrast polarity (Butler et al., 2008). Further, individuals with schizophrenia show a decrease in contrast sensitivity and deficits in contrast gain control (Butler et al., 2008). In Chubb, Sperling, and Solomon (1989), a small textured disc was presented with an intermittent presentation of a high-contrast disc surrounding it. It was hypothesized that the small disc would appear reduced when a high-contrast disc surrounded it, as opposed to when the small disc was presented on its own. The study showed that individuals with schizophrenia were less susceptible to the illusion.

Temporal manipulations

Traditional backward masking tasks mainly utilize temporal perception. Temporal perception refers to a relationship with time, the time intervals between masking and stimulus. Usually, masking tasks employs vernier offsets, where the vernier stimulus is the two vertical bars that slightly offset in the horizontal direction. In each trial, the vernier is randomly offset either to the left or the right, and participants indicate the direction of the offset. Generally, when verniers are presented with long duration, individuals with schizophrenia experience very little or no deficits.

The results of previous studies suggested that there is a general temporal processing deficit in schizophrenia (Chkonia et al., 2010; Davalos, Kisley, & Ross, 2002; Herzog et al., 2013; Peterburs et al., 2013). For instance, patients with schizophrenia showed impaired temporal processing as compared to controls as they consistently underestimated the time a visual stimulus needed to complete a horizontal movement towards the target position (Davalos et al., 2002). On the other hand, Carroll, Boggs, O'Donnell, Shekhar, and Hetrick (2008) found that patients with schizophrenia have less temporal accuracy than controls in the perception of auditory durations.

Spatial manipulations

Spatial perception refers to the spatial distance between target and stimulus. There are only few studies focusing on spatial manipulation in schizophrenia (Dakin et al., 2005; Herzog et al., 2013). For instance, one study found that individuals with schizophrenia were not susceptible to the contrast illusion, with 12 of 15 patients with schizophrenia were more accurate than the most accurate controls (Dakin et al., 2005). On the other hand, Barch et al. (2012) got similar results but not the same magnitude. This could be due to several factors such as sample size, the difference in methodology, and so forth (Slavin & Smith, 2009). Despite methodological differences, these findings were consistent with gain control literature, that is, an expected decrease in center-surround antagonism (CSA) decreased gain control in individuals with schizophrenia. Thus, it can be expected that individuals with schizophrenia or at-risk populations that have been shown to obtain similar performance patterns show little to no effects in relation to spatial manipulations while showing a clear deficit in temporal manipulations testing working memory and visual perception.

Conclusions

Visual masking techniques provide an accurate framework to analyze at millisecond precision the earliest stages of visual processing in patients with schizophrenia. Techniques such as backward masking provide neurobiological insights into the nature of the deficit and thereby improve our understanding of the clinical and functional features of schizophrenia. In addition, one can observe that visual masking tasks are highly connected to well-identified neural processes, namely the parvocellular and magnocellular visual pathways. This chapter has established that patients with schizophrenia require more time than healthy individuals to ascertain the target stimulus in backward masking tests due to the hypoactivation of the magnocellular pathway. Furthermore, patients with schizophrenia exhibited deficits in both spatial and temporal manipulations between targets and stimuli.

In sum, the implications of these findings suggest the existence of disturbances in the early processing of visual information that provide the substrate for higher-level cognitive deficits in working memory, executive functioning, and attention, as well as positive and negative schizophrenia symptomology. To this end, the current chapter is consistent with the generalized theories of visual perceptual deficits in individuals with schizophrenia, and in particular, with a magnocellular pathway impairment.

References

Adhan, I., Lizano, P., Bannai, D., Lutz, O., Dhaliwal, K., Zeng, V., … Keshavan, M. (2020). Visual cortical alterations and their association with negative symptoms in antypsychotic-naïve first episode psychosis. *Psichiatry Research*, *288*, 112957. https://doi.org/10.1016/j.psychres.2020.112957.

American Psychiatric Association. (2013). *Diagnostic and statistical manual of mental disorders* (5th ed.). Arlington, VA: American Psychiatric Publishing.

Ansorge, U., Francis, G., Herzog, M. H., & Ögmen, H. (2007). Visual masking and the dynamics of human perception, cognition, and consciousness. A century of progress, a contemporry synthesis, and future directions. *Advances in Cognitive Psychology*, *3*(1–2), 1–8. https://doi.org/10.2478/v10053-008-0009-0.

Bakanidze, G., Roinishvili, M., Chkonia, E., Kitzrow, W., Richter, S., Neumann, K., … Puls, I. (2013). Association of the nicotinic receptor α7 subunit gene (CHRNA7) with schizophrenia and visual backward masking. *Frontiers in Psychiatry*, *4*, 1–10. https://doi.org/10.3389/fpsyt.2013.00133.

Barch, D. M., Carter, C. S., Dakin, S. C., Gold, J., Luck, S. J., Macdonald, A., III, … Strauss, M. E. (2012). The clinical translation of a measure of gain control: The contrast-contrast effect task. *Schizophrenia Bulletin*, *38*(1), 135–143. https://doi.org/10.1093/schbul/sbr154.

Bedwell, J. S., & Donnelly, R. S. (2005). Schizotypal personality disorder or prodromal symptoms of schizophrenia? *Schizophrenia Research*, *80*(2), 263–269. https://doi.org/10.1016/j.schres.2005.07.023.

Bedwell, J. S., & Orem, D. M. (2008). The effect of red light on backward masking in individuals with psychometrically defined schizotypy. *Cognitive Neuropsychiatry*, *13*(6), 491–504. https://doi.org/10.1080/13546800802605755.

Bedwell, J. S., Rassovsky, Y., Orem, D. M., & Kamath, V. (2011). The backward masking red light effect in schizophrenia: Relationship to clinical features and neurocognitive performance. *Journal of Abnormal Psychology*, *120*(2), 490–496. https://doi.org/10.1037/a0022302.

Bedwell, J. S., Chan, C. C., Trachik, B. J., & Rassovsky, Y. (2013). Changes in the visual-evoked P1 potential as a function of schizotypy and background color in healthy young adults. *Journal of Psychiatric Research*, *47*(4), 542–547. https://doi.org/10.1016/j.jpsychires.2012.12.012.

Braver, T. S., Barch, D. M., & Cohen, J. D. (1999). Cognition and control in schizophrenia: A computational model of dopamine and prefrontal function. *Biological Psychiatry*, *46*(3), 312–328. https://doi.org/10.1016/s0006-3223(99)00116-x.

Butler, P. D., & Javitt, D. C. (2005). Early-stage visual processing deficits in schizophrenia. *Current Opinion in Psychiatry*, *18*(2), 151–157. https://doi.org/10.1097/00001504-200503000-00008.

Butler, P. D., DeSanti, L. A., Maddox, J., Harkavy-Friedman, J. M., Amador, X. F., Goetz, R. R., … Gorman, J. M. (2003). Visual backward-masking deficits in schizophrenia: Relationship to visual pathway function and symptomatology. *Schizophrenia Research*, *59*(2–3), 199–209. https://doi.org/10.1016/s0920-9964(01)00341-3.

Butler, P. D., Silverstein, S. M., & Dakin, S. C. (2008). Visual perception and its impairment in schizophrenia. *Biological Psychiatry*, *64*(1), 40–47. https://doi.org/10.1016/j.biopsych.2008.03.023.

Butler, M. G., McGuire, A. B., Masoud, H., & Manzardo, A. M. (2016). Currently recognized genes for schizophrenia: High-resolution chromosome ideogram representation. *American Journal of Medical Genetics Neuropsychiatic Genetics, Part B*, *171B*, 181–202. https://doi.org/10.1002/ajmg.b.32391.

Cadenhead, K. S., Perry, W., & Braff, D. L. (1996). The relationship of information-processing deficits and clinical symptoms in schizotypal personality disorder. *Biological Psychiatry*, *40*(9), 853–858. https://doi.org/10.1016/0006-3223(95)00547-1.

Cadenhead, K. S., Serper, Y., & Braff, D. L. (1998). Transient versus sustained visual channels in the visual backward masking deficits of schizophrenia patients. *Biological Psychiatry*, *43*(2), 132–138. https://doi.org/10.1016/s0006-3223(97)00316-8.

Cadenhead, K. S., Dobkins, K., McGovern, J., & Shafer, K. (2013). Schizophrenia spectrum participants have reduced visual contrast sensitivity to chromatic (red/green) and luminance (light/dark) stimuli: New insights into information processing, visual channel function, and antipsychotic effects. *Frontiers in Psychology*, *4*, 1–8. https://doi.org/10.3389/fpsyg.2013.00535.

Callaway, D. A., Cohen, A. S., Matthews, R. A., & Dinzeo, T. (2014). Schizotypal personality questionnaire-brief revised: Psychometric replication and extension. *Personality Disorders*, *5*(1), 32–38. https://doi.org/10.1037/per0000041.

Cappe, C., Herzog, M. H., Herzig, D. A., Brand, A., & Mohr, C. (2012). Cognitive disorganisation in schizotypy is associated with deterioration in visual backward masking. *Psychiatry Research*, *200*(2), 652–659. https://doi.org/10.1016/j.psychres.2012.07.001.

Carroll, C. A., Boggs, J., O'Donnell, B. F., Shekhar, A., & Hetrick, W. P. (2008). Temporal processing dysfunction in schizophrenia. *Brain and Cognition*, *67*(2), 150–161. https://doi.org/10.1016/j.bandc.2007.12.005.

Chieffi, S. (2019). Dysfunction of magnocellular/dorsal processing stream in schizophrenia. *Current Psychiatry Research and Reviews*, *15*, 26–36. https://doi.org/10.2174/1573400515666190119163522.

Chkonia, E., Roinishvili, M., Makhatadze, N., Tsverava, L., Stroux, A., Neumann, K., … Brand, A. (2010). The Shine-through masking paradigm is a potential Endophenotype of schizophrenia. *PLoS One*, *5*(12), 1–7. https://doi.org/10.1371/journal.pone.0014268.

Chubb, C., Sperling, C., & Solomon, J. A. (1989). Texture interactions determine perceived contrast (spatial vision/perception/lateral inhibition). *Proceedings of the National Academy of Sciences of the United States of America*, *86*, 9631–9635.

Cicero, D. C., Martin, E. A., Becker, T. M., Docherty, A. R., & Kerns, J. G. (2014). Correspondence between psychometric and clinical high risk for psychosis in an undergraduate population. *Psychological Assessment*, *26*(3), 901–915. https://doi.org/10.1037/a0036432.

Cohen, A. S., Callaway, D. A., Najolia, G. M., Larsen, J. T., & Strauss, G. P. (2012). On "risk" and reward: Investigating state anhedonia in psychometrically defined schizotypy and schizophrenia. *Journal of Abnormal Psychology*, *121*(2), 407–415. https://doi.org/10.1037/a0026155.

Crouse, J. J., Moustafa, A. A., Bogaty, S. E. R., Hickie, I. B., & Hermens, D. F. (2018). Parcellating cognitive heterogeneity in early psychosis-spectrum illness: A cluster analysis. *Schizophrenia Research*, *202*, 91–98. https://doi.org/10.1016/j.schres.2018.06.060.

da Cruz, J. R., Shaqiri, A., Roinishvili, M., Favrod, O., Chkonia, E., Brand, A., … Herzog, M. H. (2020). Neural compensation mechanisms of siblings of schizophrenia patients as revealed by high-density EEG. *Schizophrenia Bulletin*, *46*(4), 1009–1018. https://doi.org/10.1093/schbul/sbz133.

Dakin, S., Carlin, P., & Hemsley, D. (2005). Weak suppression of visual context in chronic schizophrenia. *Current Biology: CB*, *15*(20), R822–R824. https://doi.org/10.1016/j.cub.2005.10.015.

Davalos, D. B., Kisley, M. A., & Ross, R. G. (2002). Deficits in auditory and visual temporal perception in schizophrenia. *Cognitive Neuropsychiatry*, *7*(4), 273–282. https://doi.org/10.1080/13546800143000230.

Demmin, D. L., Fradkin, S. I., & Silverstein, S. M. (2019). Remediation of visual processing impairments in schizophrenia: Where we are and where we need to be. *Current Behavioral Neuroscience Reports*, *6*, 13–20. https://doi.org/10.1007/s40473-019-00171-8.

Deng, Y., Liu, K., Cheng, D., Zhang, J., Chen, H., Chen, B., … Wen, G. (2019). Ventral and dorsal visual pathways exhibit abnormalities of static and dynamic connectivities, respectively, in patients with schizophrenia. *Schizophrenia Research*, *206*, 103–110. https://doi.org/10.1016/j.schres.2018.12.005.

Dux, P. E., Visser, T. A., Goodhew, S. C., & Lipp, O. V. (2010). Delayed reentrant processing impairs visual awareness: An object-substitution-masking study. *Psychological Science*, *21*(9), 1242–1247. https://doi.org/10.1177/0956797610379866.

Elshaikh, A. A., Sponheim, S. R., Chafee, M. V., & MacDonald, A. W. (2015). Spatial attentional control is not impaired in schizophrenia: Dissociating specific deficits from generalized impairments. *Journal of Abnormal Psychology*, *124*(2), 302–308. https://doi.org/10.1037/a0038537.

Enns, J. T., & di Lollo, V. (2000). What's new in visual masking? *Trends in Cognitive Sciences*, *4*(9), 345–352. https://doi.org/10.1016/S1364-6613(00)01520-5.

Ettinger, U., Meyhöfer, I., Steffens, M., Wagner, M., & Koutsouleris, N. (2014). Genetics, cognition, and neurobiology of schizotypal personality: A review of the overlap with schizophrenia. *Frontiers in Psychiatry*, *5*(18), 1–16. https://doi.org/10.3389/fpsyt.2014.00018.

Ettinger, U., Mohr, C., Gooding, D. C., Cohen, A. S., Rapp, A., Haenschel, C., & Park, S. (2015). Cognition and brain function in schizotypy: A selective review. *Schizophrenia Bulletin*, *41*(suppl_2), S417–S426. https://doi.org/10.1093/schbul/sbu190.

Fan, F., Xiang, H., Tan, S., Yang, F., Fan, H., Guo, H., … Tan, Y. (2019). Subcortical structures and cognitive dysfunction in first episode schizophrenia. *Psychiatry Research: Neuroimaging*, *286*, 69–75. https://doi.org/10.1016/j.pscychresns.2019.01.003.

Favrod, O., Sierro, G., Roinishvili, M., Chkonia, E., Mohr, C., Herzog, M. H., & Cappe, C. (2017). Electrophysiological correlates of visual backward masking in high schizotypic personality traits participants. *Psychiatry Research*, *254*, 251–257. https://doi.org/10.1016/j.psychres.2017.04.051.

Fernandes, T. M. P., Silverstein, S. M., Butler, P. D., Kéri, S., Santos, L. G., Nogueira, R. L., & Santos, N. A. (2019). Color vision impairments in schizophrenia and the role of antipsychotic medication type. *Schizophrenia Research*, *204*, 162–170. https://doi.org/10.1016/j.schres.2018.09.002.

Flückiger, R., Michel, C., Grant, P., Ruhrmann, S., Vogeley, K., Hubl, D., … Schultze-Lutter, F. (2019). The interrelationship between schizotypy, clinical high risk for psychosis and related symptoms: Cognitive disturbances matter. *Schizophrenia Research*, *210*, 188–196. https://doi.org/10.1016/j.schres.2018.12.039.

Ganguly, P., Soliman, A., & Moustafa, A. A. (2018). Holistic management of schizophrenia symptoms using pharmachological and non-pharmacological treatment. *Frontiers in Public Health*, *6*, 166. https://doi.org/10.3389/fpubh.2018.00166.

Granholm, E., Holden, J. L., Mikhael, T., Link, P. C., Swendsen, J., Depp, C., … Harvey, P. D. (2020). What do people with schizophrenia do all day? Ecological momentary assessment of real-world functioning in schizophrenia. *Schizophrenia Bulletin*, *46*(2), 242–251. https://doi.org/10.1093/schbul/sbz070.

Green, M. F., Hugdahl, K., & Mitchell, S. (1994). Dichotic listening during auditory hallucinations in patients with schizophrenia. *The American Journal of Psychiatry*, *151*(3), 357. Retrieved from https://www.ncbi.nlm.nih.gov/pubmed/8109643.

Green, M. F., Nuechterlein, K. H., & Mintz, J. (1994). Backward masking in schizophrenia and mania. I. Specifying a mechanism. *Archives of General Psychiatry*, *51*(12), 939–944. https://doi.org/10.1001/archpsyc.1994.03950120011003.

Green, M. F., Nuechterlein, K. H., & Breitmeyer, B. (1997). Backward masking performance in unaffected siblings of schizophrenic patients. Evidence for a vulnerability indicator. *Archives of General Psychiatry*, *54*(5), 465–472. https://doi.org/10.1001/archpsyc.1997.01830170091012.

Green, M. F., Nuechterlein, K. H., Breitmeyer, B., & Mintz, J. (1999). Backward masking in unmedicated schizophrenic patients in psychotic remission: Possible reflection of aberrant cortical oscillation. *The American Journal of Psychiatry*, *156*(9), 1367–1373. https://doi.org/10.1176/ajp.156.9.1367.

Green, M. F., Nuechterlein, K. H., Breitmeyer, B., & Mintz, J. (2006). Forward and backward visual masking in unaffected siblings of schizophrenic patients. *Biological Psychiatry*, *59*(5), 446–451. https://doi.org/10.1016/j.biopsych.2005.06.035.

Green, M. F., Lee, J., Wynn, J. K., & Mathis, K. I. (2011). Visual masking in schizophrenia: Overview and theoretical implications. *Schizophrenia Bulletin*, *37*(4), 700–708. https://doi.org/10.1093/schbul/sbr051.

Gross, M. E., Araujo, D. B., Zedelius, C. M., & Schooler, J. W. (2019). Is perception the missing link between creativity, curiosity and schizotypy? Evidence from spontaneous eye-movements and responses to auditory oddball stimuli. *NeuroImage*, *202*, 116125. https://doi.org/10.1016/j.neuroimage.2019.116125.

Gruzelier, J. H. (1994). Syndromes of schizophrenia and schizotypy, hemispheric imbalance and sex differences: Implications for developmental psychopathology. *International Journal of Psychophysiology*, *18*(3), 167–178. https://doi.org/10.1016/0167-8760(94)90002-7.

Grzeczkowski, L., Roinishvili, M., Chkonia, E., Brand, A., Mast, F. W., Herzog, M. H., & Shaqiri, A. (2018). Is the perception of illusions abnormal in schizophrenia? *Psychiatry Research*, *270*, 929–939. https://doi.org/10.1016/j.psychres.2018.10.063.

Hazlett, E. A., Lamade, R. V., Graff, F. S., McClure, M. M., Kolaitis, J. C., Goldstein, K. E., … Moshier, E. (2014). Visual-spatial working memory performance and temporal gray matter volume predict schizotypal personality disorder group membership. *Schizophrenia Research*, *152*(2–3), 350–357. https://doi.org/10.1016/j.schres.2013.12.006.

Herzog, M. H., & Brand, A. (2015). Visual masking & schizophrenia. *Schizophrenia Research: Cognition*, *2*(2), 64–71. https://doi.org/10.1016/j.scog.2015.04.001.

Herzog, M. H., Roinishvili, M., Chkonia, E., & Brand, A. (2013). Schizophrenia and visual backward masking: A general deficit of target enhancement. *Frontiers in Psychology*, *4*, 1–9. https://doi.org/10.3389/fpsyg.2013.00254.

Jahshan, C., Wolf, M., Karbi, Y., Shamir, E., & Rassovsky, Y. (2017). Probing the magnocellular and parvocellular visual pathways in facial emotion perception in schizophrenia. *Psychiatry Research*, *253*, 38–42. https://doi.org/10.1016/j.schres.2006.09.004.

Jurišic, D., Ćavar, I., Sesar, A., Vukojević, J., & Ćurković, M. (2020). New insights into schizophrenia: A look at the eye and related structures. *Psychiatria Danubina*, *32*(1), 60–69. https://doi.org/10.24869/psyd.2020.60.

Kendler, K. S., McGuire, M., Gruenberg, A. M., O'Hare, A., Spellman, M., & Walsh, D. (1993). The Roscommon family study. I. Methods, diagnosis of probands, and risk of schizophrenia in relatives. *Archives of General Psychiatry*, *50*(7), 527–540. https://doi.org/10.1001/archpsyc.1993.01820190029004.

Keri, S., Kelemen, O., Benedek, G., & Janka, Z. (2001). Different trait markers for schizophrenia and bipolar disorder: A neurocognitive approach. *Psychological Medicine*, *31*(5), 915–922. https://doi.org/10.1017/s0033291701004068.

Kim, J., & Park, S. (2011). Visual perception deficits associated with the magnocellular pathway in schizophrenia. *Korean Journal of Schizophrenia Research*, *14*, 61–75. Retrieved from https://www.researchgate.net/publication/229593828_Visual_Perception_Deficits_Associated_with_the_Magnocellular_Pathway_in_Schizophrenia.

Kogata, T., & Iidaka, T. (2018). A review of impaired visual processing and the daily visual world in patients with schizophrenia. *Nagoya Journal of Medical Science*, *80*(3), 317–328. https://doi.org/10.18999/nagjms.80.3.317.

Koychev, I., El-Deredy, W., Haenschel, C., & Deakin, J. F. W. (2010). Visual information processing deficits as biomarkers of vulnerability to schizophrenia: An event-related potential study in schizotypy. *Neuropsychologia*, *48*(7), 2205–2214. https://doi.org/10.1016/j.neuropsychologia.2010.04.014.

Koychev, I., Deakin, J. F., Haenschel, C., & El-Deredy, W. (2011). Abnormal neural oscillations in schizotypy during a visual working memory task: Support for a deficient top-down network? *Neuropsychologia*, *49*(10), 2866–2873. https://doi.org/10.1016/j.neuropsychologia.2011.06.012.

Langdon, R., Connors, M. H., & Connaughton, E. (2014). Social cognition and social judgment in schizophrenia. *Schizophrenia Research: Cognition*, *1*(4), 171–174. https://doi.org/10.1016/j.scog.2014.10.001.

Lauffs, M. M., Shaqiri, A., Brand, A., Roinishvili, M., Chkonia, E., Ogmen, H., & Herzog, M. H. (2016). Local versus global and retinotopic versus non-retinotopic motion processing in schizophrenia patients. *Psychiatry Research*, *246*, 461–465. https://doi.org/10.1016/j.psychres.2016.09.049.

Lenzenweger, M. F. (2018). Schizotypy, schizotypic psychopathology and schizophrenia. *World Psychiatry*, *17*(1), 25–26. https://doi.org/10.1002/wps.20479.

Lima, F. B. V., Gracitellia, C. P. B., Junior, A. P., & Bressan, R. A. (2013). Evaluation of magnocellular pathway abnormalities in schizophrenia: A frequency doubling tecnology study and clinical implications. *Arquivos Brasileiros de Oftalmologia*, *76*(2), 85–89. https://doi.org/10.1590/S0004-27492013000200006.

Loh, P. R., Bhatia, G., Gusev, A., Finucane, H. F., Bulik-Sullivan, B. K., Pollack, S. J., … Price, A. L. (2015). Contrasting genetic architectures of schizophrenia and other complex diseases using fast variance-components analysis. *Nature Genetics*, *47*(12), 1385–1395. https://doi.org/10.1038/ng.3431.

Luber, B., Stanford, A. D., Malaspina, D., & Lisanby, S. H. (2007). Revisiting the backward masking deficit in schizophrenia: Individual differences in performance and modeling with transcranial magnetic stimulation. *Biological Psychiatry*, *62*(7), 793–799. https://doi.org/10.1016/j.biopsych.2006.10.007.

Marosi, C., Fodor, S., & Csukly, G. (2019). From basic perception deficits to facial affect recognition impairments in schizophrenia. *Scientific Reports*, *9*, 8958. https://doi.org/10.1038/s41598-019-45231-x.

Martínez, A., Hillyard, S. A., Dias, E. C., Hagler, D. J., Jr., Butler, P. D., Guilfoyle, D. N., … Javitt, D. C. (2008). Magnocellular pathway impairment in schizophrenia: Evidence from functional magnetic resonance imaging. *The Journal of Neuroscience*, *28*(30), 7492–7500. https://doi.org/10.1523/jneurosci.1852-08.2008.

McClure, R. K. (2001). The visual backward masking deficit in schizophrenia. *Progress in Neuro-Psychopharmacology and Biological Psychiatry*, *25*(2), 301–311. https://doi.org/10.1016/S0278-5846(00)00166-4.

McClure, M. M., Harvey, P. D., Bowie, C. R., Iacoviello, B., & Siever, L. J. (2013). Functional outcomes, functional capacity, and cognitive impairment in schizotypal personality disorder. *Schizophrenia Research*, *144*(1–3), 146–150. https://doi.org/10.1016/j.schres.2012.12.012.

Meehl, P. E. (1962). Schizotaxia, schizotypy schizophrenia. *American Psychologist*, *17*(12), 827–838. https://doi.org/10.1037/h0041029.

Mikanmaa, E., Grent-'t-Jong, T., Hua, L., Recasens, M., Thune, H., & Uhlhaas, P. J. (2019). Towards a neurodynamical understanding of the prodrome in schizophrenia. *NeuroImage*, *190*, 144–153. https://doi.org/10.1016/j.neuroimage.2017.11.026.

Misiak, B., Stramecki, F., Gaweda, L., Prochwicz, K., Sasiadek, M. M., Moustafa, A. A., & Frydecka, D. (2018). Interactions between variation in cadidate genes and environmental factors in the etiology of schizophrenia and bipolar disorder: A systemic review. *Molecular Neurobiology*, *55*(6), 5075–5100. https://doi.org/10.1007/s12035-017-0708-y.

Modinos, G., Mechelli, A., Ormel, J., Groenewold, N., Aleman, A., & McGuire, P. (2010). Schizotypy and brain structure: A voxel-based morphometry study. *Psychological Medicine*, *40*(9), 1423–1431. https://doi.org/10.1017/S0033291709991875.

Moustafa, A. A., Garami, J. K., Mahlberg, J., Golembieski, J., Keri, S., Misiak, B., & Frydecka, D. (2016). Neural and cognitive function in schizophrenia: Conflicting findings and future directions. *Reviews in the Neurosciences*, *27*(4), 435–438. https://doi.org/10.1515/revneuro-2015-0060.

Myamlin, V. V., Kirenskaya, A. V., & Novototsky-Vlasov, V. Y. (2016). Use of backward masking test for the study of visual information processing in healthy subjects and schizophrenic patients. *Human Physiology*, *42*(5), 492–498. https://doi.org/10.1134/S036211971605011X.

Nimgaonkar, V. L., Prasad, K. M., Chowdari, K. V., Severance, E. G., & Yolken, R. H. (2017). The complement sytem: A gateway to gene-environment interactions in schizophrenia pathogenesis. *Molecular Psychiatry*, *22*(11), 1554–1561. https://doi.org/10.1038/mp.2017.151.

Nishikawa, Y., Takahashi, T., Takayanagi, Y., Furuichi, A., Kido, M., Nakamura, M., … Suzuki, M. (2016). Orbitofrontal sulcogyral pattern and olfactory sulcus depth in the schizophrenia spectrum. *European Archives of Psychiatry and Clinical Neuroscience*, *266*(1), 15–23. https://doi.org/10.1007/s00406-015-0587-z.

Nuechterlein, K. H., Asarnow, R. F., Subotnik, K. L., Fogelson, D. L., Payne, D. L., Kendler, K. S., … Mintz, J. (2002). The structure of schizotypy relationships between neurocognitive and personality disorder features in relatives of schizophrenic patients in the UCLA family study. *Schizophrenia Research*, *54*(1–2), 121–130. https://doi.org/10.1016/s0920-9964(01)00359-0.

Olivier, R. M., Kilian, S., Chiliza, B., Asmal, L., Oosthuizen, P. P., Emsley, R., & Kidd, M. (2017). Cognitive-perceptual deficits and symptom correlates in first-episode schizophrenia. *The South African Journal of Psychiatry: SAJP: The Journal of the Society of Psychiatrists of South Africa*, *23*, 1049. https://doi.org/10.4102/sajpsychiatry.v23i0.1049.

Pariyadath, V., Gowin, J. L., & Stein, E. A. (2016). Resting state functional connectivity analysis for addiction medicine: From individual loci to complex networks. In H. Ekhtiari, & M. P. Paulus (Eds.), *Neuroscience for addiction medicine: From prevention to rehabilitation-methods and interventions* (pp. 155–173). Amsterdam, NL: Elsevier.

Peterburs, J., Nitsch, A. M., Miltner, W. H. R., & Straube, T. (2013). Impaired representation of time in schizophrenia is linked to positive symptoms and cognitive demand. *PLoS One*, *8*(6), e67615. https://doi.org/10.1371/journal.pone.0067615.

Racioppi, A., Sheinbaum, T., Gross, G. M., Ballespi, S., Kwapil, T. R., & Barrantes-Vidal, N. (2018). Prediction of prodromal symptoms and schizophrenia-spectrum personality disorder traits by positive and negative schizotypy: A 3-year prospective study. *PLoS One*, *13*(11), 1–18. https://doi.org/10.1371/journal.pone.0207150.

Rassovsky, Y., Green, M. F., Nuechterlein, K. H., Breitmeyer, B., & Mintz, J. (2004). Paracontrast and metacontrast in schizophrenia: Clarifying the mechanism for visual masking deficits. *Schizophrenia Research*, *71*(2–3), 485–492. https://doi.org/10.1016/j.schres.2004.02.018.

Rassovsky, Y., Horan, W. P., Lee, J., Sergi, M. J., & Green, M. F. (2011). Pathways between early visual processing and functional outcome in schizophrenia. *Psychological Medicine*, *41*(3), 487–497. https://doi.org/10.1017/s0033291710001054.

Roy, M., Grondin, S., & Roy, M. A. (2012). Time perception disorders are related to working memory impairment in schizophrenia. *Psychiatry Research*, *200*, 159–166.

Rund, B. R., Oie, M., & Sundet, K. (1996). Backward-masking deficit in adolescents with schizophrenic disorders or attention deficit hyperactivity disorder. *The American Journal of Psychiatry*, *153*(9), 1154–1157. https://doi.org/10.1176/ajp.153.9.1154.

Rund, B. R., Egeland, J., Sundet, K., Asbjornsen, A., Hugdahl, K., Landro, N. I., … Stordal, K. I. (2004). Early visual information processing in schizophrenia compared to recurrent depression. *Schizophrenia Research*, *68*(2–3), 111–118. https://doi.org/10.1016/s0920-9964(03)00193-2.

Silverstein, S. M. (2016). Visual perception disturbances in schizophrenia: A unified model. In M. Li, & W. D. Spaulding (Eds.), *The neuropsychopathology of schizophrenia* (pp. 77–132). Switzerland: Springer International Publishing.

Slaghuis, W. L., & Bakker, V. J. (1995). Forward and backward visual masking of contour by light in positive- and negative-symptom schizophrenia. *Journal of Abnormal Psychology*, *104*(1), 41–54. https://doi.org/10.1037/0021-843X.104.1.41.

Slavin, R., & Smith, D. (2009). The relationship between sample sizes and effect sizes in systematic reviews in education. *Educational Evaluation and Policy Analysis*, *31*(4), 500–506. https://doi.org/10.3102/0162373709352369.

Snowden, A. W., & Buhusi, C. (2019). Neural correlates of interval deficits in schizophrenia. *Frontiers in Human Neuroscience*, *13*(9). https://doi.org/10.3389/fnhum.2019.00009.

Stramecki, F., Kotowicz, K. D., Piotrowski, P., Frydecka, D., Rymaszewska, J., Beszlej, J. A., … Misiak, B. (2018). Assessment of the association between cigarette smoking and cognitive performance in patients with schizophrenia-spectrum disorders: A case-control study. *Frontiers in Psychiatry*, *9*, 642. https://doi.org/10.3389/fpsyt.2018.00642.

Tadin, D., Kim, J., Doop, M. L., Gibson, C., Lappin, J. S., Blake, R., & Park, S. (2006). Weakened center-surround interactions in visual motion processing in schizophrenia. *The Journal of Neuroscience*, *26*(44), 11403–11412. https://doi.org/10.1523/jneurosci.2592-06.2006.

Takayanagi, Y., Sasabayashi, D., Takahashi, T., Komori, Y., Furuichi, A., Kido, M., … Suzuki, M. (2018). Altered brain gyrification in deficit and non-deficit schizophrenia. *Psychological Medicine*, *49*(4), 573–580. https://doi.org/10.1017/S0033291718001228.

Tamminga, C. A., & Medoff, D. R. (2002). Studies in schizophrenia: Pathophysiology and treatment. *Dialogues in Clinical Neuroscience*, *4*(4), 432–437.

Tarbox, S. I., Almasy, L., Gur, R. E., Nimgaonkar, V. L., & Pogue-Geile, M. F. (2012). The nature of schizotypy among multigenerational multiplex schizophrenia families. *Journal of Abnormal Psychology*, *121*(2), 396–406. https://doi.org/10.1037/a0026787.

Thoenes, S., & Oberfeld, D. (2017). Meta-analysis of time perception and temporal processing in schizophrenia: Differential effects on precision and accuracy. *Clinical Psychology Review*, *54*, 44–64. https://doi.org/10.1016/j.cpr.2017.03.007.

Thormodsen, R., Jensen, J., Holmen, A., Juuhl-Langseth, M., Emblem, K. E., Andreassen, O. A., & Rund, B. R. (2011). Prefrontal hyperactivation during a working memory task in early-onset schizophrenia spectrum disorders: An fMRI study. *Psychiatry Research*, *194*(3), 257–262. https://doi.org/10.1016/j.pscychresns.2011.05.011.

Thormodsen, R., Juuhl-Langseth, M., Holmèn, A., & Rishovd Rund, B. (2012). Visual backward-masking performance in a longitudinal study of early onset schizophrenia. *Psychiatry Research*, *200*(2–3), 153–158. https://doi.org/10.1016/j.psychres.2012.05.014.

Tripathi, A., Kar, S. K., & Shukla, R. (2018). Cognitive dificits in schizophrenia: Understading the biological correlates and remediation strategies. *Clinical Psychopharmachology and Neuroscience*, *16*(1), 7–17. https://doi.org/10.9758/cpn.2018.16.1.7.

Tucci, V., Buhusi, C. V., Gallistel, R., & Meck, W. H. (2014). Towards an integrated understanding of the biology of timing. *Philosophical Transactions of the Royal Society B*, *369*, 20120470. https://doi.org/10.1098/rstb.2012.0470.

Türközer, H. B., Hasoglu, T., Chen, Y., Norris, L. A., Brown, M., Delaney-Busch, N., … Öngür, D. (2018). Integrated assessment of visual perception abnormalities in psychotic disorders and relationship with clinical characteristics. *Psychological Medicine*, *49*, 1740–1748. https://doi.org/10.1017/S0033291718002477.

Ueda, N., Maruo, K., & Sumiyoshi, T. (2018). Positive symptoms and time perception in schizophrenia: A meta-analysis. *Schizophrenia Research: Cognition*, *13*, 3–6. https://doi.org/10.1016/j.scog.2018.07.002.

Uhlhaas, P. J., & Silverstein, S. M. (2005). Perceptual organization in schizophrenia spectrum disorders: Empirical research and theoretical implications. *Psychological Bulletin*, *131*(4), 618–632. https://doi.org/10.1037/0033-2909.131.4.618.

Veit, J., Hakim, R., Jadi, M., Sejnowski, T., & Adesnik, H. (2017). Cortical gamma band synchronization through somatostatin interneurons. *Nature Neuroscience*, *20*, 951–959. https://doi.org/10.1038/nn.4562.

Yang, E., Tadin, D., Glasser, D. M., Hong, S. W., Blake, R., & Park, S. (2013). Visual context processing in schizophrenia. *Clinical Psychological Science: A Journal of the Association for Psychological Science*, *1*(1), 5–15. https://doi.org/10.1177/2167702612464618.

Working-memory impairment in schizophrenia and schizotypal personality disorder

2

Ahmed A. Moustafa[a,b], *Shadi Gray*[c], *Alejandro Morris*[a], *Glessia Matar*[c], *Anchal Garg*[c], *Ahmed A. Helal*[d], *Alaa Eldin A. Ayoub*[e], *and Eid Abo Hamza*[d,e]
[a]School of Psychology & Marcs Institute for Brain and Behaviour, Western Sydney University, Sydney, NSW, Australia, [b]Department of Human Anatomy and Physiology, the Faculty of Health Sciences, University of Johannesburg, South Africa, [c]School of Psychology, Western Sydney University, Sydney, NSW, Australia, [d]Faculty of Education, Department of Mental Health, Tanta University, Egypt, [e]College of Graduate Studies, Arabian Gulf University, Bahrain

Chapter outline

Working memory

The early detection of psychosis-spectrum disorders and individuals at risk for psychosis has become a well-established goal in clinical treatment since early interventions can reduce the risk of development of a disorder (Kamiński & Rutishauser, 2020; Park & Gooding, 2014; Pflueger, Gschwandtner, Stieglitz, & Riecher-Rössler, 2007). Risk assessment of psychosis has focused on prodromal symptoms such as unusual perceptual experiences or marked social withdrawal (George, Maheshwari, Chandran, Manohar, & Rao, 2017), as well as family history of psychosis. Nevertheless, only 20%–40% of individuals identified as being at risk progress to psychosis in a 12-month period (Riecher-Rössler et al., 2007). It is therefore necessary to explore other vulnerability markers for psychosis-spectrum disorders. One prominent area of research is

Cognitive and Behavioral Dysfunction in Schizophrenia. https://doi.org/10.1016/B978-0-12-820005-6.00007-4

cognitive markers as they are purported to be a contributing factor in the underlying etiopathogenesis of disorders such as schizophrenia, dementia, and depression (Coleman, Krastoshevsky, Tu, Mendell, & Levy, 2012; Kraguljac, Srivastava, & Lahti, 2013). More specifically, WM deficits have been repeatedly found throughout the literature in psychosis-spectrum disorders (Eryilmaz et al., 2016; Kamiński et al., 2020; Snellenberg et al., 2016). However, WM is not seen as a unitary construct, but rather split into an executive component and two storage subsystems (Baddeley, 2018). One processes speech and sound, while the other is visuo-spatial (Milas & Milas, 2019). All three systems are linked to perception and long-term memory, enabling guidance of behavior in day-to-day activities. WM is therefore crucial for a well-adapted daily life functioning. It may be the case that difficulties are found in one subsystem of WM and not another depending on the psychosis disorder. The current chapter aims to analyze whether two of the most prevalent psychosis-spectrum disorders (Morgan et al., 2010), schizotypal personality disorder (SPD), and schizophrenia, have any quantitative and qualitative differences in WM deficits. Research suggests both disorders lie on a continuum as genetic and linkage studies (i.e., genetic mapping of Mendelian and complex traits with familial aggregation) have showed considerable overlap between both genetic association profiles (Fanous et al., 2007; Walter, Fernandez, Snelling, & Barkus, 2016). Many authors believe that the profile of WM impairment is similar across schizophrenia and SPD (Ettinger, Meyhöfer, Steffens, Wagner, & Koutsouleris, 2014; Pedrero & Debanné, 2017). However, longitudinal trajectory of WM deterioration in schizophrenia is different to the one found in SPD individuals which casts doubts on the similarity in WM deficits of both disorders (Kirchner, Roeh, Nolden, & Hasan, 2018).

The current chapter aims to analyze the literature on WM impairment in schizophrenia and SPD using the N-Back Paradigm (N-BP; Schoofs, Preub, & Wolf, 2008; Owen, McMillan, Laird, & Bullmore, 2005) and AX-Continuous Performance Test (AX-CPT; Umbricht et al., 2003; Ballard, 2001) as a means to determine if both groups show similar WM deficits, or whether they show marked differences which would suggest the existence of different underlying mechanisms.

Schizophrenia

Schizophrenia is a severe chronic psychiatric disorder that is estimated to affect 23 million individuals worldwide (Abohamza, Weickert, Ali, & Moustafa, 2020; Nuechterlein et al., 2012; World Health Organization [WHO], 2018). Although outcomes are not uniformly negative, more than 50% of people who are diagnosed with schizophrenia have intermittent to long-term psychiatric problems that will require medical assistance, and around 20% will have chronic symptoms and disability (Owen, Sawa, & Mortensen, 2016). In Australia, schizophrenia is the most prevalent psychotic disorder (47%), affecting primarily males (56.3%) between the ages of 25 and 34, and is estimated to cost $1.44 billion in medical treatment and societal costs (Morgan et al., 2010).

Schizophrenia can include the following symptoms: positive symptoms (hallucinations, delusions, thought disorder, disorganized behavior such as catatonia), negative symptoms (social withdrawal, apathy) and cognitive symptoms (poor executive function and memory) (Meyer & MacCabe, 2016). An individual with schizophrenia will exhibit impairment in one or more major areas such as work, interpersonal relationships, or self-care and continuous signs of disturbance lasting for at least 6 months, including 1 month of active phase of symptoms (American Psychiatric Association [APA], 2013). Positive psychotic symptoms include catatonic behavior such as posturing or waxy flexibility, as well as delusions (irrational beliefs) and/or hallucinations (i.e., sensory experiences without causal external events (Haro et al., 2018; Meyer & MacCabe, 2016; Tandon et al., 2013). Negative symptoms refer to emotional and social withdrawal, poverty of speech or thought, and apathy (Galletly et al., 2016; Mitra, Mahintamani, Kavoor, & Nizamie, 2016). Moreover, schizophrenia patients exhibit disorganized or abnormal motor behavior (including catatonia) that ranges from childlike "silliness" to unpredictable agitation (American Psychiatric Association, 2013). Cognitive symptoms involve deficits in frontal lobe function, attention, processing speed and disorganized thinking and speech (i.e. derailment). In many cases, such cognitive symptoms are chronic and independent of positive symptoms and can significantly impact the individual's social and occupational life (Meyer & MacCabe, 2016). The etiology of schizophrenia has been linked to the *neuro-developmental hypothesis* (Owen, O'Donovan, Thapar, & Craddock, 2011), which states that the pathogenesis of the illness is an interplay between genetic vulnerability, and environmental and social factors. The genetic predisposition theory is based on genome-wide associations studies (GWAS) which found common genetic variants with small individual effect sizes contributed to the risk of schizophrenia (International Schizophrenia Consortium et al., 2009; Smeland, Frei, Dale, & Andreassen, 2020; Stefansson et al., 2009). Aside from genetic vulnerability, there is expanding literature that suggests substance abuse (i.e., cannabis and methamphetamines) and social adversity (i.e., urbanicity and immigration) increase the risk of developing schizophrenia (Kelly et al., 2010; Meyer & MacCabe, 2016). Genetic and environmental factors are of aetiological importance in the development of schizophrenia, and therefore current treatments focus on pharmacological interventions (i.e., antipsychotics such as clozapine and chlorpromazine to reduce positive symptoms) and non-pharmacological interventions such as Cognitive-Behavioral Treatment (CBT) (Ganguly, Soliman, & Moustafa, 2018) and Phenomenological Psychotherapy, which emphasizes alleviating distress, strengthening self-integration, and promoting recovery of functioning (Škodlar & Henriksen, 2019).

Schizotypal personality disorder

SPD is a condition that stems from two areas of research: (1) borderline personality conditions, which incorporates a series of pervasive disturbances in function, cognition, affect and behavioral control and (2) studies of nonpsychotic family members who exhibited chronic peculiarities of thought and communication (Lenzenweger, 2018; McClure, Harvey, Bowie, Iacoviello, & Siever, 2013; Racioppi et al., 2018; Rosell, Futterman, McMaster, & Siever, 2014). The diagnosis of schizotypal personality disorder follows a categorical approach as a minimum threshold of symptoms must be met in order to be diagnosed with the disorder. Furthermore, it is conceptualized along three constructs: interpersonal (social anxiety), cognitive-perceptual (perceptual disturbances), and disorganized-oddness (odd speech and affect) (Rosell et al., 2014). The diagnostic of SPD consists of ideas of reference, odds beliefs, or magical thinking; unusual perceptual experiences and bodily illusions; odd thinking and speech; suspiciousness or paranoid ideation; inappropriate affect; eccentric behavior and a lack of close friends, as well as excessive social anxiety that does not diminish with familiarity and tends to be associated with paranoid fears. Five of nine criteria are required for a diagnosis (Kirchner et al., 2018). Moreover, individuals must demonstrate multi-contextual impairments in areas such as work or social environments (APA, 2013). Studies found that relatives of individuals with schizophrenia show increased rates of schizotypal personality traits and were at a greater risk for the development of schizophrenia (Barch et al., 2004; Callaway, Cohen, Matthews, & Dinzeo, 2014; Tarbox, Almasy, Gur, Nimgaonkar, & Pogue-Geile, 2012). However, when compared to schizophrenia symptomology, SPD individuals experience less magical thinking, ideas of reference, as well as perceptual distortions such as illusions (Lener et al., 2015). Many SPD individuals show adequate personal and community functioning without any treatment (Debbané & Mohr, 2015).

Cognitive deficits in schizophrenia and schizotypal personality disorder

Past research has shown that individuals with schizophrenia suffer executive functional impairments in domains such as attention (Addington et al., 2017; Gjini, Burroughs, & Boutros, 2011; Nestor et al., 2020), context integration (Brébion, Stephan-Otto, Cuevas-Esteban, Usall, & Ochoa, 2020; Chun, Ciceron, & Kwapil, 2018), episodic memory (Guo, Ragland, & Carter, 2019; Kanchanatawan et al., 2018), and working memory (WM) (Cho et al., 2018; Corigliano et al., 2014; Liu et al., 2019; Nielsen et al., 2017). These deficits have shown to interfere in an individual's performance at work and in academic environments, as well as social relationships, the ability to self-care and develop independent living skills (Chang et al., 2018; Haro et al., 2018; Kaneko, 2018).

SPD individuals share similar cognitive deficits as schizophrenia patients (Breeze, Kirkham, & Marí-Beffa, 2011). However, less is known regarding the extent to which such deficits impact functional capacity and real-world functioning. Studies sought to identify the relationship between schizotypal personality disorder symptoms dimensions and cognitive dysfunctions (Rosell et al., 2014). For instance, omission errors in sustained attention span tasks were positively correlated with interpersonal schizotypal traits such as restricted affect or social anxiety, whereas disorganization traits were associated with false alarms and errors in sustained attention (Bedwell, Kamath, & Compton, 2009). Furthermore, selective attention was found to be poorer in a sample of schizotypal individuals compared to healthy controls in task-switching tests. SPD individuals showed greater sensitivity to irrelevant information that translated into greater switching times, especially in incongruent tasks (Breeze et al., 2011). The results would support the view that SPD traits may represent a risk factor in the regulation of attention under increased perceptual load. It is hypothesized that, due to these attentional difficulties, SPD individuals perform less accurately on short-term visual recognition memory tasks such as Delayed Matching to Sample (DMS) (Goldstein et al., 2016; Sahakyan & Kwapil, 2019). Furthermore, there is evidence indicating that SDP individuals perform worse than controls in free-recall memory tasks and episodic memory tests (Sahakyan & Kwapil, 2018a, 2018b). However, these studies have been unable to identify the role these cognitive deficits play in the etiology of SPD, and thus further research will help understand the degree to which each cognitive impairment represents a pre-morbid disease marker.

WM in schizophrenia and schizotypal personality disorder

There is ample research suggesting that the cognitive deficits seen in schizophrenia patients are largely due to a deficit in visuospatial and verbal WM and the inability to store and apprehend new information (Garcia-Laredo, 2018; Milas & Milas, 2019; Neu, Gooren, Niebuhr, & Schlattmann, 2019). Similarly, SPD individuals show impaired visuospatial WM (Rosell et al., 2014; Siever et al., 2002) and verbal WM (Harvey et al., 1996; Rosell et al., 2014) that hinders their ability to flexibly process and update new environmental stimuli or to control interfering information. Visuospatial WM is where 2D and 3D representations are temporarily stored while verbal WM is where linguistic and numeric information is briefly stored while being processed (Wang, Bolin, Lu, & Carr, 2018).

Verbal WM deficits have been observed consistently in schizophrenia patients (Botero et al., 2013; Kustermann, Popov, Miller, & Rockstroh, 2018; Li et al., 2018; Silver & Bilker, 2015) and SPD individuals (Marsh, Vachon, & Sörqvist, 2017; Siddi, Petretto, & Preti, 2017). This deficit is hypothesized to be linked to restricted syntactic complexity in language production and comprehension. Specifically, experimental studies such as Li et al. (2018) found that schizophrenia patients had poor syntactic familiarity which hindered their ability to recall familiar (e.g., adjective-noun) and nonfamiliar (e.g., noun-adjective) pairs of words compared to healthy individuals. Likewise, Marsh et al. (2017) found that SPD participants showed worse performance on a verbal serial recall task. One possible explanation is SPD individuals have inchoate, less fluent rehearsal abilities that hinders their performance on verbal tasks.

A study by Quee, Van Der Heijden, Eling, and Hildebrandth (2011) also analyzed verbal WM using pseudo-characters and found that schizophrenia patients were significantly slower than healthy controls at recalling such words, yet no differences were found on accuracy levels. Possibly, patients required more time to process the unfamiliar verbal information, which in turn yielded similar accuracy results as the healthy control group. These findings suggest possible deficits at verbal encoding and retrieval, as well as lack of lexical depth in schizophrenia patients which, for instance, prevented them from encoding by association (i.e., associating pseudo-character to a morphologically or semantically similar real word). Similar findings were yielded in McClure et al.'s (2007) study assessing SPD individuals on verbal and visuospatial WM capabilities. SPD participants showed less verbal memory and recognition after a short delay compared to healthy controls. These findings would support the notion that verbal WM is a core deficit that is prominent across the schizophrenia spectrum and would validate the ongoing examination of verbal WM as a central factor for understanding cognition in psychosis-spectrum disorders.

In addition, several studies (Horan et al., 2008; Silver & Bilker, 2015; Trapp et al., 2017) employed the forward and backward digit span test from the Wechsler Adult Intelligence Scale (WAIS) to measure verbal WM and found individuals with schizophrenia showed greater impairment at recalling digits than healthy controls. These findings corroborate the notion that as verbal WM load increases and more cognitive flexibility is required, schizophrenia patients have significantly greater difficulty at completing the task compared to healthy participants and other clinical groups such as individuals with unipolar depression (Trapp et al., 2017).

There are studies that employed span tasks which required schizophrenia participants to solve arithmetic tests while remembering a set of unrelated words (Cassetta, Tomfohr-Madsen, & Goghari, 2018; Mammarella et al., 2012). Participants were tested on their verbal WM and the degree to which they could memorize it while performing a distraction task. The results showed impaired working-memory performance in terms of greater number of intrusions for schizophrenia participants. These findings indicate that as cognitive load and task complexity increase, schizophrenia patients' verbal WM performance decreases significantly compared to healthy participants. Processing speed deficits in WM tasks might underlie these findings as schizophrenia patients exhibit difficulty coordinating an assembly of elementary operations such as verbal memory and arithmetic operations.

As observed in previous research, there are two predominant working-memory paradigms that are utilized in schizophrenia research. One involves transient, short-term memory requiring no manipulation of the stored information and the other involves manipulation and maintenance of verbal and numeric information (Chari et al., 2019). Individuals with schizophrenia show a higher deficit in maintaining and manipulating information which might be related to poor attentional capabilities and hypervigilance to redundant stimuli (McClure et al., 2007).

Neural substrates of working-memory deficits in schizophrenia and schizotypal personality disorder

Schizophrenia symptoms result from a disruption in brain functionality and, in some cases, of subtle brain structural dysfunction (Chari et al., 2019; Neu et al., 2019). This disruption is specifically prominent in the prefrontal cortex, which has been associated with working-memory deficits in individuals with schizophrenia (Bleich-Cohen et al., 2014; Liu et al., 2019; Neu et al., 2019). It has been suggested that alternatively working-memory deficits in individuals with schizophrenia may be due to hypoactivity of the prefrontal cortex in comparison to nonclinical populations (Barch et al., 2001; DiBiase, Cropley, Baune, Olver, & Amminger, 2017; Ebmeier, Lawrie, Blackwood, Johnstone, & Goodwin, 1995). Poor working-memory performance may rather reflect a lack motivation or effort, employment of inappropriate strategy, or a high level of task difficulty, and for these reasons possibly resulting in hypofrontality

(Chari et al., 2019; Frith et al., 1995). Although it has been shown by using magnetic resonance imaging (MRI) that the activation of the right dorsolateral prefrontal cortex, which is believed to support the maintenance of information; was matching with non-clinical control, as opposed to the activation of the left dorsolateral prefrontal cortex that was higher than the nonclinical control (Chari et al., 2019; Manoach et al., 1999). Further, the dorsolateral prefrontal cortex is believed to support the ability to hold and represent context-specific information required to direct appropriate task behaviors (Braver, Barch, & Cohen, 1999). This may include instructions, preceding stimuli, or processing a combination of letters or words preceding stimuli, such as a sentence (Barch et al., 2001). Thus, it is postulated that dorsolateral prefrontal cortex actively maintains and performs manipulations that place information into context-specific representations (Barch et al., 2001). In this way, it would be expected that working-memory impairments in individuals with schizophrenia reflect impaired context processing due to disturbed functioning of the dorsolateral prefrontal cortex (Chari et al., 2019; Cohen & Servan-Schreiber, 1992). This proposition is further corroborated by behavioral studies that have recorded observations of pattern of individuals with schizophrenia deficits in tasks sensitive to accurate processing of context (Servan-Schreiber, Cohen, & Steingard, 1996). Moreover, a growing body of work has been conducted to display the evidence of deficits in WM for schizophrenia through several different tasks (Braver et al., 1999; Chari et al., 2019; Lee & Park, 2005). This impairment is often cited as a central feature of vulnerability (Garcia-Laredo, 2018; Silver, Feldman, Bilker, & Gur, 2003). In addition, it is proposed that medication has not attributed to these deficits (Barch, 2005; Barch et al., 2001).

A disturbance in dopamine function in the dorsolateral prefrontal cortex and anterior cingulate cortex (ACC) is a critical neurobiological contributor to context-processing deficits in schizophrenia (Barch et al., 2004; Berger et al., 2016; Stäblein et al., 2018). The disturbances in the dorsolateral prefrontal cortex have been linked to working-memory deficits that are evident in individuals with schizophrenia (Barch et al., 2001). The dorsolateral prefrontal cortex is involved in manipulating the content of an individuals' WM, interrupting an individuals' ability to maintain and represent context information necessary to guide appropriate behavior during a task (Barch et al., 2004). Individuals with schizophrenia have a specific impairment in the ability to actively represent and maintain context information due to an underlying neurophysiological disturbance in the dorsolateral prefrontal cortex (Barch et al., 1997). In one study, individuals with schizophrenia demonstrated the disturbance of processing context, which refers to information that must be retained so it can be used to reconcile task appropriate behavior in a single underling information processing mechanism using various tasks. Patterns of performance were predicated within both schizophrenia and control and correlations in performance were seen across the different tasks. Furthermore, the study demonstrated that there was an association between disturbance of processing of context and formal thought disorder (Cohen, Barch, Carter, & Servan-Schreiber, 1999).

Furthermore, evidence shows that there are impairments in a cognitive task related functional activation in working-memory deficits for schizophrenia (Barch et al., 2001). The study examined dorsolateral prefrontal context using MRI with first episode schizophrenic patients performing a working-memory task that has used isolated context processing. The results suggested that there is a disturbance of the prefrontal cortex for task involved in active representation and maintenance of context information. Also, it is concluded that due to the study using first episode psychosis patients that have not taken any medication, it can be concluded that these effects are not the result of medication. Implications of this study were that patients IQ's were not accounted for and it could be important to determine how the variables related to context processing a dorsolateral prefrontal cortex are correlated. Also, alternative interpretation of the study cannot be ruled out, like patients having impairments in any type of information and not just context information. Further studies brain function on nonmedicated patients in context processing were related to disorganized symptoms however instead of context-processing tasks, patients used an encoding and retrieval strategy (MacDonald et al., 2005).

This has been explicitly shown in the form of connectionist computational models where individuals with schizophrenia display specific cognitive deficits (Braver et al., 1999). Such models provide a conceptual map between the impaired psychological processes in schizophrenia and its neurobiological foundations (Braver et al., 1999). That is, they demonstrate how cognitive control may appear from the biased influence of representations of contextual information that is actively maintained in dorsolateral prefrontal cortex on added posterior pathways that are responsible for task performance (Braver et al., 1999). Moreover, it demonstrates how dopamine can have a neuromodulatory influence on the function of dorsolateral prefrontal cortex and such disturbances in the function of neuromodulatory creates disturbances in cognitive performance that are similar to those perceived in individuals with schizophrenia (Braver et al., 1999).

As such, it has been suggested that the dopamine serves as a "gate" function in the dorsolateral prefrontal cortex, whereby it regulates access of contextual representations into active memory (Braver et al., 1999; Kindermann, Brown, Zorrilla, Olsen, & Jeste, 2004). Thus, dopamine plays an important role in control functioning because it is accountable for the flexible updating of active memory, as such; an increase in dopamine creates disturbances in the updating and maintenance of contextual information in the WM (Braver et al., 1999). In particular, schizophrenia patients display deficits on the ability to perform a cognitive task. (Braver et al., 1999; Kim et al., 2003). There is considerable evidence that show that reduced network activity appears to be adequate substrate for cognitive dysfunction and schizophrenia symptoms (Glahn et al., 2005; Honey et al., 1999, 2003; Honey, Bullmore, & Sharma, 2002). That is, individuals with schizophrenia fail to activate dorsolateral prefrontal cortex on a number of WM tasks, such as Wisconsin Card-Sorting Task, Tower of London, n-back task, and verbal fluency, with more studies (see Table 1 for further details) emphasizing that dorsolateral prefrontal cortex activation is linked to performance (Callicott et al., 2000; Glahn et al., 2005). Good performance has been associated with more activity in the dorsolateral prefrontal cortex and marked behavioral impairments has been linked to reduced activity in the dorsolateral prefrontal cortex, medial and inferior frontal gyrus, and inferior parietal lobe (Bleich-Cohen et al., 2014; Glahn et al., 2005; Stäblein et al., 2018).

Table 1 Summary of studies analyzing neural substrates in WM dysfunction in schizophrenia.

	Schizophrenia/control sample						
Study	***n***	**Mean age (years)**	**Males (%)**	**Medication**	**Neural substrate(s)**	**Working-memory task**	**Findings**
Chari et al. (2019)	16/18	26/29	78/68	Antipsychotics: typical (25%), atypical (63%) and none (12%)	Lateral PFC and visual cortex	Variant of Stenberg Task	Schizophrenia patients less accurate and slower than controls on WM tasks
Stäblein et al. (2018)	25/25	37/35	68/48	Antipsychotic medication (99%)	Anterior cingulate cortex (ACC), medial and inferior frontal gyrus, and inferior parietal lobe	Mask- Change detection task	Hypoactivation in prefrontal regions and inferior parietal lobe compared to controls
DiBiase et al. (2017)	64/87	31/30	70/64	Antipsychotics: typical (60%), atypical (4.4%) and none (4.4%)	White matter connectivity in orbital-PFC and precentral gyrus	–	Diminished white matter connectivity in OPFC and precentral gyrus compared to healthy controls
Snellenberg et al. (2016)	30/45	36/34	57/47	Antipsychotic medication (100%)	DLPFC	Self-Ordered WM task	Dysfunction in DLPFC compared to controls
Berger et al. (2016)	10/10	33/33	80/60	Typical and atypical antipsychotics	ACC and fronto-parietal region	Visuospatial delayed-match-to-sample WM task	Overactivation of theta power in the ACC in schizophrenia patients, but not controls
Bleich-Cohen et al. (2014)	17/20	26/26	65/60	Antipsychotics (100%)	DPFC and right caudate nucleus	N-Back	Diminished activation of DPFC and right caudate nucleus compared to controls

Continued

Table 1 Continued

Study	Schizophrenia/control sample				Neural substrate(s)	Working-memory task	Findings
	n	Mean age (years)	Males (%)	Medication			
Ebmeier et al. (1995)	60/20	33/34	46/60	Had not received neuroleptics for at least 2 weeks	PFC and mesial frontal/ cingulate cortex	–	Dissociation between prefrontal and anterior cingulate structures in schizophrenia patients
MacDonald et al. (2005)	18/28	28/25	72/64	Non-medicated	Middle frontal gyrus, prefrontal cortical areas (anterior and inferior)	AX-CPT	Prefrontal cortical dysfunction and increased activity in anterior and inferior prefrontal cortices in schizophrenia patients
Kindermann et al. (2004)	8/12	58/64	50/67	Typical antipsychotics (1005)	DLPFC, anterior cingulate gyrus,	Spatial WM task	No significant difference in brain activation of DLPFC nor task performance between both groups
Honey et al. (2003)	30/27	24/37	90/78	Typical antipsychotic drug (100%)	Left Lingual gyrus, left superior temporal gyrus and PFC	Verbal WM task (11 letters)	Dysfunction of left lingual gyrus, left superior temporal gyrus, and left temporal lobe in general
Kim et al. (2003)	12/12	26/26	50/50	Atypical neuroleptics	Right Ventrolateral PFC and right dorsolateral PFC	N-Back sequential-picture task	Right Ventrolateral PFC disconnected to inferior parietal cortex resulting in worse performance in schizophrenia group

Honey et al. (2002)	20/20	34/39	100/100	Typical antipsychotic drug (100%)	DPFC, left and right parietal lobe and supplementary motor area (SMA)	Verbal N-Back task	Hyperactivation of DPFC, bilateral posterior parietal cortex and SMA
Barch et al. (2001)	14/12	24/25	57/75	Neuroleptic naïve	Dorsolateral PFC	AX-CPT	Dorsolateral PFC dysfunction in schizophrenia group compared to healthy controls
Callicott et al. (2000)	13/18	34/30	77/61	Antipsychotic medication	Dorsolateral PFC	N-Back	Overactivation of DPFC during WM task
Braver et al. (1999)	16/16	24/25	56/50	Neuroleptic naïve	PFC	AX-CPT	Reduced dopamine activity in PFC
Honey et al. (1999)	10/10	37/38	100/100	Typical antipsychotic drug (100%)	DPFC, Posterior Parietal Cortex (PPC), Inferior frontal Gyrus	Verbal WM-Block periodic design	Enhanced activation of DPFC and PPC in schizophrenia group compared to controls.
Servan-Schreiber et al. (1996)	11/21	32/36	76/27	Neuroleptic medication (100%)	PFC	AX-CPT	Memory and inhibition deficits related to PFC functioning in schizophrenia group

It has been argued that tasks related to dorsolateral prefrontal cortex may be second to methodological issues or motivational differences or to between-group performance (Glahn et al., 2005). This suggests that understanding the exact role of the dorsolateral prefrontal cortex in WM ought to be better defined. Interpretation of reduced network activation in the dorsolateral prefrontal cortex in schizophrenia to be momentarily confounded (Glahn et al., 2005). It is understood that working-memory tasks, like most complex behaviors, activate a spatially distributed large-scale network or cortical and sub-cortical regions (Glahn et al., 2005). However, it is postulated that regions within dorsolateral prefrontal cortex and the parietal cortex are involved in WM (Barch et al., 2004). Studies indicate (see Table 1) that dorsolateral prefrontal cortex, left inferior frontal cortex, Broca's area, and the left parietal cortex demonstrated that all areas are precisely engaged WM demands, the precise function that each of these areas contribute is yet to be identified (Barch et al., 2004). It has been stipulated that delay manipulation engages WM because dorsolateral prefrontal cortex, Brocca's area, and parietal cortex because delay manipulation has been identified to affect (Barch et al., 2004). Brocca's area and dorsolateral prefrontal cortex demonstrated higher activation in the long delay conditions supports that dorsolateral prefrontal cortex and schizophrenia characteristics impairment may be influenced by a dysfunction in the dorsolateral prefrontal cortex, but parietal cortex increased activity as a function of delay (Berger et al., 2016; Callaway et al., 2014).

As such, dorsolateral prefrontal cortex plays a role in various subcomponents of WM that represent and maintain necessary context information and preserve context information necessary to guide appropriate task behavior (Callaway et al., 2014; Snellenberg et al., 2016). However, much controversy surrounds the functioning of specific regions that are involved in the process of WM (Barch et al., 2001, 2004; Callaway et al., 2014). Particularly, not understanding the components in WM and being able to identify its specific processes that are disturbed in individuals with schizophrenia has been related to the types of tasks that have been used in studies that are either prefrontal cortex dysfunction sensitive or tap more than one component of WM (Callaway et al., 2014). The tasks that have been used to involve WM have been increasingly difficult and in turn may be influencing the poor performance of the participants (Callaway et al., 2014). This may be because working-memory tasks require more effort to perform, and as such dorsolateral prefrontal cortex activation may just be a reflection of this increase in mental arousal, as opposed to a specific role in working-memory function (Barch, 2005). This is a fundamental and limiting concern in research in dorsolateral prefrontal cortex that needs to be addressed for research to progress on the information processing function that is subserved by this particular brain region (Barch et al., 2004). There are also possibilities that those specific processes that are involved in manipulations that increase task difficulty, even if manipulation has no influence on WM (Barch, 2005). Such processes may be dissociable from another that is directly influenced to the functioning of WM (Barch, 2005).

N-Back Paradigm

The N-Back Paradigm is a task in which stimulus sequences are presented to participants (e.g., a sequence of letters or images) (Bakanidze et al., 2013; Butler et al., 2002; Butler, Silverstein, & Dopaminekin, 2008). For each item in the sequence, individuals are required to determine if the presented stimulus matches the presented stimulus "n" items ago (Thormodsen et al., 2011). Perlstein, Dixit, Carter, Noll, and Cohen (2003) explored the processes involved in the active maintenance and manipulation of information in WM and the preparation to override response tendencies through fMRI of the dorsolateral prefrontal cortex. The behavioral performance and brain activity were examined in individuals with schizophrenia and healthy control comparisons using the 2-back task. It was hypothesized that WM and preparation to override pre-potent response tendencies would activate the dorsolateral prefrontal cortex; however, individuals with schizophrenia would show altered activity and decrease task performance. Results supported their predictions that individuals with schizophrenia had less activation in the dorsolateral prefrontal cortex under conditions of high working-memory load compared to healthy controls. Individuals with schizophrenia and SPD were also more impaired compared to healthy controls in the n-back task. Thormodsen et al. (2011) investigated the activation levels of the dorsolateral prefrontal cortex in individuals with early onset schizophrenia and healthy controls using an fMRI while participants completed a 2-back task. Their results indicated that the activation of the dorsolateral prefrontal cortex did not deviate between individuals with schizophrenia and healthy controls. It was suggested that the lack of deviation could be due to the schizophrenia group having used compensatory strategy during the working-memory task. Barch et al. (2004) employed a 2-back task to determine if individuals with schizophrenia exhibited a deficit in the representation and maintenance of context information processing. Their results showed no significant interaction between schizotypal personality disorder and healthy controls on the 2-back task.

In SPD individuals, research that employed the n-back task to assess WM performance indicated that this patient group performed worse than healthy controls (Carrigan, Barkus, Ong, & Wei, 2017; McClure, Barch, Flory, Harvey, & Siever, 2008). It was found that as the task demands increased, performance worsened which suggested deficits in context processing and management of cognitive load. Together, these findings suggest reduced efficiency of working-memory resources along the psychosis continuum for handling high cognitive loads in short time spans.

AX-Continuous Performance Task

The Continuous Performance Test (CPT) had been used extensively in psychiatric research and was initially designed to measure impairments in brain injuries (Barch et al., 1997). However, the test has been modified for wide use in schizophrenia in order to probe the mechanism within context processing (Cohen et al., 1999). According to Cohen et al. (1999), context processing refers to the information that is stored temporarily in the mind to facilitate task performance behaviors. The task that has been used from the original version is the AX-CPT, which has been used in a number of previous studies known as the AX-CPT (Cohen et al., 1999; Hazlett et al., 2014; Moustafa, Sherman, & Frank, 2008). Barch et al., 2001; Barch et al., 2004; Bleich-Cohen et al., 2014; Polizzotto, Hill-Jarrett, Walker, & Cho, 2018). A commonly used working-memory task that isolates context processing: is the AX-CPT (Braver et al., 1999) which is an "AX" adopamineptation of the original CPT (Rosvold, Mirsky, Sarason, Bransome, & Beck, 1956). In the AX-CPT task, participants are presented with a sequence of letters and instructed to respond to a prespecified probe stimuli (X) only in the event it followed a specific contextual cue (A) with (A-X) being the target trials (Polizzotto et al., 2018). In the AX-CPT, two nontarget trials, B-X and A-Y, selectively probe context processing (Braver et al., 1999). In B-X trials, context of the (B) would inhibit the tendency to make a target response to the subsequent (X) (Braver et al., 1999). Alternatively, in A-Y trials, the context of the (A) creates an expectancy that an (X) would occur next, leading to a tendency to false alarm to the probe (Braver et al., 1999). Failure to represent and maintain context in this task would be expected to manifest as an increase in B-X false alarms with either no change, or decrease, in A-Y false alarms (Braver et al., 1999). This task also involves a temporal manipulation varying the delay between the cue and probe onset (Barch et al., 2001). Using functional magnetic resonance imaging (fMRI) during the AX-CPT, it was shown that individuals with SZ demonstrated a pattern of responding expected with dorsolateral prefrontal cortex disruption, yielding fewer A-Y errors and more B-X behavioral performance errors then the nonclinical control group (Barch et al., 2001). The findings suggested a deficit in the ability to actively hold and represent context-specific information for individuals with SZ (Barch et al., 2001). During this task subjects were presented with a sequence of letters (e.g., A, B, X, Y), and they were instructed to respond to a specified probe (e.g., X) but only if it preceded a particular contextual cue (e.g., A) (Barch et al., 2001). Throughout this task context processing was selectively probed in two types of nontargets (e.g., B-X and A-Y) (Barch et al., 2001). In B-X trials context was required to inhibit prepotent tendency to make a target response to the X whereas, in the A-Y trials, the context created expectancy that the X will occur, leading to a tendency to false alarm to the probe (Barch et al., 2001).

Cohen et al. (1999) investigated context-processing deficits that are present in individuals with schizophrenia, and how a disturbance of this function contributes to cognitive deficits. They modified three tasks, which included the AX-CPT, Stroop, and Lexical disambiguation to explore if a disturbance of context-processing could account for performance deficits among individuals with schizophrenia (Cohen et al., 1999). The results indicated that individuals with SZ displayed the greatest deficits in the task conditions that drew heavily on the use of context information to support the execution of weaker but task-appropriate responses (Cohen et al., 1999). Barch et al. (2004) studied deficits in context processing which are evident in both schizotypal personality disorder and schizophrenia. They administered three versions of the AX-CPT tasks to determine if individuals' performance on context-processing tasks deviated as well on N-back task and the Eriksen Flanker Task to determine if context-processing deficits were evident in other domains such as WM and selective attention (Barch et al., 2004). It was predicted that individuals with schizotypal personality disorder would show context-processing deficits similar to those seem in individuals with schizophrenia (Barch et al., 2004). Additionally, individuals with schizotypal personality disorder would display deficits in the WM and selective attention tasks (Barch et al., 2004). The results indicated that individuals with schizotypal personality disorder demonstrated similar deficits in the ability to represent context information (Barch et al., 2004). Moreover, individuals with SPD demonstrated deficits in WM but not in selective attention compared to healthy controls (Barch et al., 2004).

Yoon et al. (2012) measured fMRI responses in a cohort of subjects with first episode schizophrenia and a healthy control group while they completed an AX-CPT. It was predicted that individuals with schizophrenia would exhibit a greater cognitive and behavioral disorganization than healthy individuals (Yoon et al., 2012). Their results demonstrated individual with schizophrenia exhibited greater behavioral disorganization compared to the healthy individuals (Yoon et al., 2012). However, there was no difference between cognitive disorganization in individuals with schizophrenia compared to the control, as indicated by the fMRI results yielding similar brain activation (Yoon et al., 2012). It has been suggested that these insignificant results may be due to the study of individuals with first episode schizophrenia, as it is a possibility that the neurophysiological markers of this disorder may not be evident in first episode patients compared to patients with their illness being more established (Yoon et al., 2012).

Niendam et al. (2014) explored the relationship between functional deficits, cognitive and psychosocial impairments during the period in which they are at risk for psychosis. They employed an AX version of the Continuous Performance Task (AX-CPT), to examine high-risk individuals and determine if cognitive control deficits are associated with clinical symptoms and functional disability (Niendam et al., 2014). It was predicted that reduced dorsolateral prefrontal cortex (DLPFC) activation in response to cognitive control demands was associated with poorer task performance and global functioning at baseline in first episode schizophrenia and high-risk individuals (Niendam et al., 2014). Their findings were consistent with their hypothesis, as individuals with high risk for schizophrenia show a specific behavioral pattern of impaired cognitive control as well as failure to engage the DLPFC during high control conditions (Niendam et al., 2014).

Barch et al. (1997) sought to establish whether the activation of the dorsolateral prefrontal cortex was due to the difficulty of the task or the demand of an individuals' WM during a task (Barch et al., 1997). They employed fMRI to monitor activation within the dorsolateral prefrontal cortex, while individuals completed a version of the AX-CPT, which they manipulated delay as well as visual degrades to significantly decrease performance in the task and allow them to demonstrate a dissociation between task difficulty and demands of WM (Barch et al., 1997). It was predicted that the dorsolateral prefrontal cortex, which had increased activation activity in response to the delay manipulation would not increase activity in response to the delay manipulation (Barch et al., 1997). The results indicated a significantly greater activity in the long compared to the short delay conditions of the task, but did not show greater activity as a function on the task difficulty manipulation (Barch et al., 1997). Thus, suggesting that dorsolateral prefrontal cortex is engaged by working-memory demands rather than other cognitive processes which could be affected by increases in task difficulty (Barch et al., 1997).

Braver et al. (1999) suggested that dopamine serves as a gating function in the prefrontal cortex, regulating access of context representation into active memory. This gives dopamine important control responsible for the flexible updating of memory in the prefrontal cortex, while retaining protection against interference (Braver et al., 1999). They predicted that an important component of schizophrenia may increase the noise in the dopamine system, and that this increased variability leads to disturbances in both the updating and maintenance of context information within an individual's WM (Braver et al., 1999). Their results indicated that performance of individuals with schizophrenia demonstrated impairment in both representation and maintenance of context information (Braver et al., 1999). Furthermore, it was demonstrated that their deficit was specific to cognitive control rather than a general deficit (Braver et al., 1999). This pattern can be observed from the context disturbance exhibited by individuals with SZ as they responded less to A-Y trials relative to B-Y trials (Braver et al., 1999). Context information must be used on B-X trials to inhibit the tendency to make a target response to the X (Braver et al., 1999). In contrast, context acts as a bias for the incorrect responding on A-Y trials, because the presence of the A sets up a strong expectancy to make a target response to the probe (Braver et al., 1999).

Barch et al. (2001) examined the prefrontal cortex activation using a fMRI in medication naive individuals with first episode schizophrenia. An AX-CPT task was employed to examine the relationship between maintaining context information within the task and the activation in the dorsolateral prefrontal cortex of the individuals with schizophrenia. Individuals with schizophrenia displayed impairment in their ability to actively represent and maintain context information. The deficit in context information has been shown to be due to an underlying neurophysiological disturbance in the dorsolateral prefrontal cortex. A specific pattern was demonstrated in the patients with both better (e.g., fewer A-Y trial errors) and worse behavior performance (e.g., more B-X trial errors). Individuals with schizophrenia demonstrated a selective deficit in the ability to appropriately activate the dorsolateral prefrontal cortex in response to the demands for the maintenance of context. The deficits in the dorsolateral prefrontal cortex are present at the onset of the first acute exacerbation of this disorder; medication naïve patients demonstrate this, as previous medication effects do not confound the results.

Dopamine plays a major role in the cognitive impairment in individuals with schizophrenia (Braver et al., 1999). Disturbances caused by abnormal dopamine activity results in abnormal modulation of prefrontal cortex (Braver et al., 1999). Individuals with schizophrenia have a wide range of cognitive deficits, meaning a disturbance in their ability to represent, maintain, and update context information (Haro et al., 2018). Braver et al. (1999) was able to link the physiological disturbances with psychological deficits in individuals with schizophrenia. This link is demonstrated through the dysfunction of dopamine levels that effected the modulation of the prefrontal cortex and hence caused deficits in maintaining and updating of internally represented context information.

Context is defined as prior task-relevant information, which is represented in such a way that it can bias selection of appropriate behavior response. Individuals with schizophrenia show an increase in context-processing deficits at the long delay compared to short delay (McClure et al., 2008). However, the same increases in context-processing deficits were found in some studies on a normal control population (Cohen et al., 1999). Individuals who experience early onset of schizophrenia tend not to have such significant deficits compare to chronic patients (Javitt, Shelley, Silipo, & Lieberman, 2000). These selective deficits in context processing were also found in unaffected siblings of individuals with schizophrenia (Barch et al., 2004). Such findings support the notion that deficit like these are associated with schizophrenia. Evidence that specifically links schizophrenia with the context-processing deficits illustrates, those individuals with nonpsychotic major depressive disorder did present with the same pattern of deficits.

Active maintenance of contextual information is controlled by prefrontal cortex mechanism, and that context processing is a component of WM (Cohen et al., 1999). Performance in the AX-CPT task heavily rely on the representation and maintenance of contextual information, meaning participant's response to "X" depends on whether the previous stimulus is "A" or not A (Cohen et al., 1999). Participants need to be able to maintain the information before the target "X" so that they can respond correctly. However, individuals with schizophrenia consistently show increased errors on this task, therefore there is a deficit in context processing among the schizophrenia population. Results from Cohen et al. (1999) found that individuals with schizophrenia displayed the greatest deficits in the task condition, which heavily rely on context information to elicit task appropriate responses. As demonstrated in the AX- CPT task, individuals with schizophrenia experience more AX misses and BX false alarm compared to the control population. Consistent with previous studies, Barch et al. (2004) demonstrated that individuals with SPD would exhibit deficits in the ability to represent contextual information. However, such deficits did not interfere with their ability to maintain context representation over a long delay. Furthermore, they also found that individuals with SPD also experienced deficits on working-memory tasks but no deficits were found on selective attention task.

Additionally, chronically hospitalized individuals with schizophrenia were found to have deficits performing the traditional AX-CPT task, meaning they also have difficulty with short-term memory (Chen, Hsiao, Hsiao, & Hwu, 1998). Alternatively, nonpsychotic relatives of individuals with SZ schizophrenia have been found to have some level of deficits on the similar AX-CPT tasks. Similarly, more difficult AX-CPT task, which require high processing load, could detect deficits in children of mothers with schizophrenia (Chen et al., 1998). These results indicate that a deficit on the high processing load form of CPT possibly a marker of schizophrenia.

A study conducted by Yoon et al. (2012), fMRI was conducted while participants performed the AX-CPT task. "A" cue in the AX condition represents a low cognitive control where as "B" cue in the BX condition represents high cognitive control. Results in this study shows that individuals with schizophrenia displayed impaired overall performance in the AX-CPT task. Comparison between AX to BX condition shows individuals with SZ where slower and less accurate in the BX high cognitive control condition. When BX condition was considered alone, individuals with SZ were less accurate and slower compared to the control sample. fMRI contrast between B cue and A cue results reveals activation within the left dorsolateral prefrontal cortex.

Across different phases of psychotic illness, cognitive neuroscience-based imaging reveal dorsolateral prefrontal cortex deficits (Niendam et al., 2014). Reduced dorsolateral prefrontal cortex activation is identified as the underlie impairment in cognitive control in schizophrenia population. Clinically high-risk individuals also show structural and functional abnormalities, including deficits in the cognitive control network. Cognitive dysfunction may represent a clear marker for future deterioration for high-risk individuals. Niendam et al. (2014)'s study provides supporting evidence that high-risk individuals show specific behavioral patterns of impaired cognitive process as well as low activation of dorsolateral prefrontal cortex during high control condition. Moreover, consistent with other studies, high-risk individual as well as individuals with first episode schizophrenia both exhibit disruption in dorsolateral prefrontal cortex modulation, which was significantly associated with impaired task performance (Niendam et al., 2014).

All these results all point to a conclusion that context-processing deficits are trait like deficits associated with schizophrenia (Barch et al., 2004). It also suggests that schizotypal personality disorder is part of the schizophrenia spectrum as similar deficits are shown in individuals with schizotypal personality disorder compared to those with schizophrenia.

Moreover, the AX-CPT task also provides a way to look at how context processing is maintained by manipulating both the probe and the cue. Meaning, that when the cue and probe delay is extended by 5 in comparison to 1 s, this information must be actively preserved within the WM (Barch et al., 2001, 2004). According to the contextual processing framework, it has been suggestive that there is an effect of delay that interacts with performance in the AY and BX trials (Barch et al., 2004). That is, studies indicate that when context can be maintained in the WM the strength of the contextual representation should remain the same or it should increase with a delay (Barch et al., 2004). As such, BX performance remains the same or it may improve in longer delays, as opposed to AY performance that may get worse, because the contextual representations are accessible over the delay to assist processing (Barch et al., 2004). On the contrary, if there is impairment in context maintenance, as is found in individuals with schizophrenia, then BX performance has been shown to get worse with a delay, but the AY performance has been shown to improve (Barch et al., 2004).

Moreover, various studies indicate that individuals with schizophrenia show an increase in contextual processing impairments at the long delays as opposed to the short delays (Barch et al., 2004), and yet other studies have not (Barch et al., 2001). Interestingly, studies on individuals with schizophrenia commonly find that they perform worse at long delays as opposed to short delays; however, such a finding has been found in various studies where such performance worsened in long delays as opposed to short delays among the controls (but no information mentioned if the schizotypal traits were investigated) (Barch et al., 2004). It should be mentioned that studies with individuals that were at the early stages of onset of schizophrenia did not display greater deficits at long delays compared to short delays (Barch et al., 2004). However, in studies where small increases in deficits at long delays were demonstrated they were relatively smaller as compared to individuals with chronic schizophrenia (Barch et al., 2004).

Moreover, it has been proposed that correct responding to AXCPT could be due to two different approaches, which include a proactive control strategy characterized by pre-emptive engagement of task-relevant representations for efficient responding, and a reactive strategy involving the retrieval of task representations at the time of responding only (Braver, 2012). Numerous studies have provided support regarding context deficits in schizophrenia using the AXCPT task. One study showed that performance deficits among individuals with schizophrenia were due to disturbance in context processes (Cohen et al., 1999).

Barch et al. (1997) explored the neural substrates of WM, especially the prefrontal cortex and the dorsolateral prefrontal cortex. WM is needed to successfully perform the AXCPT task. Within the study participants observed letters on a screen and responded to an X only when it followed an A. WM was influenced by the delay between the letters on the screen. They used a factorial analysis with two levels of memory and two levels of task difficulty. They stated that the AXCPT did not require maintenance of sequential order information. They found that manipulating task difficulty (making features of stimuli either easy or hard) affected the anterior cingulate. Changing the working-memory delay affected the prefrontal cortex only. The current study will also be manipulating the delay interval; that is the time between the A and the X.

Barch et al. (2001) investigated AXCPT task performance in individuals with schizophrenia. This study also examined the dorsolateral prefrontal cortex and WM. They proposed that the dorsolateral prefrontal cortex supports a part of the WM, specifically the ability to represent and maintain context information that is used to guide task behavior. Context information includes instructions, prior stimuli, or processing a sequence of prior stimuli. They used an example of a sentence that participants were required to know and remember the context of the sentence to be able to make sense of it or any story or instructions formulated by the sentence. They hypothesized that the discrepancies in WM in schizophrenia reflects an impairment in context processing due to the functioning of the dorsolateral prefrontal cortex being disturbed. Within the AXCPT task participants were presented with a sequence of letters and were instructed to only respond to the probe (the letter X) if it comes after the cue (A). The targets occurred frequently at 70%, which then made the participants more likely to respond to an X and be expected to make a response after seeing an A. This often led to a false alarm of the probe (X). They varied the delay between the cues (A) and probe (X) and thus manipulated contextual memory demands. The current study has equal number of trials and therefore equals probabilities of the targets occurring.

In the Cohen et al. (1999) study, participants also completed a Lexical Disambiguation task and an AXCPT task. Within all of the tasks participants with schizophrenia showed the most deficits in the conditions that relied on the use of context information to support the weaker but task-appropriate responses. There was more AX misses and BX false alarms within the AXCPT. Their results showed that deficits in context processing are associated with the disorganization symptoms of schizophrenia.

Within Yoon et al. (2012) study, it was found that individuals with schizophrenia exhibited levels of disorganization significantly greater than those of the control group. This was found using an fMRI study whilst participants performed an AXCPT task. Participants with schizophrenia exhibited deficits in cognitive control within the task.

Barch et al. (2004) also included context information. There is a deficit within schizophrenia in the ability to be able to represent and maintain context information. The main neurobiological contributor to context-processing deficits within schizophrenia is the disturbance in dopamine functioning within the dorsolateral prefrontal cortex. Individuals with SPD have some of the same cognitive deficits that are found in individuals with schizophrenia. They found that individuals with SPD have deficits in being able to represent context information and processing. They did not find any deficits in maintaining context representations over a delay. The researchers administered the same AXCPT task as observed in Barch et al. (2001). Their target AX trials occurred 70% of the time which created two biases, the first being on a BX trial (B being a non-A cue) where they had to use the context provided by seeing the B cue to inhibit the bias to respond to an X. The second bias was when participants saw an A cue and expected to make a target response because most of the time an X will follow. But when it the X did not precede (such as with AY trials, where Y is a non-X probe) it created false alarms. Individuals with deficits in context processing showed worse within BX performances but better within AY performances, compared to healthy individuals.

Chen et al. (1998) found that poor performance on the CPT (attentional test) was associated with severity of schizotypy. They used the Perceptual Aberration Scale (PAS) as well as the schizotypal personality questionnaire to measure schizotypy within individuals. The PAS also involved a self-report and consisted of 35 true or false questions measuring nonpsychotic body image and perceptual distortions (Chapman, Chapman, & Raulin, 1978). Chapman, Chapman, Kwapil, Eckblad, and Zinser (1994) found students high on the PAS also had a higher risk of schizotypal symptoms. The difference between the two questionnaires is that the schizotypal personality questionnaire involves the nine criteria in the DSM-5-TR of schizotypal personality disorder whereas the PAS has a focus on perceptual abnormalities within schizotypy. A limitation of the study is that they did not screen for a family history of psychosis. As demonstrated in previous studies (Geng et al., 2013; Kendler, 2005; Kendler et al., 1993; Kim, Jang, & Kim, 2015) there has been evidence that non-diagnosed family members can display schizotypy, and schizophrenia is genetic.

Conclusions and future directions

The current chapter examined the verbal and visuospatial working-memory deficits that exist in two highly prevalent psychosis spectrum disorders, namely schizophrenia and SPD. Multiple research sources were used to assess the extent to which WM deficits are present in both populations and the neuroanatomical underpinnings of these deficits. Compared to healthy controls, schizophrenia and SPD patients showed heightened vulnerability to cognitive failures as the cognitive demands increased. In schizophrenia patients, the neural substrates that were found to be most affected were pre-frontal cortex regions, anterior cingulate cortex, and frontal and inferior gyrus. The impairment was characterized by hypoactivation of these regions which hindered their ability to encode and retrieve information during the working-memory tasks. Taken together, the current data suggests a dysfunction in both bottom-up sensory processing regions in the visual cortex as well as in top-down higher cortical storage areas involved in the active maintenance of information during short delay intervals. Moreover, detailed assessment was provided of the N-Back test and AX-CPT as a means to understand qualitatively and quantitatively the WM deficits found in both psychosis-spectrum disorders.

This current chapter highlights the need to increment research on verbal and visuospatial WM in SPD in order to understand whether certain cognitive constructs such as WM can be considered an endophenotypic marker of SPD. Similarly, more research comparing SPD and schizophrenia on the same working-memory tasks is required as a means to better understand whether the cognitive impairments observed in both disorders lie on a continuum of impairment severity. To this end, the current chapter points towards the need to understand WM as an area of impairment that is crucial to understanding the pathology of SPD in its own right, as cognitive impairments may relate to the chronic and debilitating social inappropriateness and interpersonal isolation of SPD, and psychosis-spectrum disorders in general.

References

Abohamza, E., Weickert, T., Ali, M., & Moustafa, A. A. (2020). Reward and punishment learning in schizophrenia and bipolar disorder. *Behavioural Brain Research*, *381*, 112298. https://doi.org/10.1016/j.bbr.2019.112298.

Addington, J., Liu, L., Perkins, D. O., Carrion, R. E., Keefe, R. S., & Woods, S. W. (2017). The role of cognition and social functioning as predictors in the transition to psyhcosis for youth with attenuated psychotic symptoms. *Schizophrenia Bulletin*, *43*(1), 57–63. https://doi.org/10.1093/schbul/sbw152.

American Psychiatric Association. (2013). *Diagnostic and statistical manual of mental disorders* (5th ed.). Washington: American Psychiatric Association. https://doi.org/10.1176/appi.books.9780890425596.070363.

Baddeley, A. (2018). *Exploring working memory: Selected works of Alan Baddeley*. Routledge.

Bakanidze, G., Roinishvili, M., Chkonia, E., Kitzrow, W., Richter, S., Neumann, K., … Puls, I. (2013). Association of the nicotinic receptor alpha7 subunit gene (CHRNA7) with schizophrenia and visual backward masking. *Frontiers in Psychiatry*, *4*, 133. https://doi.org/10.3389/fpsyt.2013.00133.

Ballard, J. C. (2001). Assessing attention: Comparison of response-inhibition and traditional continuous performance tests. *Journal of Clinical and Experimental Neuropsychology*, *23*(3), 331–350. https://doi.org/10.1076/jcen.23.3.331.1188.

Barch, D. M. (2005). The cognitive neuroscience of schizophrenia. *Annual Review of Clinical Psychology*, *1*, 321–353.

Barch, D. M., Braver, T. S., Nystrom, L. E., Forman, S. D., Noll, D. C., & Cohen, J. D. (1997). Dissociating working memory from task difficulty in human prefrontal cortex. *Neuropsychologia*, *35*(10), 1373–1380. https://doi.org/10.1016/S0028-3932(97)00072-9.

Barch, D. N., Carter, C. S., Braver, T. S., Sabb, F. W., MacDonald, A., Noll, D. C., & Cohen, J. D. (2001). Selective deficits in prefrontal cortex function in medication - naive patients with schizophrenia. *Archives of General Psychiatry*, *58*, 280–288. https://doi.org/10.1001/archpsyc.58.3.280.

Barch, D. M., Mitropoulou, V., Harvey, P. D., New, A. S., Silverman, J. M., & Siever, L. J. (2004). Context-processing deficits in schizotypal personality disorder. *Journal of Abnormal Psychology*, *113*(4), 556–568. https://doi.org/10.1037/0021-843x.113.4.556.

Bedwell, J. S., Kamath, V., & Compton, M. T. (2009). The relationship between interview-based schizotypal personality dimension scores and the continuous performance test. *Schizophrenia Research*, *108*(1-3), 158–162. https://doi.org/10.1016/j.schres.2008.11.020.

Berger, B., Minarik, T., Griesmayr, B., Stelzing-Schoeler, R., Aichhorn, W., & Sauseng, P. (2016). Brain oscillatory correlates of altered executive functioning in positive and negative symptomatic schizophrenia patients and healthy controls. *Frontiers in Psychology*, *7*, 705. https://doi.org/10.3389/fpsyg.2016.00705.

Bleich-Cohen, M., Hendler, T., Weizman, R., Faragian, S., Weizman, A., & Poyurovsky, M. (2014). Working memory dysfunction in schizo phrenia patients with obsessive-compulsive symptoms: An fMRI study. *European Psychiatry*, *29*(3), 160–166. https://doi.org/10.1016/j.eurpsy.2013.02.004.

Botero, S., Muñoz, C. C., Ocampo, M. V., Escobar, M., Rangel, A., Quintero, C., … García, J. (2013). Verbal working memory in individuals with schizophrenia and their first degree relatives: Relationship with negative and disorganized symptoms. *Actas Españolas de Psiquiatría*, *41*(2), 106–114.

Braver, T. S. (2012). The variable nature of cognitive control: A dual mechanisms framework. *Trends in Cognitive Sciences*, *16*(2), 106–113.

Braver, T. S., Barch, D. M., & Cohen, J. D. (1999). Cognition and control in schizophrenia: A computational model of dopamine and prefrontal function. *Journal of Biological Psychiatry*, *46*(3), 312–328. https://doi.org/10.1016/S0006-3223(99)00116-X.

Brébion, G., Stephan-Otto, C., Cuevas-Esteban, J., Usall, J., & Ochoa, S. (2020). Impaired memory for temporal context in schizophrenia patients with hallucinations and thought disorganisation. *Schizophrenia Research*, *220*, 225–231. https://doi.org/10.1016/j.schres.2020.03.014.

Breeze, J. M. B., Kirkham, A. J., & Marí-Beffa, P. (2011). Evidence of reduced selective attention in schizotypal personality disorder. *Journal of Clinical and Experimental Neuropsychology*, *33*(7), 776–784. https://doi.org/10.1080/13803395.2011.558495.

Butler, P. D., DeSanti, L. A., Maddox, J., Harkavy-Friedman, J. M., Amador, X. F., Goetz, R. R., … Gorman, J. M. (2002). Visual backward-masking deficits in schizophrenia: Relationship to visual pathway function and symptomatology. *Schizophrenia Research*, *59*(2–3), 199–209. https://doi.org/10.1016/S0920-9964(01)00341-3.

Butler, P. D., Silverstein, S. M., & Dopaminekin, S. C. (2008). Visual perception and its impairment in schizophrenia. *Biological Psychiatry*, *64*(1), 40–47. https://doi.org/10.1016/j.biopsych.2008.03.023.

Callaway, D., Cohen, A., Matthews, R., & Dinzeo, T. (2014). Schizotypal personality questionnaire-brief revised: Psychometric replication and extension. *Personality Disorders, Theory, Research, and Treatment*, *5*(1), 32–38. https://doi.org/10.1037/per0000041.

Callicott, J. H., Bertolino, A., Mattat, V. S., Langheim, F. J., Duyn, J., Coppola, R., ... Weinberger, D. R. (2000). Physiological dysfunction of the dorsolateral prefrontal cortex in schizophrenia revisited. *Cerebral Cortex, 10*(11), 1078–1092. https://doi.org/10.1093/cercor/10.11.1078.

Carrigan, N., Barkus, E., Ong, A., & Wei, M. (2017). Do complaints of everyday cognitive failures in high schizotypy relate to emotional working memory deficits in the lab? *Comprehensive Psychiatry, 78*, 115–129. https://doi.org/10.1016/j.comppsych.2017.06.016.

Cassetta, B. D., Tomfohr-Madsen, L. M., & Goghari, V. M. (2018). A randomized controlled trial of working memory and processing speed training in schizophrenia. *Psychological Medicine, 49*(12), 2009–2019. https://doi.org/10.1017/S0033291718002775.

Chang, W. C., Chu, A. O. K., Wong, C. S. M., Hui, C. L. M. N., Chan, S. K. W., Lee, E. H. M., & Chen, E. Y. H. (2018). Patterns and predictors of trajectories for social and occupational functioning in patient with first episode non-affective psychosis: A three-year follow-up study. *Schizophrenia Research, 197*, 131–137. https://doi.org/10.1016/j.schres.2018.01.021.

Chapman, L. J., Chapman, J. P., Kwapil, T. R., Eckblad, M., & Zinser, M. C. (1994). Putatively psychosis-prone subjects 10 years later. *Journal of Abnormal Psychology, 103*, 171–183.

Chapman, L. J., Chapman, J. P., & Raulin, M. L. (1978). Body-image aberration in schizophrenia. *Journal of Abnormal Psychology, 87*, 399–407.

Chari, S., Minzenberg, M. J., Solomon, M., Ragland, J. D., Nguyen, Q., Carter, C. S., & Yoon, J. H. (2019). Impaired prefrontal functional connectivity associated with working memory task performance and disorganization despite intact activations in schizophrenia. *Psychiatry Research: Neuroimaging, 287*, 10–18. https://doi.org/10.1016/j.pscychresns.2019.01.013.

Chen, W. J., Hsiao, C. K., Hsiao, L.-L., & Hwu, H.-G. (1998). Performance of the continuous performance test among community samples. *Schizophrenia Bulletin, 24*(1), 163–174.

Cho, M., Lam, N. H., Starc, M., Santamauro, N., Savic, A., Diehl, C. K., ... Anticevic, A. (2018). Effects of reward on spatial working memory in schizophrenia. *Journal of Abnormal Psychology, 127*(7), 695–709. https://doi.org/10.1037/abn0000369.

Chun, C. A., Ciceron, L., & Kwapil, T. R. (2018). A meta-analysis of context integration deficits across the schizotypy spectrum using AX-CPT and DPX tasks. *Journal of Abnormal Psychology, 127*(8), 789–806. https://doi.org/10.1037/abn0000383.

Cohen, J. D., Barch, D. M., Carter, C., & Servan-Schreiber, D. (1999). Context-processing deficits in schizophrenia: Converging evidence from three theoretically motivated cognitive tasks. *Journal of Abnormal Psychology, 108*(1), 120–133. https://doi.org/10.1037/0021-843X.108.1.120.

Cohen, J. D., & Servan-Schreiber, D. (1992). Context, cortex, and dopamine: A connectionist approach to behavior and biology in schizophrenia. *Psychological Review, 99*(1), 45.

Coleman, M. J., Krastoshevsky, O., Tu, X., Mendell, N. R., & Levy, D. L. (2012). The effects of perceptual encoding on the magnitude of object working memory impairment in schizophrenia. *Schizophrenia Research, 139*(1–3), 60–65. https://doi.org/10.1016/j.schres.2012.05.003.

Corigliano, V., De Carolis, A., Trovini, G., Dehning, J., Di Pietro, S., Curto, M., ... Comparelli, A. (2014). Neurocognition in schizophrenia: From prodrome to multi-episode illness. *Psychiatry Research, 220*(12), 129–134.

Debbané, M., & Mohr, C. (2015). Integration and development in schizotypy research: An introduction to the special supplement. *Schizophrenia Bulletin, 41*(2), 363–365. https://doi.org/10.1093/schbul/sbv003.

DiBiase, M. A., Cropley, V. L., Baune, B. T., Olver, J., & Amminger, G. P. (2017). White matter connectivity disruptions in early and chronic schizophrenia. *Psychological Medicine, 47*(16), 2797–2810. https://doi.org/10.1017/S003329171001313.

Ebmeier, K. P., Lawrie, S. M., Blackwood, D. H., Johnstone, E. C., & Goodwin, G. M. (1995). Hypofrontality revisited: A high resolution single photon emission computed tomography study in schizophrenia. *Journal of Neurology, Neurosurgery, and Psychiatry*, *58*(4), 452–456.

Eryilmaz, H., Tanner, A. S., Ho, N. F., Nitenson, A. Z., Silverstein, N. J., Petruzzi, L. J., … Roffman, J. L. (2016). Disrupted working memory circuitry in schizophrenia: Disentangling fMRI markers of core pathology vs other aspects of impaired performance. *Neuropsychopharmachology*, *41*, 2411–2420. https://doi.org/10.1038/npp.2016.55.

Ettinger, U., Meyhöfer, I., Steffens, M., Wagner, M., & Koutsouleris, N. (2014). Genetics, cognition, and neurobiology of schizotypal personality: A review of the overlap with schizophrenia. *Frontiers in Psychology*, *5*, 18. https://doi.org/10.3389/fpsyt.2014.00018.

Fanous, A. H., Neale, M. C., Gardner, C. O., Webb, B. T., Straub, R. E., O'Neill, F. A., … Kendler, K. S. (2007). Significant correlation in linkage signals from genome-wide scans of schizophrenia and schizotypy. *Molecular Psychiatry*, *12*, 958–965. https://doi.org/10.1038/sj.mp.4001996.

Frith, C. D., Friston, K. J., Herold, S., Silbersweig, D., Fletcher, P., Cahill, C., … Liddle, P. F. (1995). Regional brain activity in chronic schizophrenic patients during the performance of a verbal fluency task. *The British Journal of Psychiatry: the Journal of Mental Science*, *167*(3), 343–349.

Galletly, C. A., Castle, D., Dark, F., Humberstone, V., Jablensky, A., Killackey, E., … Tran, N. (2016). Royal Australian and New Zealand College of Psychiatrists practice guidelines for the management of schizophrenia and related disorders. *Australian and New Zealand Journal of Psychiatry*, *50*(5), 1–117.

Ganguly, P., Soliman, A., & Moustafa, A. A. (2018). Holistic management of schizophrenia symptoms using pharmacological non-pharmacological treatment. *Frontiers in Public Health*, *6*, 166. https://doi.org/10.3389/fpubh.2018.00166.

Garcia-Laredo, E. (2018). Cognitive impairment in schizophrenia: Description and cognitive familiar endophenotypes. A review of the literature. In *Psychosis: Biopsychosocial and relational perspectives*. Madrid: IntechOpen. doi:10.5772/intechopen.78948.

Geng, F., Xu, T., Wang, Y., Shi, H., Yan, C., Neumann, D. L., … Chan, R. C. (2013). Developmental trajectories of schizotypal personality disorder-like behavioural manifestations: A two-year longitudinal prospective study of college students. *BMC Psychiatry*, *13*, 323.

George, M., Maheshwari, S., Chandran, S., Manohar, J. S., & Rao, T. S. S. (2017). Understanding the schizophrenia prodrome. *Indian Journal of Psychiatry*, *59*(4), 505–509. https://doi.org/10.4103/psychiatry.IndianJPsychiatry_464_17.

Gjini, K., Burroughs, S., & Boutros, N. N. (2011). Relevance of attention in auditory sensory gating paradigms in schizophrenia: A pilot study. *Journal of Psychophysiology*, *25*(2), 60–66. https://doi.org/10.1027/0269-8803/a000042.

Glahn, D. C., Ragland, J. D., Abramoff, A., Barnett, J., Laird, A. R., Bearden, C. E., & Velligand, D. I. (2005). Beyond hypofrontality: A quantitative meta-analysis of cuntional neuroimaging studies of working memory in schizophrenia. *Human Brain Mapping*, *25*(1), 60–69.

Goldstein, K. E., Berlin, H. A., Hamilton, H. K., Mitsis, E. M., McClure, M. M., Savage, K. R., … Hazlett, E. A. (2016). Cognitive and mood functioning in borderline and schizotypal personality disorders. *Psychology Faculty Publication*, *7*(3), 292–299. https://doi.org/10.4236/psych.2016.73032.

Guo, J. Y., Ragland, J. D., & Carter, C. S. (2019). Memory and cognition in schizophrenia. *Molecular Psychiatry*, *24*, 633–642. https://doi.org/10.1038/s41380-018-0231-1.

Haro, J. M., Altamura, C., Corral, R., Elkis, R., Evabs, H., Krebs, M., … Nordstroen, A. (2018). Understanding the course of persistent symptoms in schizophrenia: Longitudinal findings from the pattern of study. *Psychiatry Research*, *267*, 56–62. https://doi.org/10.1016/j.psychres.2018.04.005.

Harvey, P. D., Keefe, R. S. E., Mitroupolou, V., DuPre, R., Roitman, S. L., Mohs, R. C., & Siever, L. J. (1996). Information-processing markers of vulnerability to schizophrenia: Performance of patients with schizotypal and nonschizotypal personality disorders. *Psychiatry Research*, *60*(1), 49–56. https://doi.org/10.1016/0165-1781(95)02764-5.

Hazlett, E. A., Lamade, R. V., Graff, F. S., McClure, M. M., Kolaitis, J. C., Goldstein, K. E., & Moshier, E. (2014). Visual-spatial working memory performance and temporal gray matter volume predict schizotypal personality disorder group membership. *Schizophrenia Research*, *152*(2–3), 350–357.

Honey, G. D., Bullmore, E. T., & Sharma, T. (2002). De-coupling of cognitive performance and cerebral functional response during working memory in schizophrenia. *Schizophrenia Research*, *53*, 45–56. https://doi.org/10.1016/S0920-9964(01)00154-2.

Honey, G. D., Bullmore, E. T., Soni, W., Varatheesan, M., Williams, S. C., & Sharma, T. (1999). Differences in frontal cortical activation by a working memory task after substitution of risperidone for typical antipsychotic drugs in patients with schizophrenia. *Proceedings of the National Academy of Sciences of the United States of America*, *96*(23), 13432–13437. https://doi.org/10.1073/pnas.96.23.13432.

Honey, G. D., Sharma, T., Suckling, J., Giampietro, V., Soni, W., Williams, S. C. R., & Bullmore, E. T. (2003). The functional neuroanatomy of schizophrenic syndromes. *Psychological Medicine*, *33*(6), 1007–1018. https://doi.org/10.1017/s0033291703007864.

Horan, W. P., Braff, D. L., Nuechterlein, K. H., Sugar, C. A., Cadenhead, K. S., Calkins, M. E., … Green, M. F. (2008). Verbal working memory impairments in individuals with schizophrenia and their first-degree relatives: Findings from the consortium on the genetics of schizophrenia. *Schizophrenia Research*, *103*(1–3), 218–228. https://doi.org/10.1016/j.schres.2008.02.014.

International Schizophrenia Consortium, Purcell, S. M., Wray, N. R., Stone, J. L., Visscher, P. M., O'Donovan, M. C., … Sklar, P. (2009). Common polygenic variation contributes to risk of schizophrenia and bipolar disorder. *Nature*, *460*(7256), 748–752. https://doi.org/10.1038/nature0818.

Javitt, D. C., Shelley, A., Silipo, G., & Lieberman, J. A. (2000). Deficits in auditory and visual context processing in schizophrenia. *Archives of General Psychiatry*, *57*, 1131–1137.

Kamiński, J., Gleich, T., Fukuda, Y., Katthagen, T., Gallinat, J., Heinz, A., & Schlangenhauf, F. (2020). Association of cortical glutamate and working memory activation in patients with schizophrenia: A multimodal proton magnetic resonance spectroscopy and functional magnetic resonance imaging study. *Biological Psychiatry*, *87*(3), 225–233. https://doi.org/10.1016/j.biopsych.2019.07.011.

Kamiński, J., & Rutishauser, U. (2020). Between persistently active and activity-silent frameworks: Novel vistas on the cellular basis of working memory. *Annals of the New York Academy of Sciences*, *1464*(1), 64–75. https://doi.org/10.1111/nyas.14213.

Kanchanatawan, B., Hemrungrojn, S., Thika, S., Sirivichayakul, S., Ruxrungtham, K., Carvalho, A. F., … Maes, M. (2018). Changes in tryptophan catabolite (TRYCAT) pathway patterning are associated with mild impairments in declarative memory in schizophrenia and deficits in semantic and episodic memory coupled with increased false-memory creation in deficit schizophrenia. *Molecular Neurobiology*, *55*, 5184–5201. https://doi.org/10.1007/s12035-017-0751-8.

Kaneko, K. (2018). Negative symptoms and cognitive impairments in schizophrenia: Two key symptoms negatively influencing social functioning. *Journal of Medical Sciences*, *61*(2), 91–102. https://doi.org/10.33160/yam.2018.06.001.

Kelly, B. D., O'Callaghan, E., Waddington, J. L., Feeney, L., Browne, S., Scully, P. J., … Larkin, C. (2010). Schizophrenia and the city: A review of literature and prospective study of psychosis and urbanicity in Ireland. *Schizophrenia Research*, *116*, 75–89. https://doi.org/10.1016/j.schres.2009.10.015.

Kendler, K. S. (2005). 'A gene for..': The nature of gene action in psychiatric disorders. *The American Journal of Psychiatry*, *162*(7), 1243–1252. https://doi.org/10.1176/appi.ajp.162.7.1243.

Kendler, K. S., McGuire, M., Gruenberg, A. M., O'Hare, A., Spellman, M., & Walsh, D. (1993). The roscommon family study. Methods, diagnosis of probands, and risk of schizophrenia in relatives. *Archives of General Psychiatry*, *50*(7), 527–540.

Kim, S., Jang, K., & Kim, M. (2015). Deficits in error- monitoring by college students with schizotypal traits: An event-related potential study. *PLoS One*, *10*(3), e0122861.

Kim, J., Kwon, S., Park, J., Youn, T., Kang, D. H., Kim, M. S., … Lee, M. C. (2003). Functional disconnection between the prefrontal and parietal cortices during working memory processing in schizophrenia: A[^{15}O]H_2O PET study. *American Journal of Psychiatry*, *160*(5), 919–923. https://doi.org/10.1176/appi.ajp.160.5.919.

Kindermann, S. S., Brown, G. G., Zorrilla, L. E., Olsen, R. K., & Jeste, D. V. (2004). Spatial working memory among middle-aged and older patients with schizophrenia and volunteers using fMRI. *Schizophrenia Research*, *68*, 203–216. https://doi.org/10.1016/j.schres.2003.08.010.

Kirchner, S. K., Roeh, A., Nolden, J., & Hasan, A. (2018). Diagnosis and treatment of schizotypal personality disorder: Evidence from systematic review. *NPJ Schizophrenia*, *4*(20). https://doi.org/10.1038/s41537-018-0062-8.

Kraguljac, N. V., Srivastava, A., & Lahti, A. C. (2013). Memory deficits in schizophrenia: A selective review of functional magnetic resonance imaging (fMRI) studies. *Behavioral Science*, *3*, 330–347. https://doi.org/10.3390/bs3030330.

Kustermann, T., Popov, T., Miller, G. A., & Rockstroh, B. (2018). Verbal working memory-related neural network communication in schizophrenia. *Psychophysiology*, *55*(9), e13088. https://doi.org/10.1111/psyp.13088.

Lee, J., & Park, S. (2005). Working memory impairments in schizophrenia: A meta-analysis. *Journal of Abnormal Psychology*, *114*(4), 599–610.

Lener, M. S., Wong, C. Y., Tang, W., Byne, K. E., Goldstein, Blair, N. J., … Hazlett, E. A. (2015). White matter abnormalities in schizophrenia and schizotypal personality disorder. *Schizophrenia Bulletin*, *41*(1), 300–310. https://doi.org/10.1093/schbul/sbu093.

Lenzenweger, M. F. (2018). Schiztoty, schizotypic, psychopathology and schizophrenia. *World Psychiatry*, *17*(1), 25–27.

Li, A. W. Y., Viñas-Guasch, N., Hui, C. L. M., Chang, W. C., Chan, S. K. W., Lee, E. H. M., & Chen, E. Y. H. (2018). Verbal working memory in schizophrenia: The role of syntax in facilitating serial recall. *Schizophrenia Research*, *192*, 294–299. https://doi.org/10.1016/j.schres.2017.04.008.

Liu, Y., Wang, G., Jin, H., Lyu, H., Liu, Y., Guo, W., … Dopaminevis, J. (2019). Cognitive deficits in subjects at risk for psychosis, first-episode and chronic schizophrenia patient. *Psychiatry Research*, *274*, 235–242. https://doi.org/10.1016/j.psychres.2019.01.089.

MacDonald, A. W., Carter, C. S., Kerns, J. G., Ursu, S., Barch, D. M., Holmes, A. J., … Cohen, J. D. (2005). Specificity of prefrontal dysfunction and context processing deficits to schizophrenia in never-medicated patients with first-episode psychosis. *American Journal of Psychiatry*, *162*(3), 475–484.

Mammarella, N., Fairfield, B., De Leonardis, V., Carretti, B., Borella, E., Frisullo, E., & Di Domenico, A. (2012). Is there an affective working memory deficit in patients with chronic schizophrenia? *Schizophrenia Research*, *138*(1), 99–101.

Manoach, D. S., Press, D. Z., Thangaraj, V., Searl, M. M., Goff, D. C., Halpern, E., … Warach, S. (1999). Schizophrenic subjects activate dorsolateral prefrontal cortex during a working memory task, as measured by fMRI. *Biological Psychiatry*, *45*(9), 1128–1137.

Marsh, J. E., Vachon, F., & Sörqvist, P. (2017). Increased distractibility in schizotypy: Independent of individual differences in working memory capacity? *The Quaterly Journal of Experimental Psychology*, *70*(3), 565–578. https://doi.org/10.1080/17470218.2016.1172094.

McClure, M., Barch, D., Flory, J., Harvey, P., & Siever, L. (2008). Context processing in schizotypal personality disorder: Evidence of specificity of impairment to the schizophrenia spectrum. *Journal of Abnormal Psychology*, *117*(2), 342–354.

McClure, M. M., Harvey, P. D., Bowie, C. R., Iacoviello, B., & Siever, L. J. (2013). Functional out- comes, functional capacity, and cognitive impairment in schizotypal personality disorder. *Schizophrenia Research*, *144*, 146–150.

McClure, M. M., Romero, M. J., Bowie, C. R., Reichenberg, A., Harvey, P. D., & Siever, L. J. (2007). Visual-spatial learning and memory in schizotypal personality disorder: Continued evidence for the importance of working memory in the schizophrenia spectrum. *Archives of Clinical Neuropsychology*, *22*, 109–116. https://doi.org/10.1016/j.acn.2006.11.004.

Meyer, N., & MacCabe, J. H. (2016). Schizophrenia. *Medicine*, *44*(11), 649–653. https://doi.org/10.1016/j.mpmed.2016.08.003.

Milas, D. Z., & Milas, G. (2019). Working memory in patients with schizophrenia and bipolar affective disorder: Quantitative or qualitative differences? *Psychiatria Danubina*, *31*(1), 54–61. https://doi.org/10.24869/psyd.2019.54.

Mitra, S., Mahintamani, T., Kavoor, A. R., & Nizamie, S. H. (2016). Negative symptoms in schizophrenia. *Industrial Psychiatry Journal*, *25*(2), 135–144.

Morgan, V. A., Waterreus, A., Jablensky, A., Mackinnon, A., McGrath, J. J., Carr, V., … Saw, S. (2010). People living with psychotic illness 2010: The second Australian national survey of psychosis. *The Australian and New Zealand Journal of Psychiatry*, *46*(8), 735–752. https://doi.org/10.1177/0004867412449877.

Moustafa, A. A., Sherman, S. J., & Frank, M. J. (2008). A dopaminergic basis for working memory, learning and attentional shifting in parkinsonism. *Neuropsychologia*, *46*(13), 3144–3156. https://doi.org/10.1016/j.neuropsychologia.2008.07.011.

Nestor, P. G., Forte, M., Ohtani, T., Levitt, J. J., Newell, D. T., Shenton, M. E., … McCarley, R. W. (2020). Faulty executive attention and memory interactions in schizophrenia. *Prefrontal Gray Matter Volume and Neuropsychological Impairment*, *51*(4), 267–274. https://doi.org/10.1177/1550059419881529.

Neu, P., Gooren, T., Niebuhr, U., & Schlattmann, P. (2019). Cognitive impairment in schizophrenia and depression: A comparison of stability and course. *Journal of Applied Neuropsychology*, *26*(3), 215–228. https://doi.org/10.1080/23279095.2017.1392962.

Nielsen, J. D., Madsen, K. H., Wang, A., Liu, A., Friston, K. J., & Zhou, Y. (2017). Working memory modulation of frontoparietal network connectivity in first-episode schizophrenia. *Cerebral Cortex*, *27*(7), 3832–3841. https://doi.org/10.1093/cercor/bhx050.

Niendam, T. A., Lesh, T. A., Yoon, J., Westphal, A. J., Hutchison, N., Dopamineniel Ragland, J., … Carter, C. S. (2014). Impaired context processing as a potential marker of psychosis risk state. *Psychiatry Research: Neuroimaging*, *221*(1), 13–20. https://doi.org/10.1016/j.pscychresns.2013.09.001.

Nuechterlein, K. H., Kenneth, L. S., Ventura, J., Green, M. F., Gretchen-Doorly, D., & Asarnow, R. F. (2012). The puzzle of schizophrenia: Tracking the core role of cognitive deficits. *Development and Psychopathology*, *24*, 529–536. https://doi.org/10.1017/S0954579412000132.

Owen, A. M., McMillan, K. M., Laird, A. R., & Bullmore, E. (2005). N-back working memory paradigm: A meta-analysis of normative functional neuroimaging studies. *Human Brain Mapping*, *25*(1), 46–59. https://doi.org/10.1002/hbm.20131.

Owen, M. J., O'Donovan, M. C., Thapar, A., & Craddock, N. (2011). Neurodevelopmental hypothesis of schizophrenia. *The British Journal of Psychiatry*, *198*(3), 173–175. https://doi.org/10.1192/bjp.bp.110.084384.

Owen, M. J., Sawa, A., & Mortensen, P. B. (2016). Schizophrenia. *The Lancet*, *10039*(388), 86–97. https://doi.org/10.1016/S0140-6736(15)01121-6.

Park, S., & Gooding, D. C. (2014). Working memory impairment as an endophenotypic marker of a schizophrenia diathesis. *Schizophrenia Research: Cognition*, *1*(3), 127–136. https://doi.org/10.1016/j.scog.2014.09.005.

Pedrero, E. F., & Debanné, M. (2017). Schizotypal traits and psychotic-like experiences during adolescence: An update. *Psicothema*, *29*(1), 5–17. https://doi.org/10.7334/psicothema2016.209.

Perlstein, W. M., Dixit, N. K., Carter, C. S., Noll, D. C., & Cohen, J. D. (2003). Prefrontal cortex dysfunction mediates deficits in working memory and prepotent responding in schizophrenia. *Biology Psychiatry*, *53*(1), 25–38.

Pflueger, M. O., Gschwandtner, U., Stieglitz, R. D., & Riecher-Rössler, A. (2007). Neuropsychological deficits in individuals with an at risk mental state for psychosis- working memory as a potential trait marker. *Schizophrenia Research*, *97*(1–3), 14–24. https://doi.org/10.1016/j.schres.2007.09.003.

Polizzotto, N. R., Hill-Jarrett, T., Walker, C., & Cho, R. Y. (2018). Normal development of context processing using the AXCPT paradigm. *PLoS One*, *13*(5), e0197812. https://doi.org/10.1371/journal.

Quee, P. J., Van Der Heijden, F. M. A., Eling, P., & Hildebrandth, H. (2011). Working memory in schizophrenia: A systematic study of specific modalities and processes. *Psychiatry Research*, *185*(1–2), 54–59.

Racioppi, A., Sheinbaum, T., Gross, G. M., Ballespi, S., Kwapil, T. R., & Barrantes-Vidopaminel, N. (2018). Prediction of prodromal symptoms and schizophrenia-spectrum personality disorder traits by positive and negative schizotypy: A 3-year prospective study. *PLoS One*, *13*(11), e0207150. https://doi.org/10.1371/journal.pone.0207150.

Riecher-Rössler, A., Gschwandtner, U., Aston, J., Borgwardt, S., Drewe, M., Fuhr, P., … Stieglitz, R. D. (2007). The Basel early-detection-of-psychosis (FEPSY)-study—Design and preliminary results. *Acta Psychiatrica Scandinavica*, *115*(2), 114–125. https://doi.org/10.1111/j.1600-0447.2006.00854.x.

Rosell, D. R., Futterman, S. E., McMaster, A., & Siever, L. J. (2014). Schizotypal personality disorder: A current review. *Current Psychiatry Reports*, *16*(4), 452. https://doi.org/10.1007/s11920-014-0452-1.

Rosvold, H. E., Mirsky, A. F., Sarason, I., Bransome, E. D. J., & Beck, L. H. (1956). A continuous performance test of brain image. *Journal of Consulting Psychology*, *20*(5), 343–350. https://doi.org/10.1037/h0043220.

Sahakyan, L., & Kwapil, T. R. (2018a). Episodic memory retrieval is impaired in negative schizotypy under fast response deadline. *Schizophrenia Research*, *201*, 167–171. https://doi.org/10.1016/j.schres.2018.05.039.

Sahakyan, L., & Kwapil, T. R. (2018b). Moving beyond summary scores: Decomposing free recall performance to understand episodic memory deficits in schizotypy. *Journal of Experimental Psychology: General*, *147*, 1919–1930. https://doi.org/10.1037/xge0000401.

Sahakyan, L., & Kwapil, T. R. (2019). Hits and false alarms in recognition memory show differential impairment in positive and negative schizotypy. *American Psychological Association*, *128*(6), 633–643. https://doi.org/10.1037/abn0000441.

Schoofs, D., Preub, D., & Wolf, O. T. (2008). Psychosocial stress induces working memory impairments in an *n*-back paradigm. *Psychoneuroendocrinology*, *33*, 643–653. https://doi.org/10.1016/j.psyneuen.2008.02.004.

Servan-Schreiber, D., Cohen, J. D., & Steingard, S. (1996). Schizophrenic deficits in the processing of context. A test of a theoretical model. *Archives of General Psychiatry*, *53*(12), 1105–1112.

Siddi, S., Petretto, D. R., & Preti, A. (2017). Neuropsychological correlates of schizotypy: A systemic review and meta-analysis of cross-sectional studies. *Cognitive Neuropsychiatry*, *22*(3), 186–212. https://doi.org/10.1080/13546805.2017.1299702.

Siever, L. J., Koenigsberg, H. W., Harvey, P., Mitropoulou, V., Laruelle, M., Abi-Dargham, A., … Buchsbaum, M. (2002). Cognitive and brain function in schizotypal personality disorder. *Schizophrenia Research*, *54*(1–2), 157–167. https://doi.org/10.1016/S0920-9964(01)00363-2.

Silver, H., & Bilker, W. B. (2015). Similar verbal memory impairments in schizophrenia and healthy aging. Implications for understanding of neural mechanisms. *Psychiatry Research*, *226*, 227–283. https://doi.org/10.1016/j.psychres.2014.12.062.

Silver, H., Feldman, P., Bilker, W. B., & Gur, R. C. (2003). Working memory deficit as a core neuropsychological dysfunction in schizophrenia. *American Journal of Psychiatry*, *160*, 1809–1816.

Škodlar, B., & Henriksen, M. G. (2019). Toward a phenomenological psychotherapy for schizophrenia. *Psychopathology*, *52*, 117–125. https://doi.org/10.1159/000500163.

Smeland, O. B., Frei, O., Dale, A. M., & Andreassen, O. A. (2020). The polygenic architecture of schizophrenia – Rethinking pathogenesis and nosology. *Nature Reviews Neurology*, *16*, 366–379. https://doi.org/10.1038/s41582-020-0364-0.

Snellenberg, J. X. V., Girgis, R. R., Horga, G., van de Giessen, E., Slifstein, M., Ojeil, N., … Abi-Dargham. (2016). Mechanisms of working memory impairment in schizophrenia. *Biological Psychiatry*, *80*(8), 617–626. https://doi.org/10.1016/j.biopsych.2016.02.017.

Stäblein, M., Storchak, H., Ghinea, D., Kraft, D., Knöchel, C., Prvulovic, D., … Oertel-Knöchel, V. (2018). Visual working memory encoding in schizophrenia and first-degree relatives: Neurofunctional abnormalities and impaired consolidation. *Psychological Medicine*, *49*, 75–83. https://doi.org/10.1017/S003329171800051X.

Stefansson, H., Ophoff, R. A., Steinberg, S., Andreassen, O. A., Cichon, S., Rujescu, D., … Collier, D. A. (2009). Common variants conferring risk of schizophrenia. *Nature*, *460*(7256), 744–747. https://doi.org/10.1038/nature08186.

Tandon, R., Gaebel, W., Barch, D. M., Bustillo, J., Gur, R. E., Heckers, S., … Carpenter, W. (2013). Definition and description of schizophrenia in the DSM-5. *Schizophrenia Research*, *150*(1), 3–10. https://doi.org/10.1016/j.schres.2013.05.028.

Tarbox, S. I., Almasy, L., Gur, R. E., Nimgaonkar, V. L., & Pogue-Geile, M. F. (2012). The nature of schizotypy among multigenerational multiplex schizophrenia families. *Journal of Abnormal Psychology*, *121*(2), 396–406. https://doi.org/10.1037/a0026787.

Thormodsen, R., Jensen, J., Holmèn, A., Juuhl-Langseth, M., Emblem, K. E., Andreassen, O. A., & Rund, B. R. (2011). Prefrontal hyperactivation during a working memory task in early-onset schizophrenia spectrum disorders: An fMRI study. *Psychiatry Research: Neuroimaging*, *194*(3), 257–262. https://doi.org/10.1016/j.pscychresns.2011.05.011.

Trapp, W., Dotterweich, S., Hintner, L., Wollny, H., Lautenbacher, S., & Hajak, G. (2017). Speed and capacity of working memory and executive function in schizophrenia compared to unipolar depression. *Schizophrenia Research: Cognition*, *10*, 1–6. https://doi.org/10.1016/j.scog.2017.07.002.

Umbricht, D., Vollenweider, F. X., Schmid, L., Grübel, C., Skrabo, A., Huber, T., & Koller, R. (2003). Effects of the 5-HT_{2A}agonist psilocybin on mismatch negativity generation and AX-continuous performance task: Implications for the neuropharmachology of cognitive deficits in schizophrenia. *Neuropsychopharmacology*, *28*, 170–181. https://doi.org/10.1038/sj.npp.1300005.

Walter, E. E., Fernandez, F., Snelling, M., & Barkus, E. (2016). Genetic consideration of schizotypal traits: A review. *Frontiers in Psychology*, *7*, 1769. https://doi.org/10.3389/fpsyg.2016.01769.

Wang, L., Bolin, J., Lu, Z., & Carr, M. (2018). Visuospatial working memory mediates the relationship between executive functioning and spatial ability. *Frontiers in Psychology*, *9*, 2302. https://doi.org/10.3389/fpsyg.2018.02302.

World Health Organization. (2018). *Mental health, schizophrenia.*

Yoon, J. H., Nguyen, D. V., McVay, L. M., Deramo, P., Minzenberg, M. J., Ragland, J. D., … Carter, C. (2012). Automated classification of fMRI during cognitive control identifies more severely disorganised subjects with schizophrenia. *Schizophrenia Research*, *135*, 28–33. https://doi.org/10.1016/j.schres.2012.01.001.

Deductive reasoning abilities in schizophrenia and related disorders: A systematic review

3

Ahmed A. Moustafa[a,b], *Anchal Garg*[c], *Ahmed A. Helal*[d], *and Eid Abo Hamza*[d,e]
[a]School of Psychology & Marcs Institute for Brain and Behaviour, Western Sydney University, Sydney, NSW, Australia, [b]Department of Human Anatomy and Physiology, the Faculty of Health Sciences, University of Johannesburg, South Africa, [c]School of Psychology, Western Sydney University, Sydney, NSW, Australia, [d]Faculty of Education, Department of Mental Health, Tanta University, Egypt, [e]College of Graduate Studies, Arabian Gulf University, Bahrain

Chapter outline

Introduction

According to the Diagnostic and Statistical Manual for Mental Disorders, Fifth Edition (DSM-V), schizophrenia spectrum and other psychotic disorders are characterized by abnormalities in one or more of the following domains: delusions, hallucinations, disorganized thinking (speech), grossly disorganized behavior (including catatonia), and negative symptoms (American Psychiatric Association, 2013). This spectrum includes

Cognitive and Behavioral Dysfunction in Schizophrenia. https://doi.org/10.1016/B978-0-12-820005-6.00004-9

schizophrenia, schizophreniform disorder, schizotypal personality disorder, delusional disorder, schizoaffective disorder, and unspecified schizophrenia spectrum and other psychotic disorders, among others. Schizophrenia is a disorder that includes two or more of the following symptoms: delusions, hallucinations, disorganized speech, grossly disorganized or catatonic behavior, and negative symptoms, whereas delusional disorder is characterized by at least 1 month of delusions but no other psychotic symptoms. On the other hand, schizotypal personality disorder is characterized by a pervasive pattern of social and interpersonal deficits including reduced capacity for close relationships, cognitive or perceptual distortions, and eccentricities of behavior usually beginning in early adulthood but in some cases, it becomes apparent in childhood and adolescence.

Reasoning: Definition and tasks

Reasoning can be defined as a logical thinking process that results in a conclusion (Northrop, 1977) or a process whose goal is to enable the reasoner to make the best decision about a particular issue, in particular circumstances, within a particular forum and enterprise (Toulmin & Rieke, 1984). In other words, reasoning involves the process of inferring information from an existing body of knowledge and/or assumptions. Deductive reasoning is defined as an inference process based on existing premises, in which the conclusion is either right or wrong. There have been several tasks that investigate reasoning processes in schizophrenia spectrum and other psychotic disorders including Transitive Inference, Wason Card Selection, Syllogism, Aha! Sentences Task, and Thematic Selection tasks. Below, we briefly define each of these tasks.

Deductive reasoning tasks

There are deductive reasoning tasks that have been used in the field which involve an inference process that is either true or false (see definition above). Further, in deductive reasoning, no information other than that which incorporated into the task is needed to solve the inference problem. For example, the transitive inference task is used infer a relationship between the items that have not been explicitly compared before (Lazareva & Wasserman, 2012; Silverman, Gastrell, Karras, Solomon, & Crawley, 2015). This task consists of inferring the relationship between two items based on their shared relationship with a third item (Gazes, Chee, & Hampton, 2012). For example, knowing that Ben is taller than Emily and Emily is taller than Dina, one can infer that Ben is taller than Dina. In a typical laboratory tests of transitive inference, participants are trained on a set of overlapping two-choice conditional discriminations (A+B-, B+C-, C+D-, D+*E*-, E+F-, F+G-) consistent with an implicit order (A>B>C>D>E>F>G). After which, the participants evaluate the relationship between non-adjacent (i.e., novel) pairings (e.g., BD) (Gazes et al., 2012; Ranganath, Minzenberg, & Ragland, 2008).

The Wason Card Selection Task (WCST) is used to assess following the rules of logical inference (Foss, 1966; Wason, 1968). In other words, this task assesses reasoning abilities through the application of deductive reasoning rule. In its original format, participants are given four cards, with only one side visible. On each card, either: "P", "not P", "Q", or "not Q" is written. Participants are then given a conditional rule concerning the information written on both sides of the cards, which conforms to the following conditional format: if “P” is on one side, then the other side must be “Q”. Then, participants are asked to test the validity of this rule, by turning the cards in the most economical way to confirm or disconfirm the conditional rule using the least amount of turns possible. A correct response requires that participants to turn both the cards “P” and “not Q” that is, turning the card “P” would test the rule to see if the other side is indeed “Q”, confirming the conditional rule. Similarly, the “not Q” card is required to be turned, as reviling “A” would break the rule in this condition. Presenting the task in this abstract format has proven rather difficult for most people, with only about 10% of participants reporting correct responses. Interestingly, the performance on the Wason Card Selection Task improves as the content became more realistic or familiar.

The thematic selection task is a variant of The Wason Card Selection Task (Corcoran & Frith, 2005). In this task, performance can be facilitated by using thematic materials (Johnson-Laird, Legrenzi, & Legrenzi, 1972; Wason & Shapiro, 1971). For instance, Wason and Shapiro (1971) used rules about four journeys made by them. It consisted of cities and modes of transportation such as “Everytime I go to Miami, I travel by car” which is presented on note card. Following instructions are given to the subject by the experimenter “I will now present you with four cards; the test you are about to do concerns only these four cards. These cards show cities and modes of transportation for four journeys that I took on four different days, with the city to which I travelled on one side and the mode of transportation on the other side. I am going to make a claim about a city to which I travel and mode of transportation I use, and your task is to say which of the cards would need to be turned over to decide whether that claim is true or false. You may choose any or all of the cards. Take your time and make your choice carefully” (Griggs & Cox, 1982). Thus, a particular subject receives one of the four possible rules formed by permuting the two city names (Miami and Atlanta) and the two modes of transportation (plane and car). Each variation of the rule is presented four times in each group to control any bias about the relationship between a city and a mode of transportation that subjects might entertain. Each of the four stimulus cards has a separate day of the week appearing in smaller type on the top of the card. The order of the four cards in the presentation array is randomized for each subject (Griggs & Cox, 1982). In addition to The Wason Card Selection Task and thematic selection tasks, there are other tasks that also test conditional reasoning rules which takes the form of “If A, then B”, where A and B are often different sentences. Participatns are often tested on the truth of various sentences of these structure.

Syllogism is a form of a deductive reasoning in which validity of the conclusion depends on the validity of the preceding premises (that is, the truth of the conclusion depends on the truth of the premises) (Forbes, 1994; Revsbech et al., 2015). One example of syllogistic reasoning is “All ice (P) is water (Q). All ice (P) is frozen (R)” therefore some water (Q) is frozen (R). On the other hand, invalid syllogims will be All ice (P) is water (Q), some water (Q) is frozen (R); therefore, ice (P) is frozen (R). Syllogism reflects a certain logical structure or a blueprint, which can be applied to any verbal content. Research has shown that the error rate in this task is affected by the semantic embodiment (content) of the sentences. Such embodiment can be ordinary or unusual: Ordinary content refers to the instance where the content of the syllogism is congruent with what would be typically familiar to us from the experience, whereas unsual syllogisms consists of unusual presentations such as blue concepts or buildings that sings (Revsbech et al., 2015).

There have some reviews and theoretical analysis of deductive reasoning tasks in schizophrenia (Mujica-Parodi, Malaspina, & Sackeim, 2000), showing evidence that impaired deductive reasoning is related to impaired emotional processing (Mirian, Heinrichs, & Vaz, 2011). One other study has provided a theoretical analysis (as well as review of prior studies) on kinds of fallacies underlying impaired and sometimes intact reasoning abilities in schizophrenia (Selesnick & Owen, 2012).

Neural correlates of reasoning

Heckers, Zalesak, Weiss, Ditman, and Titone (2004) tested whether the hippocampus plays a role in the integration of memories in transitive inference tasks by studying brain activation during the discrimination of a series of overlapping and nonoverlapping arbitrary visual stimulus pairs in healthy subjects. Results showed that transitive inference about overlapping pairs was associated with right anterior hippocampal activation. Further, the recognition of nonoverlapping stimulus pairs was associated with bilateral medial temporal lobe activation centered in the anterior parahippocampal gyrus. A more recent study has also found support for the role of the hippocampus in relational memory and transitive inference (Avery, Rogers, & Heckers, 2018).

All the brain areas activated in reasoning tasks as described in this section are also implicated in schizophrenia, including midbrain (presumably dopamine), striatum, hippocampus, and prefrontal cortex (Abi-Dargham et al., 2002; Moustafa et al., 2016; Moustafa & Gluck, 2011; Moustafa, Keri, Herzallah, Myers, & Gluck, 2010; Moustafa, Misiak, & Frydecka, 2017). The findings that several brain areas are involved in reasoning suggest that they are complex process. The complex network underlying reasoning also suggests that this could be due the impact of other emotional and cognitive processes, such as stress, working memory, theory of mind, and others, on reasoning. However, these relationships should be investigated in future studies.

Goal and hypotheses

The purpose of the present review is to discuss and compare deductive reasoning abilities in schizophrenia spectrum patients. Specifically, this review will discuss whether schizophrenia patients show impairment on which kinds of deductive reasoning tasks. We hypothesize that schizophrenia patients will be impaired on deductive reasoning tasks, as compared to healthy normal controls. Further, we hypothesize that impairment in deductive reasoning tasks is related to theory of mind and working memory.

Methods

In this study, we provide a systematic review on reasoning deficits in schizophrenia and related disorders. Further, we aim to understand the relationship between reasoning and symptoms in schizophrenia and related disorders. Our search strategy included the following combination of two key words from two sets. The first set included schizophrenia, delusional disorder, and so on. The second set included Wason Selection

Tasks, and other reasoning task. The list of key words are as follows: schizophrenia, deductive reasoning, transitive inference, Wason Card selection task, syllogism (or syllogistic reasoning), and conditional reasoning. We have searched previous studies assessing the reasoning anomalies in schizophrenia a in Pubmed, PsychoInfo, and also Google. Further, we have examined each paper carefully to make sure the goal of the study is studying a form of reasoning in schizophrenia spectrum disorder. Studies that did not address a reasoning task as well as a schizophrenia spectrum disorder were excluded. Below, we review studies that have employed the reasoning tasks in schizophrenia and related disorders. Some of these studies have compared schizophrenia spectrum disorder patients with other clinical disorders and normal controls. We present our review on the following tasks, respectively: Transitive Inference Task, Wason Card Selection Task, Thematic Selection Task, conditional reasoning, and syllogism.

Deductive reasoning

Below, we discuss several studies discussing deductive reasoning abilities in schizophrenia and related disorders. For example, Selesnick and Owen (2012) argue that delusional beliefs can stem from impaired deductive reasoning abilities. In one case study, a schizophrenia patient reported he is against wars. He found out that Switzerland is against wars. The patient then identified himself with Switzerland (Arieti, 1974). In another case study, the patient argues that she is unkillable and thus supernatural. And given that Virgin Mary is supernatural, then the patient herself is Virgin Mary (Bandinelli, Palma, Penna, & Pessa, 2006). These findings are in agreement with arguments made by Von Domarus (1944).

Transitive inference

Table 1 summarizes studies that have used the Transitive Inference Task in schizophrenia and related disorders.

Titone et al. (2004) assessed the transitive inference in schizophrenia patients and healthy controls by training them on a series of learned discriminations that were hierarchically organized (A > B, B > C, C > D, and D > E). Later, they were assessed on each training pair and two novel "inference pairs": AE was evaluated without consideration of hierarchical relationships, and BD was evaluated by hierarchical relations. Results indicated that schizophrenia patients and controls successfully learnt the training pairs and correctly responded to the nonrelational AE pairs. However, schizophrenia patients were less accurate than controls in answering to the relational BD pair consistent with the hypothesis (that higher-level memory processes associated with relational memory are impaired in schizophrenia patients). In one older study, Sinha and Nelson (1993) found that schizophrenia patients are more impaired than patients with alcohol use disorders on transitivity tasks. One example is if A is B, and B is C, then one can conclude that A is C. Building on prior work, Coleman et al. (2010) aimed to disambiguate the transitive inference deficits from the effects of ambiguous reinforcement history and novelty in schizophrenia and healthy control subjects. A newly developed transitive inference and

Table 1 Summary of the previous studies on deductive reasoning.

Author (s)	Groups and scales	Results
Transitive inference		
Titone, Ditman, Holzman, Eichenbaum, and Levy (2004)	Transitive inference was assessed by training schizophrenia patients and healthy controls on a series of learned discriminations that were hierarchically organized (A > B, B > C, C > D and D > E)	Schizophrenia patients were less accurate in answering to the relational BD pair than controls. Results were consistent with the hypothesis that higher-level memory processes are associated with relational memory (which were impaired in schizophrenia patients)
Sinha and Nelson (1993)	Schizophrenia patients and alcohol use disorder individuals	Schizophrenia patients show impaired performance in comparison to other groups
Coleman et al. (2010)	Investigating the effects of ambiguous reinforcement history and novelty in schizophrenia and healthy control subjects	Schizophrenia patients performed significantly worse than controls on transitive inference task. However, schizophrenia patients were able to make equivalently difficult nontransitive judgments as compared to controls
Wason Card Selection Task		
Peters, Thornton, Siksou, Linney, and MacCabe (2008)	Participants were divided into deluded versus non-deluded individuals	There were no differences on Wason's 2–4-6 task, and Wason's selection task when
Mirabilio et al. (2006)	Investigating impact of neurocognitive, clinical and community functioning variables on reasoning in schizophrenia patients	Global functioning was the strong predictor of social reasoning, whereas community functioning and neurocognitive measures (attention and contextual reasoning) had no effect
Dudley, Young, John, and Over (1998)	Reasoning ability was examined in individuals with delusions and non-deluded individuals	Individuals with delusions performed poorly on certain reasoning tasks because of the impairments in working memory as compared to non-deluded individuals

Table 1 Continued

Author (s)	Groups and scales	Results
Thematic selection task		
Corcoran and Frith (2005)	The relationship between theory of mind and social conditioning reasoning among schizophrenia patients and normal controls was examined	The extent of facilitation afforded social reasoning and the performance on the hinting task (measure of theory of mind) in schizophrenia sample are related
Conditional if rules		
Mellet et al. (2006)	Schizophrenia patients and healthy controls were compared on various "if... then" logic rules	In certain logic sentences, especially when the antecedent has a negation, schizophrenia patients have outperformed the healthy control group
Syllogism		
Owen, Cutting, and David (2007)	Schizophrenia patients and healthy controls	Schizophrenia patients reasoned more logically as compared to healthy individuals in certain syllogistic reasoning problems
Mirian et al. (2011)	Deductive reasoning in schizophrenia patients and healthy controls with special reference to whether accuracy varies across the type of stimulus problem was assessed	Schizophrenia patients performed lower in all reasoning task conditions as compared to healthy controls. However, group differences were nonsignificant after controlling the IQ
Von Domarus (1944)	Schizophrenia patients and controls	Both patients and controls were impaired on performing syllogistic reasoning tasks
Kemp, Chua, McKenna, and David (1997)	Disordered reasoning in deluded patients and healthy controls was examined	Both groups frequently made logical errors with conditional statements. Further, deluded subjects endorsed fallacies more than normal volunteers. The effect of emotional content on endorsement of unbelievable responses was increased slightly in the deluded group

nontransitive inference tasks were used. They found that schizophrenia patients performed significantly worse than controls on transitive inference task but were able to make equivalently difficult nontransitive judgments. Further, novelty and reinforcement did not account for selective deficits of patients on the transitive inference task. In a recent study, it was found that biological relatives of patients with schizophrenia are also impaired at transitive inference task performance (Onwuameze, Titone, & Ho, 2016).

The Wason Card Selection Task

Table 1 summarizes studies that have used the Wason Card Selection Task in schizophrenia, (deluded and non-deluded group) and normal controls.

Peters et al. (2008) reported no group differences on Wason's 2–4-6 task, and Wason's selection task when participants were grouped into deluded versus nondeluded individuals.

Mirabilio et al. (2006) assessed the neurocognitive, clinical, and community functioning variables to predict social reasoning in schizophrenia patients. In this study, Wason Selection Task, Continuous Performance Test, Cognitive Bias Task, Positive and Negative Syndrome Scale, DSM-IV Global Assessment of Functioning, and Life-Skills Profile were used. They found that global functioning was a strong predictor of the social reasoning, whereas community functioning and neurocognitive measures (in terms of attention and contextual reasoning) had no predictive effect on social reasoning. In one earlier study, Dudley et al. (1998) assessed the differences in the reasoning among deluded and nondeluded individuals when the content of the task was manipulated (by changing the material gradually from being neutral to being more realistic in the content). Wason Selection Task was administered on the three groups: individuals with delusions, depression, and nonclinical control subjects. In Experiment 1, the subjects were presented with four Wason Selection Tasks (that were varied in the realism of the content), whereas in Experiment 2, the purpose was to replicate and understand the findings of Experiment 1 (in which four cards use was conditional). Results of Experiment 1 indicated that on three of the conditionals, performance between groups was equivalently poor, whereas on realistic and conditional tasks, individuals with delusions performed worse than the two control groups. On other hand, in Experiment 2, individuals with delusions performed less well than psychiatric and non-clinical control participants on a variant of Wason Selection Tasks, which reflected the inefficiency in reasoning rather than inability to reason at all. As the tasks became more realistic, performance in normal subjects typically improved. These findings indicated that individuals with delusions perform poorly on certain reasoning tasks because of the impairments in the working memory.

In another study, it was found that patients were schizophrenia were more impaired on Wason Selection Tasks compared to healthy controls and patients with major depressive disorder (Kornreich et al., 2017). However, Kornreich and colleagues also found that the performance of schizophrenia patients in these tasks depends on the content, such that patients' performance was better in social contract and precaution ones than in purely descriptive tasks.

Thematic selection task

Corcoran and Frith (2005) examined the relationship between theory of mind and social reasoning in schizophrenia patients and normal controls using the thematic selection task. They found a relationship between theory of mind and social reasoning in schizophrenia patients. Social reasoning was most markedly affected in schizophrenia patients with negative signs and paranoid delusions.

Conditional reasoning

In one study, Mellet and colleagues have assessed the performance of schizophrenia patients and healthy controls on truth or falseness of certain sentences. The participants were also given a set of geometric shapes, with a sentence like "If there is not a red square on the left, then there is a yellow circle on the right." (Mellet et al., 2006). They found that the patients outperformed the healthy control group on these kinds of conditioned rules. In another study, it was found that individuals who high on schizotypy were also impaired on conditional reasoning tasks (Sellen, Oaksford, & Gray, 2005). Schizotypy is a risk factor for the development of schizophrenia (Barrantes-Vidal, Grant, & Kwapil, 2015), and thus this study suggests that conditional reasoning impairment may even being before the development of schizophrenia symptoms.

One type of conditional reasoning is counterfactual thinking that involves creating alternative scenarios than what happened in real life (Van Hoeck, Watson, & Barbey, 2015). It was previously reported that patients with schizophrenia are impaired at counterfactual thinking (Contreras et al., 2016; Hooker, Roese, & Park, 2000). One study found that relatives of patients with schizophrenia were impaired at counterfactual thinking than healthy controls (Albacete et al., 2016).

Syllogism

Table 1 summarizes studies on syllogism in schizophrenia. Owen et al. (2007) assessed deductive reasoning abilities in schizophrenia patients and healthy controls. In this study, two types of syllogism were constructed: noncommon sense syllogisms and common-sense syllogisms and in each there was a conflict between deductive truth and common sense truth. Participants were asked to accept the first two sentences of each syllogism as true and then decide the truth or falsity of the third sentence. They found that schizophrenia patients reasoned more logically as compared to healthy individuals in conditions involving common sense and logic conflict. This is different from earlier results by Von Domarus (1944) who reported impairment in syllogistic reasoning in both schizophrenia patients and controls.

The reason underlying conflicting results could be the presentence of confounding factors. Accordingly, Mirian et al. (2011) analyzed deductive reasoning in schizophrenia patients and healthy controls with reference to whether accuracy varies across the type of stimulus problem. Syllogistic reasoning task consisting of five argument types varying in salience, congruence with commonly held beliefs and meaningfulness along with standard intellectual and symptom measures were used. They found that schizophrenia patients performed below control participants in all reasoning task conditions, but group differences were nonsignificant after controlling for IQ. There were no significant interactions between group and augment type in terms of reasoning accuracy and both schizophrenia patients and controls performed better when reasoning tasks consisted of commonsensical material. Thus, formal deductive reasoning abnormalities in schizophrenia are a reflection of the broadly based cognitive impairment documented in the illness.

Kemp et al. (1997) assessed disordered reasoning in deluded patients and normal controls by using standard tests consisting of Conditional Statements, Syllogisms (In these tasks, the subjects were required to choose between logically fallacious and valid responses) included neutral and emotive content. They found that both groups frequently made logical errors with conditional statements and deluded subjects endorsed more fallacies than normal controls. Similarly, with syllogism, the effect of emotional content on the endorsement of unbelievable responses increased slightly in the deluded group. In addition, the deluded patients showed a trend to be less prone to the conjunction fallacy than healthy controls.

Discussion

We first discuss a summary of results. Following that, we will discuss neural correlates of reasoning, similarities, and differences among deductive reasoning performance in different tasks in schizophrenia patients, clinical relevance of our findings, and future directions.

Summary and interpretations of results

In the current review, we have extended prior studies and reviewed existing literature on deductive reasoning tasks including Transitive Inference, Wason Card Selection, Thematic Selection Task, and Syllogistic tasks to assess reasoning performance in schizophrenia and related disorders (Corcoran, 2003; Corcoran & Frith, 2005; Dudley & Over, 2003; Gras-Vincendon et al., 1994; Mirian et al., 2011; Owen et al., 2007; So, Garety, Peters, & Kapur, 2010). Deductive reasoning is most likely related to delusions in schizophrenia patients (Arieti, 1974; Bandinelli et al., 2006; Selesnick & Owen, 2012). Further, other studies found that patients with schizophrenia are impaired at less commonly used reasoning tasks that involve verbal and arithmetic deductive questions (Smeland et al., 2017).

Several tasks have used to measure deductive reasoning. Most studies have indicated that schizophrenia patients exhibit deficits in transitive inference (Coleman et al., 2010; Heckers et al., 2004). There are, however, conflicting results on differences between the performance of controls and schizophrenia on syllogistic reasoning tasks. For example, Williams (1964) indicated that there is no difference between delusion-prone individuals and nondelusion prone individuals on syllogistic reasoning. In fact, under certain conditions, schizophrenia patients seem to perform better than normal controls. When a syllogistic reasoning task utilizes unintuitive or noncommon sense statements (e.g., all buildings speak loudly; a hospital does not speak loudly; therefore, a hospital is not a building), healthy controls seem to make more logical errors as compared to schizophrenia patients. Schizophrenia individuals are not distracted by the noncommon sense content and are able to reason, irrespectively. Other studies show that schizophrenia patients are more impaired on syllogistic reasoning than controls (see Table 1). Cardella and Gangemi (2015) argue that reasoning abilities in schizophrenia patients are not caused by a deficit but instead, somewhat of an over-application of reason and logic. Cardella and Gamgeli suggested that when controlling for factors of education and IQ, the difference between schizophrenia individuals and controls fades away.

Another paradigm utilizes the statement form, if A… then B, and require the participant to judge the validity of its content based on this structure. As discussed above, schizophrenia patients seem to perform better than healthy participants when the statement utilizes misleading content. Interestingly, no differences between groups was observed when the task contained a neutral content, while negative emotional content elicited worse performance in both groups, with the schizophrenia group performed significantly worse as compared to health controls with regard to negative emotional content. The authors draw a link between delusions and negative emotions, suggesting that the negative emotion can trigger delusional behavior. Cardella and Gangemi (2015) suggest that in this situation, schizophrenia patients' difficulties in context processing contribute to the observed improved performance. Further, the Wason Card Selection task has been administered on deluded and nondeluded individuals, schizophrenia patients, and depression group (Dudley et al., 1998; Mirabilio et al., 2006; Peters et al., 2008). Findings of these studies have shown that reasoning biases are specific to delusion and data-gathering tasks. Selesnick and Owen (2012) provided a theoretical analysis of deductive reasoning performance in schizophrenia patients. They showed that by ignoring context, schizophrenia patients can sometimes outperform healthy controls on some deductive reasoning tasks, including syllogism and conditioned If rules. Healthy individuals often show poor performance in deductive reasoning tasks, that they show floor effect (Johnson-Laird, 1995). This can possibly explain why schizophrenia patients perform at same level or even better than healthy controls.

Similarities and differences between inductive and deductive reasoning performance in schizophrenia patients

There are some similarities between inductive and deductive reasoning performance in schizophrenia patients. For example, across both deductive and inductive reasoning tasks, it was reported that the theory of mind (Brakoulias et al., 2008; Corcoran

& Frith, 2005; Langdon, Ward, & Coltheart, 2010), working memory (Dudley et al., 1998; Menon, Pomarol-Clotet, McKenna, & McCarthy, 2006), and the use of emotional stimuli (R. E. Dudley, John, Young, & Over, 1997; Fraser, Morrison, & Wells, 2006; Kemp et al., 1997) impact task performance. However, it remains to be explained how these processes exactly play a role in reasoning processes. To our knowledge, there are no theoretical model that explains the link between these cognitive processes and reasoning abilities.

However, there are some differences as well between both deductive and inductive reasoning. As discussed above, several studies show that the hippocampus plays a key role in (at least some) deductive reasoning tasks (Avery et al., 2018; Heckers et al., 2004). Unlike deductive reasoning, it was found that the prefrontal cortex and basal ganglia play a key role in inductive reasoning, including the beads (jumping to conclusions) task (Lunt et al., 2012). It is possible that both kinds of reasoning are mediated by different neural mechanisms. However, to the best of our knowledge, this was not tested empirically, but future work should investigate the neural dissociation between deductive and inductive reasoning. However, inductive reasoning tasks recruit more neural network regions than those activated during deductive reasoning performance. This is possibly the case as unlike deductive reasoning, inductive reasoning relies more on context and background information, as is the case for scientific reasoning. Conducting deductive reasoning tasks mainly relies on given premises.

Garety et al. (2011) have developed an inductive reasoning training method, which aims at correcting jumping to conclusion biases in schizophrenia patients (Waller, Freeman, Jolley, Dunn, & Garety, 2011). Importantly, unlike prior attempts at treating inductive reasoning biases, to our knowledge, there are no studies that have aimed at treating deductive reasoning in schizophrenia patients.

Future directions

Based on the review of the previous studies on utilizing reasoning tasks in schizophrenia and related disorders, there can be various avenues for future studies. For example, future studies should focus on developing techniques that aim to treat or remediate the reasoning deficits in schizophrenia and related disorders. While there have been some attempts to developing reasoning-based treatments (see above), it remains to be shown whether ameliorating reasoning deficits may help reduce delusions in schizophrenia patients.

It is also important to compare and contrast between performance on inductive and deductive reasoning tasks in schizophrenia as there is no single study assessing this phenomena. These studies will help explain which reasoning processes underlie delusions in schizophrenia. For example, studies can compare both conditional and abductive reasoning in schizophrenia. While conditional reasoning has the form of "A is true & A implies B, then we infer B", abductive reasoning has the form of "A is true & B implies A, then we infer B" Abductive reasoning is a form of deductive reasoning. Importantly, it is similar enough to (deductive) conditional reasoning, making the comparison between the plausible.

Further, more research is needed to understand neural structures underlying performance in reasoning tasks and how cognitive and emotional factors underlying reasoning affects the brain. Based on a review of prior neural studies, it is suggested that both deductive and inductive reasoning recruits different brain areas. Further, it is argued that computational neural network modeling work will help understand how complex interactions among different brain areas may explain performance in reasoning tasks.

One limitation of most prior studies is they assume reasoning deficits in schizophrenia are related to positive symptoms in the patients. However, most of these studies did not factor in any role played by negative symptoms or cognitive impairment. Several studies have reported cognitive impairment in schizophrenia, including attention (Bergman, O'Brien, Osgood, & Cornblatt, 1995; Moustafa et al., 2016; Sapir, Dobrusin, Ben-Bashat, & Henik, 2007), IQ (Kappelmann et al., 2018; van Os, Marsman, van Dam, Simons, & Investigators, 2017), and working memory (Anticevic, Repovs, & Barch, 2013; Frydecka et al., 2014; Moustafa et al., 2016). These processes are also known to impact reasoning abilities (Howe, Rabinowitz, & Powell, 1998; Ren, Schweizer, & Fen, 2013). Accordingly, it is possible that reasoning deficits in schizophrenia could be related more to cognitive impairment in the patients, rather than positive symptoms. Future research should address these methodological issues.

Conflict of interest

All authors declare no conflict of interest.

Data availability

This is a review article and does not include any data.

References

Abi-Dargham, A., Mawlawi, O., Lombardo, I., Gil, R., Martinez, D., Huang, Y., ... Laruelle, M. (2002). Prefrontal dopamine D1 receptors and working memory in schizophrenia. *The Journal of Neuroscience*, *22*(9), 3708–3719.

Albacete, A., Contreras, F., Bosque, C., Gilabert, E., Albiach, A., Menchon, J. M., ... Ayesa-Arriola, R. (2016). Counterfactual reasoning in non-psychotic first-degree relatives of people with schizophrenia. *Frontiers in Psychology*, *7*, 665. https://doi.org/10.3389/fpsyg.2016.00665.

American Psychiatric Association. (2013). *Diagnostic and statistical manual of mental disorders (DSM-5®)*. American Psychiatric Pub.

Anticevic, A., Repovs, G., & Barch, D. M. (2013). Working memory encoding and maintenance deficits in schizophrenia: Neural evidence for activation and deactivation abnormalities. *Schizophrenia Bulletin*, *39*(1), 168–178. https://doi.org/10.1093/schbul/sbr107.

Arieti, S. (1974). *Interpretation of Schizophrenia* (s. edition Ed.). Northvale, NJ, London: Jason Aronson Inc.

Avery, S. N., Rogers, B. P., & Heckers, S. (2018). Hippocampal network modularity is associated with relational memory dysfunction in schizophrenia. *Biological Psychiatry: Cognitive Neuroscience and Neuroimaging*, *3*(5), 423–432. https://doi.org/10.1016/j.bpsc.2018.02.001.

Bandinelli, P. L., Palma, C., Penna, M. P., & Pessa, E. (2006). Logic and context in schizophrenia. In G. Minati, E. Pessa, & M. Abram (Eds.), *Systemics of emergence*. New York: Springer.

Barrantes-Vidal, N., Grant, P., & Kwapil, T. R. (2015). The role of schizotypy in the study of the etiology of schizophrenia spectrum disorders. *Schizophrenia Bulletin*, *41*(Suppl 2), S408–S416. https://doi.org/10.1093/schbul/sbu191.

Bergman, A., O'Brien, J., Osgood, G., & Cornblatt, B. (1995). Distractibility in schizophrenia. *Psychiatry Research*, *57*(2), 131–140.

Brakoulias, V., Langdon, R., Sloss, G., Coltheart, M., Meares, R., & Harris, A. (2008). Delusions and reasoning: A study involving cognitive behavioural therapy. *Cognitive Neuropsychiatry*, *13*(2), 148–165.

Cardella, V., & Gangemi, A. (2015). Reasoning in schizophrenia. Review and analysis from the cognitive perspective. *Clinical Neuropschiatry*, *12*, 3–8.

Coleman, M. J., Titone, D., Krastoshevsky, O., Krause, V., Huang, Z., Mendell, N. R., … Levy, D. L. (2010). Reinforcement ambiguity and novelty do not account for transitive inference deficits in schizophrenia. *Schizophrenia Bulletin*, *36*(6), 1187–1200. https://doi.org/10.1093/schbul/sbp039.

Contreras, F., Albacete, A., Castellvi, P., Cano, A., Benejam, B., & Menchon, J. M. (2016). Counterfactual reasoning deficits in schizophrenia patients. *PLoS One*, *11*(2), e0148440. https://doi.org/10.1371/journal.pone.0148440.

Corcoran, R. (2003). Inductive reasoning and the understanding of intention in schizophrenia. *Cognitive Neuropsychiatry*, *8*(3), 223–235. https://doi.org/10.1080/13546800244000319.

Corcoran, R., & Frith, C. D. (2005). Thematic reasoning and theory of mind. Accounting for social inference difficulties in schizophrenia. *Evolutionary Psychology*, *3*(1). 147470490500300101.

Dudley, R. E., John, C. H., Young, A. W., & Over, D. E. (1997). Normal and abnormal reasoning in people with delusions. *The British Journal of Clinical Psychology*, *36*(Pt 2), 243–258.

Dudley, R., & Over, D. (2003). People with delusions jump to conclusions: A theoretical account of research findings on the reasoning of people with delusions. *Clinical Psychology & Psychotherapy*, *10*(5), 263–274.

Dudley, R. E. J., Young, A. W., John, C. H., & Over, D. E. (1998). Conditional reasoning in people with delusions: Performance on the Wason selection task. *Cognitive Neuropsychiatry*, *3*(4), 241–258. https://doi.org/10.1080/135468098396071.

Forbes, G. (1994). *Modern logic: A text in elementary symbolic logic*.

Foss, B. M. (1966). *New horizons in psychology*. Harmondsworth: Penguin.

Fraser, J., Morrison, A., & Wells, A. (2006). Cognitive processes, reasoning biases and persecutory delusions: A comparative study. *Behavioural and Cognitive Psychotherapy*, *34*(4), 421–435.

Frydecka, D., Eissa, A. M., Hewedi, D. H., Ali, M., Drapala, J., Misiak, B., … Moustafa, A. A. (2014). Impairments of working memory in schizophrenia and bipolar disorder: The effect of history of psychotic symptoms and different aspects of cognitive task demands. *Frontiers in Behavioral Neuroscience*, *8*, 416. https://doi.org/10.3389/fnbeh.2014.00416.

Garety, P., Freeman, D., Jolley, S., Ross, K., Waller, H., & Dunn, G. (2011). Jumping to conclusions: The psychology of delusional reasoning. *Advances in Psychiatric Treatment*, *17*, 332–339.

Gazes, R. P., Chee, N. W., & Hampton, R. R. (2012). Cognitive mechanisms for transitive inference performance in rhesus monkeys: Measuring the influence of associative strength and inferred order. *Journal of Experimental Psychology. Animal Behavior Processes*, *38*(4), 331.

Gras-Vincendon, A., Danion, J.-M., Grangé, D., Bilik, M., Willard-Schroeder, D., Sichel, J.-P., & Singer, L. (1994). Explicit memory, repetition priming and cognitive skill learning in schizophrenia. *Schizophrenia Research*, *13*(2), 117–126. https://doi.org/10.1016/0920-9964(94)90092-2.

Griggs, R. A., & Cox, J. R. (1982). The elusive thematic-materials effect in Wason's selection task. *British Journal of Psychology*, *73*(3), 407–420.

Heckers, S., Zalesak, M., Weiss, A. P., Ditman, T., & Titone, D. (2004). Hippocampal activation during transitive inference in humans. *Hippocampus*, *14*(2), 153–162. https://doi.org/10.1002/hipo.10189.

Hooker, C., Roese, N. J., & Park, S. (2000). Impoverished counterfactual thinking is associated with schizophrenia. *Psychiatry*, *63*(4), 326–335.

Howe, M. L., Rabinowitz, F. M., & Powell, T. L. (1998). Individual differences in working memory and reasoning-remembering relationships in solving class-inclusion problems. *Memory & Cognition*, *26*(5), 1089–1101.

Johnson-Laird, P. N. (1995). Mental models, deductive reasoning, and the brain. In M. S. Gazzaniga (Ed.), *The cognitive neurosciences* (pp. 999–1008). Cambridge, Massachusetts: MIT Press.

Johnson-Laird, P. N., Legrenzi, P., & Legrenzi, M. S. (1972). Reasoning and a sense of reality. *British Journal of Psychology*, *63*(3), 395–400.

Kappelmann, N., Khandaker, G. M., Dal, H., Stochl, J., Kosidou, K., Jones, P. B., … Karlsson, H. (2018). Systemic inflammation and intelligence in early adulthood and subsequent risk of schizophrenia and other non-affective psychoses: A longitudinal cohort and co-relative study. *Psychological Medicine*, 1–8. https://doi.org/10.1017/S0033291718000831.

Kemp, R., Chua, S., McKenna, P., & David, A. (1997). Reasoning and delusions. *The British Journal of Psychiatry*, *170*(5), 398–405.

Kornreich, C., Delle-Vigne, D., Brevers, D., Tecco, J., Campanella, S., Noel, X., … Ermer, E. (2017). Conditional reasoning in schizophrenic patients. *Evolutionary Psychology*, *15*(3). https://doi.org/10.1177/1474704917721713. 1474704917721713.

Langdon, R., Ward, P. B., & Coltheart, M. (2010). Reasoning anomalies associated with delusions in schizophrenia. *Schizophrenia Bulletin*, *36*(2), 321–330. https://doi.org/10.1093/schbul/sbn069.

Lazareva, O. F., & Wasserman, E. A. (2012). Transitive inference in pigeons: Measuring the associative values of stimuli B and D. *Behavioural Processes*, *89*(3), 244–255.

Lunt, L., Bramham, J., Morris, R. G., Bullock, P. R., Selway, R. P., Xenitidis, K., & David, A. S. (2012). Prefrontal cortex dysfunction and 'Jumping to Conclusions': Bias or deficit? *Journal of Neuropsychology*, *6*(1), 65–78. https://doi.org/10.1111/j.1748-6653.2011.02005.x.

Mellet, E., Houde, O., Brazo, P., Mazoyer, B., Tzourio-Mazoyer, N., & Dollfus, S. (2006). When a schizophrenic deficit becomes a reasoning advantage. *Schizophrenia Research*, *84*(2–3), 359–364. https://doi.org/10.1016/j.schres.2006.03.024.

Menon, M., Pomarol-Clotet, E., McKenna, P. J., & McCarthy, R. A. (2006). Probabilistic reasoning in schizophrenia: A comparison of the performance of deluded and nondeluded schizophrenic patients and exploration of possible cognitive underpinnings. *Cognitive Neuropsychiatry*, *11*(6), 521–536. https://doi.org/10.1080/13546800544000046.

Mirabilio, D., Di Tommaso, S., Riccardi, I., Marinelli, M., Daneluzzo, E., Stratta, P., … Rossi, A. (2006). Predictors of social cognition in patients with schizophrenia. *Neuropsychiatric Disease and Treatment*, *2*(4), 571.

Mirian, D., Heinrichs, R. W., & Vaz, S. M. (2011). Exploring logical reasoning abilities in schizophrenia patients. *Schizophrenia Research, 127*(1), 178–180.

Moustafa, A. A., Garami, J. K., Mahlberg, J., Golembieski, J., Keri, S., Misiak, B., & Frydecka, D. (2016). Cognitive function in schizophrenia: Conflicting findings and future directions. *Reviews in the Neurosciences*. https://doi.org/10.1515/revneuro-2015-0060.

Moustafa, A. A., & Gluck, M. A. (2011). Computational cognitive models of prefrontal-striatal-hippocampal interactions in Parkinson's disease and schizophrenia. *Neural Networks, 24*(6), 575–591. https://doi.org/10.1016/j.neunet.2011.02.006.

Moustafa, A. A., Keri, S., Herzallah, M. M., Myers, C. E., & Gluck, M. A. (2010). A neural model of hippocampal-striatal interactions in associative learning and transfer generalization in various neurological and psychiatric patients. *Brain and Cognition, 74*(2), 132–144. https://doi.org/10.1016/j.bandc.2010.07.013.

Moustafa, A. A., Misiak, B., & Frydecka, D. (2017). Computational models of schizophrenia. In A. A. Moustafa (Ed.), *Computational models of Brain and Behavior* Wiley-Blackwell.

Mujica-Parodi, L. R., Malaspina, D., & Sackeim, H. A. (2000). Logical processing, affect, and delusional thought in schizophrenia. *Harvard Review of Psychiatry, 8*(2), 73–83.

Northrop, L. C. (1977). *The definition and measurement of reasoning (technical memorandum 77–10)*. Washington, DC: US: Civil Service Commission.

Onwuameze, O. E., Titone, D., & Ho, B. C. (2016). Transitive inference deficits in unaffected biological relatives of schizophrenia patients. *Schizophrenia Research, 175*(1–3), 64–71. https://doi.org/10.1016/j.schres.2016.02.015.

Owen, G. S., Cutting, J., & David, A. S. (2007). Are people with schizophrenia more logical than healthy volunteers? *The British Journal of Psychiatry, 191*(5), 453–454. https://doi.org/10.1192/bjp.bp.107.037309.

Peters, E. R., Thornton, P., Siksou, L., Linney, Y., & MacCabe, J. H. (2008). Specificity of the jump-to-conclusions bias in deluded patients. *British Journal of Clinical Psychology, 47*(2), 239–244.

Ranganath, C., Minzenberg, M. J., & Ragland, J. D. (2008). The cognitive neuroscience of memory function and dysfunction in schizophrenia. *Biological Psychiatry, 64*(1), 18–25. https://doi.org/10.1016/j.biopsych.2008.04.011.

Ren, X., Schweizer, K., & Fen, X. (2013). The sources of the relationship between sustained attention and reasoning. *Intelligence, 41*(1), 51–58.

Revsbech, R., Mortensen, E. L., Owen, G., Nordgaard, J., Jansson, L., Sæbye, D., … Parnas, J. (2015). Exploring rationality in schizophrenia. *British Journal of Psychiatry Open, 1*(1), 98–103.

Sapir, A., Dobrusin, M., Ben-Bashat, G., & Henik, A. (2007). Neuroleptics reverse attentional effects in schizophrenia patients. *Neuropsychologia, 45*(14), 3263–3271. https://doi.org/10.1016/j.neuropsychologia.2007.06.007.

Selesnick, S. A., & Owen, G. S. (2012). Quantum-like logics and schizophrenia. *Journal of Applied Logic, 10*, 115–126.

Sellen, J. L., Oaksford, M., & Gray, N. S. (2005). Schizotypy and conditional reasoning. *Schizophrenia Bulletin, 31*(1), 105–116. https://doi.org/10.1093/schbul/sbi012.

Silverman, J. L., Gastrell, P. T., Karras, M. N., Solomon, M., & Crawley, J. N. (2015). Cognitive abilities on transitive inference using a novel touchscreen technology for mice. *Cerebral Cortex, 25*(5), 1133–1142. https://doi.org/10.1093/cercor/bht293.

Sinha, B. K., & Nelson, T. M. (1993). Transitivity of thought in schizophrenic, brain damaged and alcoholic patients. *Imagination, Cognition and Personality, 13*, 25–37.

Smeland, O. B., Frei, O., Kauppi, K., Hill, W. D., Li, W., Wang, Y., ... Neuro, C. C. W. G. (2017). Identification of genetic loci jointly influencing schizophrenia risk and the cognitive traits of verbal-numerical reasoning, reaction time, and general cognitive function. *JAMA Psychiatry*, *74*(10), 1065–1075. https://doi.org/10.1001/jamapsychiatry.2017.1986.

So, S. H., Garety, P. A., Peters, E. R., & Kapur, S. (2010). Do antipsychotics improve reasoning biases? A review. *Psychosomatic Medicine*, *72*(7), 681–693.

Titone, D., Ditman, T., Holzman, P. S., Eichenbaum, H., & Levy, D. L. (2004). Transitive inference in schizophrenia: Impairments in relational memory organization. *Schizophrenia Research*, *68*(2), 235–247.

Toulmin, S. E., & Rieke, R. D. J. (1984). *An introduction to reasoning*. Pearson.

Van Hoeck, N., Watson, P. D., & Barbey, A. K. (2015). Cognitive neuroscience of human counterfactual reasoning. *Frontiers in Human Neuroscience*, *9*, 420. https://doi.org/10.3389/fnhum.2015.00420.

van Os, J., Marsman, A., van Dam, D., Simons, C. J., & Investigators, G. (2017). Evidence that the impact of childhood trauma on IQ is substantial in controls, moderate in siblings, and absent in patients with psychotic disorder. *Schizophrenia Bulletin*, *43*(2), 316–324. https://doi.org/10.1093/schbul/sbw177.

Von Domarus, E. (1944). The specific laws of logic in schizophrenia. In J. S. Kasanin (Ed.), *Language and thought in schizophrenia* (pp. 104–114). Berkeley: University of California Press.

Waller, H., Freeman, D., Jolley, S., Dunn, G., & Garety, P. (2011). Targeting reasoning biases in delusions: A pilot study of the Maudsley review training Programme for individuals with persistent, high conviction delusions. *Journal of Behavior Therapy and Experimental Psychiatry*, *42*(3), 414–421.

Wason, P. C. (1968). Reasoning about a rule. *The Quarterly Journal of Experimental Psychology. B*, *20*(3), 273–281.

Wason, P. C., & Shapiro, D. (1971). Natural and contrived experience in a reasoning problem. *The Quarterly Journal of Experimental Psychology. B*, *23*(1), 63–71.

Williams, E. B. (1964). Deductive reasoning in schizophrenia. *The Journal of Abnormal and Social Psychology*, *69*(1), 47–61. https://doi.org/10.1037/h0044311.

A review on inductive reasoning abilities in schizophrenia and related disorders

4

Ahmed A. Moustafa[a,b] *and Anchal Garg*[c]
[a]School of Psychology & Marcs Institute for Brain and Behaviour, Western Sydney University, Sydney, NSW, Australia, [b]Department of Human Anatomy and Physiology, the Faculty of Health Sciences, University of Johannesburg, South Africa, [c]School of Psychology, Western Sydney University, Sydney, NSW, Australia

Chapter outline

Introduction

According to the Diagnostic and Statistical Manual for Mental Disorders, Fifth Edition (DSM-V), schizophrenia spectrum and other psychotic disorders are characterized by abnormalities in one or more of the following domains: delusions, hallucinations, disorganized thinking (speech), grossly disorganized behavior (including catatonia), and negative symptoms (American Psychiatric Association, 2013). This spectrum includes schizophrenia, schizophreniform disorder, schizotypal personality disorder, delusional disorder, schizoaffective disorder, and unspecified schizophrenia spectrum and other psychotic disorders, among others. Schizophrenia disorder includes two or more of the following symptoms: delusions, hallucinations, disorganized speech, grossly disorganized or catatonic behavior, and negative symptoms, whereas delusional disorder is

Cognitive and Behavioral Dysfunction in Schizophrenia. https://doi.org/10.1016/B978-0-12-820005-6.00006-2

characterized by at least 1 month of delusions but no other psychotic symptoms. On the other hand, schizotypal personality disorder is characterized by a pervasive pattern of social and interpersonal deficits including reduced capacity for close relationships, cognitive or perceptual distortions, and eccentricities of behavior usually beginning in early adulthood; however, in some cases it becomes apparent in childhood and adolescence.

Reasoning: Definition and tasks

Reasoning can be defined as a logical thinking process that results in a conclusion (Northrop, 1977), or a process whose goal is to enable the reasoner to make the best decision about a particular issue, in particular circumstances, within a particular forum and enterprise (Toulmin, 1984). In other words, reasoning involves the process of inferring information from an existing body of knowledge and/or assumptions. Inductive reasoning involves inference based on prior knowledge and information, as in scientific methods (Hayes & Heit, 2018). This kind of reasoning is not always right or wrong, but it is justified on how plausible the inference is. There are several tasks which investigate reasoning processes in schizophrenia spectrum and other psychotic disorders including The Beads Task, The Survey Task, and The Aha! Sentences Task (as explained in the next section).

Inductive reasoning tasks

The Beads Task is most commonly used to assess jumping to conclusion biases, which is a reasoning style characterized as a tendency or bias to early acceptance (Garety & Freeman, 1999). It consists of two containers with large number of different colored beads in different ratios. Moreover, participants are informed about the proportions of these beads, but the containers are hidden from the view. Then, participants are shown a sequence of beads apparently being drawn from one of the containers (the sequence is actually prespecified by the experimenter). After each draw, the experimenter asks participants if they are ready to make a decision about which container the beads are being drawn from, or if they would like to see another bead (Phillips & Edwards, 1966; Ross, McKay, Coltheart, & Langdon, 2015).

The Survey Task is a variant of the Beads Task which assesses jumping to conclusion reasoning style (Dudley, John, Young, & Over, 1997a). It consists of two new variants of the Bead Task. The first task is realistic in nature as it consists of concrete examples, but remains neutral in content that is, rather than showing beads in jars, participants are presented with a description of two schools, one that is mainly for boys (60 boys and 40 girls) and another is mainly for girls (60 girls and 40 boys). On each trial, the first names of children from one of the schools is presented one at a time, and the participant is allowed to request as many names as he/she felt necessary to make a decision. On this task, the participants have to identify whether the sample came from mainly boys or girls school (Dudley et al., 1997a; Dudley, John, Young, & Over, 1997b; Huq, Garety, & Hemsley, 1988). In the salient version of the Survey Task, stimuli are emotional in nature, in which participants are presented with a hypothetical scenario (to the effect that two surveys had been conducted that gathered comments about someone who was very similar to the participant). The intention is to allow the participant to identify with the descriptions presented. One survey is generally positive and indicates that person is well-liked by other people (60 positive comments and 40 negative) and in the other survey the person was generally disliked (60 negative comments and 40 positive). Based on the sequence of comments shown to the participants, they decide whether the survey indicates that the person is generally liked or disliked. The participants can request as many comments as necessary in order to decide whether comments originated from a mainly positive or a mainly negative survey (Dudley et al., 1997a, 1997b; Huq et al., 1988).

The Aha! Sentences Task also probes inductive reasoning. It consists of series of sentences that are read out to the participants and they have to explain what sentences actually mean. If the participant fails to comprehend the sentence in the manner intended, then a clue is given (i.e., in the form of a single word or phrase). On this task, it is assumed that to find meaning of unusual sentences, previously stored information must be invoked in order to find the context within which the sentence is comprehensible. Further, it seems likely that the difficulty of the sentences reflects the type of memory store that is being sampled. The easy sentences appear to draw on semantic memory while the more difficult ones may require information derived from personal past experiences in order for sense to be derived. In other words, the resolution of the ambiguity within these sentences requires inductive reasoning (Corcoran, 2000; Corcoran & Frith, 2005).

Prior reviews on reasoning tasks

There are several reviews mostly focusing on reviewing the Jumping to Conclusions data using standard inductive reasoning task. As discussed above, a commonly used paradigm to assess inductive reasoning is the Beads Task. For instance, Dudley and Over (2003) reviewed the previous studies on reasoning of individuals with delusions and then drew a model of normal reasoning to distinguish reasoning in line with logic and probability theory from reasoning used to achieve one‘s individual (epistemic and other) goals. Results showed that individuals with delusions are different from control groups in terms of reasoning on neutral tasks. Specifically, Dudley and Over (2003) viewed delusional reasoning as being an extension of a common reasoning style to situations that normally would not activate it. On the other hand, Fine, Gardner, Craigie, and Gold (2007) conducted a meta-analysis of studies that used the Beads Task to investigate whether jumping to conclusion bias correlate with delusions, or only with symptomatology of schizophrenia, and whether jumping to conclusions bias enhanced by emotionally salient material. Results indicated that "draws to decision" is the most reliable measure of the jumping to conclusion bias and contributes to delusional symptomatology. It was also reported that jumping to conclusion reasoning plays a casual role in the formation and/or retention of delusional beliefs. Emotional salience did not increase the hastiness of decision-making in patients with delusions, which indicates that particular delusional beliefs adopted by schizophrenia patients cannot be explained by the emotional nature of that type of belief instead, delusional patients may be hasty with respect to all types of material.

So, Garety, Peters, and Kapur (2010) reviewed 17 longitudinal studies to investigate how the reasoning biases in schizophrenia patients respond to the treatment. They found that jumping to conclusions and reduced belief flexibility were closely related to the severity of delusions, whereas theory of mind was better associated with negative symptoms and attributional style to overall psychopathology. They also reported that the jumping to conclusion bias was likely to be stable trait factor which does not change with treatment. A more recent review on the Beads Task has also discussed the role of jumping to conclusions in the treatment of schizophrenia (Evans, Averbeck, & Furl, 2015). Further, Garety and Freeman (2013) provided an update on their previous review (i.e., Garety & Freeman, 1999) highlighting the contribution that deficits in reasoning have on the formation and maintenance of delusions. They reported a positive relationship between jumping to conclusions and delusions which intensify during acute states. Furthermore, a similar positive, though attenuated effect was found between the jumping to conclusion bias and a proneness to delusional thinking in the general population, suggesting jumping to conclusion bias as a stable trait associated with delusional thinking in general.

Neural correlates of reasoning

There have been a few studies investigating neural correlates of reasoning. For example, Lunt et al. (2012) investigated the underlying mechanisms of jumping to conclusions by comparing the three groups: prefrontal lobe damaged patients, adults with attention-deficit hyperactivity disorder, and healthy controls. The jumping to conclusions bias was only found in the patients with lesions in the left prefrontal cortex. On the other hand, Esslinger et al. (2013) measured brain activation during the beads task in a group of nonclinical individuals and reported activation in the midbrain and striatum. Similarly, another study reported that reduced ventral striatum activity is related to jumping to conclusion task performance in individuals at risk of developing schizophrenia (Rausch et al., 2015).

All the brain areas activated in reasoning tasks as described earlier are also reported in schizophrenia studies including midbrain (presumably dopamine), striatum, hippocampus, and prefrontal cortex (Abi-Dargham et al., 2002; Moustafa et al., 2016; Moustafa & Gluck, 2011; Moustafa, Keri, Herzallah, Myers, & Gluck, 2010; Moustafa, Misiak, & Frydecka, 2017). These findings suggest that several brain areas are involved in reasoning indicating that it is a complex process. Further, the complex network underlying reasoning also suggests that this could be due the impact of other emotional and cognitive processes including stress, working memory, and theory of mind on reasoning. Therefore, these factors should be investigated in future studies.

Aims

The purpose of the present review is to discuss and compare inductive reasoning abilities in schizophrenia spectrum patients. Specifically, in this review we will discuss whether schizophrenia patients show impairment on different types of inductive reasoning tasks. A secondary focus of this review is to understand the relationship between reasoning and symptoms in schizophrenia and related disorders.

Methods

In this study, we provide a systematic review on reasoning deficits in schizophrenia and related disorders. Our search strategy included the following a combination of two key words from two sets. The first set included schizophrenia, delusional disorder, schizotypy, psychotic disorder, and so on. The second set included jumping to conclusions, the Beads Task, the Survey Task, and the Aha! Sentence Task. The list of key words are as follows: schizophrenia, inductive reasoning, and jumping to conclusions. We have searched previous studies assessing the reasoning anomalies in schizophrenia and related disorders on PubMed, PsychInfo, and Google Scholar. Further, we have examined each paper carefully to make sure the goal of the study is examined reasoning in schizophrenia spectrum disorders. Studies that did not include reasoning task and/or schizophrenia spectrum disorders were excluded (as explained in Fig. 1).

Below, we review studies that have employed the reasoning tasks in schizophrenia and related disorders. Some of these studies have compared schizophrenia spectrum disorder patients with other clinical disorders and normal controls. We present our review on the following tasks: The Beads Task, The Survey Task, and The Aha! Sentences Task.

The beads task

Some studies using the Beads task have mainly investigated group differences across different clinical groups (as summarized in Table 1). For instance, Garety et al. (1991) compared schizophrenia patients with patients of anxiety disorders and control group using the beads task. They found that schizophrenia patients with delusions requested less information before reaching a decision and were more ready to change their estimates of the likelihood of an event when confronted with potentially discomfirmatory information as compared to other groups. Extending prior results, Warman et al. (2007) assessed the jumping to conclusion bias in individuals with active delusions, delusion-prone, and nondelusion prone and were also asked to report their level of confidence in their decisions. Results indicated that individuals with delusions gathered significantly less information than delusion prone and nondelusion prone participants on the task. Further, individuals with delusions made less accurate

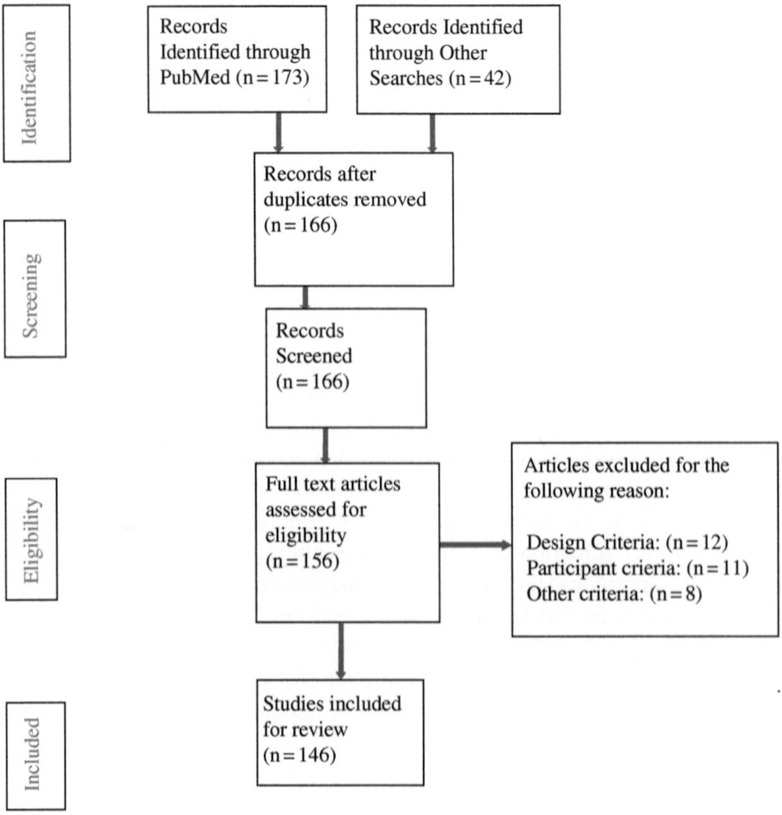

Fig. 1 Decision tree for article search and selection.

decisions as compared to delusion-prone and nondelusion prone participants on the task. Individuals with delusions and delusion-prone individuals reported higher self-confidence in their performance on self-referent task as compared to neutral task version of the Beads Task.

Using a different group, Peters et al. (2008) investigated the specificity of the jumping-to-conclusion bias in delusions among psychotic patients (i.e., deluded versus nondeluded individuals). Results showed that the deluded group made showed jumping to conclusions biases than the non-deluded group with no differences on these tasks when participants were grouped based on the diagnosis of schizophrenia. Thus, jumping to conclusion bias is specific to delusions rather than diagnosis and a general deficit in reasoning.

Using subjects from nonclinical population, Colbert and Peters (2002) studied two groups (i.e., delusion-prone vs. non-delusion-prone) formed based on the scores in the upper and lower quartiles of the Peters et al. Delusion Inventory. In this study, the need for closure was assessed as a motivational factor that may correlate with the reasoning bias (using the Beads Task). There was an evidence for the existence of the data gathering bias among the delusion-prone individuals. However,

Table 1 A summary of studies on inductive reasoning.

Study	Sample	Key findings
The beads task		
Garety, Hemsley, and Wessely (1991)	27 schizophrenia patients (with delusional disorders or delusions) 14 anxious control patients 13 healthy controls	Schizophrenia patients requested less information before reaching a decision and changed their estimates of the likelihood of an event when given potentially discomfirmatory information as compared to the other groups
Colbert and Peters (2002)	68 healthy subjects (34 delusion-prone vs. 34 non-delusion-prone)	Delusion-Prone subjects showed more jumping to conclusion bias (i.e., made their decision after few beads) as compared to non-delusion-prone subjects
Garety et al. (2005)	100 patients with non-affective psychosis (with current delusions)	Belief inflexibility and jumping to conclusions contributed to the severity and persistence of delusional conviction. Belief inflexibility mediated the relationship between jumping to conclusion and delusional conviction
Fraser, Morrison, and Wells (2006)	15 psychotic patients with persecutory delusions 15 panic disorder patients 15 healthy controls	There was no main effect of group as all participants requested significantly less information in the emotional condition
Warman, Lysaker, Martin, Davis, and Haudenschield (2007)	37 schizophrenia/schizoaffective disorder patients (with active delusions) 60 university students (delusion-prone, and non-delusion-prone)	Clinical sample gathered significantly less information and made less accurate decisions than delusion-prone and non-delusion-prone participants the task
Brakoulias et al. (2008)	16 psychotic patients	Subjects who completed the cognitive behavioral therapy program showed significant reductions in delusional conviction and preoccupation. Further, subjects showed some form of abnormal probabilistic reasoning, excessive attributional biases, and deficits in theory of mind compared to norms at baseline with no change in these cognitive mechanisms post-treatment
Freeman, Pugh, and Garety (2008)	200 subjects from local community	Jumping to conclusion bias was found in 20% of the sample and was strongly associated with the higher levels of conviction in paranoid thoughts and the occurrence of perceptual anomalies

Continued

Table 1 Continued

Study	Sample	Key findings
Peters, Thornton, Siksou, Linney, and MacCabe (2008)	37 psychotic patients (21 deluded vs. 16 non-deluded)	Deluded group showed more jumping to conclusion bias on data-gathering tasks as compared to non-deluded group
Langdon, Ward, and Coltheart (2010)	35 schizophrenia patients with a history of delusions (30 with current delusions) 34 healthy controls	Schizophrenia patients showed jumping to conclusion bias in order to over-adjust when confronted with a change of evidence on probabilistic reasoning tasks, excessive externalizing attributional bias, and performance deficits on three theory of mind tasks as compared to healthy controls
Averbeck, Evans, Chouhan, Bristow, and Shergill (2011)	33 schizophrenia patients 39 healthy controls	Schizophrenia patients with jumping to conclusion style as compared to the healthy controls
Keefe and Warman (2011)	133 undergraduate students (delusion-prone vs. non- delusion-prone)	Both groups performed similarly when there was no stress induction. However, delusion-prone individuals demonstrated reasoning biases relative to non- delusion-prone individuals when stress was induced
Waller, Freeman, Jolley, Dunn, and Garety (2011)	13 psychotic patients	There were improvements in level of jumping to conclusion bias, belief flexibility, and delusional conviction between pre and post intervention measures
Balzan, Delfabbro, Galletly, and Woodward (2012)	25 schizophrenia patients (with history of delusions) 25 non-clinical delusion-prone subjects 25 non-delusion-prone controls	Miscomprehension was a valid construct for jumping to conclusion bias and premature decisions were significantly prevalent in schizophrenia as compared to other groups
The survey task		
Dudley et al. (1997a)	15 schizophrenia patients (with delusions) 16 depression patients 15 healthy controls	Schizophrenia patients made decisions based on less evidence as compared to other groups. When the salient material was presented, all groups became hastier in their decision-making
Menon, Pomarol-Clotet, McKenna, and McCarthy (2006)	36 schizophrenia patients (18 deluded and 18 non-deluded) 18 healthy controls	All the groups performed similarly on probabilistic reasoning tasks in Study 1. Schizophrenia patients showed jumping to conclusion style as compared to controls with no difference between clinical sub-groups in Study 2 (i.e., providing a memory aid)
The Aha! Sentence task		
Corcoran (2003)	39 schizophrenia patients 44 healthy controls	There was a significant correlation between performance on inductive reasoning and language understanding in schizophrenia patients even when the role of immediate memory for narrative and intellectual ability

the probability judgment, part of the jumping to conclusion reasoning bias was not significant in the delusion-prone individuals. Moreover, delusion-prone individuals also scored significantly higher on the need for closure scale (desire of predictability, preference for order and structure, discomfort with ambiguity, decisiveness, and close-mindedness) as compared to non-delusion prone individuals. Thus, the data-gathering reasoning bias may play a role in formation rather than maintenance of delusional beliefs and need for closure may be a motivational factor involved in the formation of delusional beliefs. Similarly, another study reported that probabilistic reasoning impairment (and jumping to conclusions) in schizophrenia patients is related to delusional beliefs and impaired learning (Stuke, Stuke, Weilnhammer, & Schmack, 2017).

Other studies using the Beads Task have investigated emotional and cognitive factors underlying performance in the Beads Task. Garety et al. (2005) conducted a study of 100 individuals with current delusions to elucidate the factors that contribute to the severity and persistence of delusional conviction by assessing the associations between the general cognitive processing styles of jumping to conclusions, extreme responding, and metacognitive process of belief inflexibility. Results showed that reasoning biases (i.e., belief inflexibility, jumping to conclusions, and extreme responding) were present in about half of the sample. Further, belief inflexibility mediated the relationship between jumping to conclusions and delusional conviction and anxiety made an independent contribution to delusional conviction. In another study, Freeman et al. (2008) assessed symptoms, psychological, and social correlates of jumping to conclusions in the general population by using the Beads Task and other scales. They found that jumping to conclusions reasoning bias were present in 20% of the sample. Further, the jumping to conclusion bias was strongly associated with the higher levels of conviction in paranoid thoughts and the occurrence of perceptual anomalies but not with the presence of affective symptoms.

Langdon et al. (2010) examined relationship between attributional style questionnaires, inductive reasoning using the Beads task, and theory of mind in schizophrenia patients with a history of delusions (30 patients were currently deluded) and healthy controls. They found that deluded individuals showed jumping to conclusion bias, an excessive externalizing attributional bias, and performance deficits on the theory of mind tasks as compared to healthy controls. In addition, proneness to delusional ideation was correlated with performance in the beads tasks and theory of mind measures, while externalizing bias was unrelated to delusional ideation. Further, personalizing bias was associated specifically with paranoia across the clinical and nonclinical participants. On the other hand, Averbeck et al. (2011) assessed cognitive processes underpinning jumping to conclusion by using the beads task as well as sequence learning tasks in schizophrenia patients and healthy subjects. In this study, the participants had to learn a sequence of button presses, while receiving corrective feedback on their choices. A Bayesian Decision-Making Model was used to compare model parameters to the choice behaviors in the beads tasks in both schizophrenia patients and healthy subjects. Results indicated that schizophrenia patients with jumping to conclusion style and those who picked early in the beads task tended to learn less from positive feedback in the sequence task as compared to normal controls. Thus, likelihood of the schizophrenia patients selecting early because they have a low threshold for making decisions and they made choices on the basis of relatively little evidence.

Balzan et al. (2012) assessed the effects of miscomprehension on the jumping to conclusion bias in schizophrenia patients with a history of delusions, nonclinical delusion prone and non-delusion-prone controls. They operationalized jumping to conclusion bias in two components: "premature decisions" in which decisions were based on limited evidence and "over-adjustment" involves situations where decisions were radically altered in the face of modest accumulations of disconfirming evidence. In this study, identical versions of the beads task, distinct only by the inclusion of an extra instructional set assigned to increase comprehension was used. In Task 1, participants were presented with a picture of two containers full of red and green beads. After each trial, participants were asked to select from one of the following seven options: 1 = beads are definitely from Container A, 2 = beads very likely from Container A, 3 = beads probably from Container A, 4 = no estimate possible yet, 5 = beads from Container B, 6 = beads very likely from Container B, 7 = beads definitely from Container B. Further, Task 2 was similar to Task 1 except it also included additional instructions, which were intended to make it clear to the participants that the containers did not swap during the task. They found that miscomprehension was a valid construct and indicated that the addition of an instructional set to the second version of the task led to greater comprehension and statistically significant drop in over-adjustment. Further, both tasks showed that premature decisions were significantly prevalent in schizophrenia and were unaffected by the intervention.

Some studies using the Beads Task have investigated the role played by emotional processes. For instance, Fraser et al. (2006) investigated group differences between individuals with persecutory delusions, panic disorder and healthy controls by using the Beads Task (involving three types of material), Psychotic Symptoms Rating Scale, Structured Clinical Interview for DSM-IV, Beck Depression Inventory. They also assessed the impact of emotional content on reasoning by using emotionally salient material. They reported no main effect of group. However, all participants requested significantly less information on the two types of emotional material and the aspects of metacognition were involved with the ratings of delusions. Thus, emotional content has an equal impact on reasoning processing of all groups. On the other hand, Keefe and Warman (2011) examined impact of stress (i.e., in the form of feeling rushed) on jumping to conclusions reasoning bias in delusion-prone individuals. They used Peters et al. Delusions Inventory to assess delusion proneness among university students. Following that, the students were randomly assigned to either receiving, or not receiving stress induction in the form of a speeded subtraction task. In addition, all the participants were engaged in four trials of beads task. Results showed that delusion-prone and nondelusion-prone participants performed similarly when there was no stress induction. However, delusion-prone individuals demonstrated reasoning biases relative to nondelusion prone individuals when stress was induced.

Some studies have investigated the effects of behavioral treatments on reasoning performance. For example, Brakoulias et al. (2008) assessed the efficacy of Cognitive Behavior Therapy (CBT) in reducing delusional conviction in delusional individuals by changing the general reasoning anomalies (anomalies in probabilistic reasoning, theory of mind tasks, and attributional biases) through 8–11 week CBT program. Further, probabilistic reasoning, attributional biases, and theory of mind were assessed by using Scales for the Assessment of Positive Symptoms, Scales for Assessment of Negative Symptoms, Maudsley Assessment of Delusions Scale, Wisconsin Card Sorting Test, Beads Task, Internal Personal and Situation Attribution Questionnaire and three measures of theory of mind. The results indicated that the patients showed impairment in probabilistic reasoning, excessive attributional biases, theory of mind as compared to normal controls. Some patients completed cognitive behavioral therapy program and showed significant reductions in delusional conviction and preoccupation. Thus, CBT is effective in reducing delusional conviction in this sample without any prominent changes in the reasoning anomalies commonly associated with delusions.

In another study, Waller et al. (2011) assessed reasoning processes focusing on the jumping to conclusion bias and belief inflexibility by conducting Maudsley Review Training Package (lasting approximately 1.5 h). They administered the Beads Task (to assess jumping to conclusion reasoning style), three items from Belief Maintenance Scale of Maudsley Assessment of Delusion Schedule (to assess belief flexibility), and Visual Analogue Scale (to assess delusion conviction) on psychotic patients. Further, high levels of conviction and the outcomes were assessed at baseline, pre-intervention, post-intervention, and at 1-month follow up. Results showed that there were improvements in jumping to conclusion bias, belief flexibility, and delusional conviction between pre and post intervention measures.

The survey task

Few studies have administered the Survey Task to assess reasoning (as summarized in Table 1). For instance, Dudley et al. (1997a) examined whether hastiness will be demonstrated by individuals with delusions on neutral and abstract task as compared to other clinical and nonclinical groups. Further, the effect of reasoning due to salient or emotional material on the data gathering was also assessed. In this study, two variants of the Survey Task (i.e., realistic and salient) were administered. On both the versions, the description of two schools was same that is, one consisted of mainly boys (60 boys and 40 girls) and other consisted of mainly girls (60 girls and 40 boys). In the salient version of the task, the stimuli were emotional in content. Results showed that individuals with delusions made decisions based on less evidence as compared to other groups. Thus, hastiness in reasoning or jumping to conclusion style found on abstract probability tasks was generalized to another task which had more realistic content. Further, when the salient material was presented, all the participants became hastier in their decision-making. Thus, the impact of pre-existing hastiness biases, in combination with additional hastiness due to emotional or self-related content, leads to more errors in reasoning in individuals with delusions.

Menon et al. (2006) investigated the role of working memory performance on a range of probabilistic reasoning tasks in deluded and non-deluded schizophrenia patients. In Study 1, deluded and non-deluded schizophrenia patients and normal controls were examined on a range of probabilistic reasoning tasks (Beads Task,

Survey Task, and emotionally salient version of the task). They found that performance of three groups on all versions of the task was similar and there was no evidence of jumping to conclusions bias by both the clinical sub-groups suggesting that this reasoning style is not necessarily observed in schizophrenia patients. In Study 2, two variants of the standard beads task were used to assess the role of working memory load on task performance among deluded and nondeluded schizophrenia patients and normal controls. A working memory-aided condition was utilized in which each bead was in left view of the participant after being drawn. A significant difference was found between schizophrenia and normal controls in drawing in decision component of beads task, whereas no difference was found among deluded and nondeluded schizophrenia group. In other words, jumping to conclusion effect was related to the memory demands imposed by the task. Thus, deluded and nondeluded schizophrenia patients perform similarly on probabilistic reasoning tasks and only show "jumping to conclusions" style under some conditions.

The Aha! Sentence task

Corcoran (2003) examined the relationship between language understanding (using the Hinting Task) and inductive reasoning (using the Aha! Sentences task) in schizophrenia patients and healthy controls. Results indicated a correlation between performance on inductive reasoning and language understanding in schizophrenia patients even after controlling for immediate memory for narrative and intellectual ability and null results in normal controls. This suggests that schizophrenia patients use a different strategy to understand the meaning behind the language understanding as compared to nonclinical subjects.

Discussion

Summary and interpretations of results

In the current review, we reviewed existing literature on inductive reasoning tasks including the Beads Task, the Survey Task, and Aha! Sentences Task, to assess reasoning performance in schizophrenia and related disorders. Most studies have reported that inductive reasoning is impaired in schizophrenia patients compared to normal controls. The Beads Task is most commonly used to assess Jumping to Conclusion Bias in schizophrenia and related disorders (Freeman et al., 2004; Garety et al., 1991, 2005). Most of the studies have indicated that reasoning biases (i.e., belief inflexibility, jumping to conclusion biases, and extreme responding) are prevalent in schizophrenia and related disorders (Colbert & Peters, 2002; Freeman et al., 2004; Phillips & Edwards, 1966). Further, jumping to conclusion biases seem to play an important role in the development of delusions and are strongly associated with higher levels of conviction in paranoid thoughts or among delusion-prone individuals (Freeman et al., 2004; Garety et al., 1991, 2005; Warman et al., 2007). Overall, clinical studies have indicated that inductive reasoning biases are related to the following psychotic symptoms: delusional conviction (Dudley, Young, John, & Over, 1998; Fraser et al., 2006; Garety et al., 2005; Warman et al., 2007), paranoid thoughts (Freeman et al., 2008), and perceptual anomalies (Freeman et al., 2008; Warman et al., 2007). Apart from these clinical studies, the Beads Task has been used in nonclinical sample such as university students (who are prone to delusions), which indicated that jumping to conclusion phenomena is also present in nonclinical sample (Keefe & Warman, 2011).

Clinical relevance

Here, we argue that understanding inductive reasoning biases in schizophrenia will help in their treatment. For instance, Garety et al. (2011) developed a novel clinical treatment method called "reasoning training" based on jumping to conclusion biases in schizophrenia patients. Accordingly, its aims to correct these biases, by training patients to gather more information before making a decision. It is argued that such training will reduce positive symptoms in schizophrenia and such type of training is more beneficial than cognitive behavioral therapy (as compared to Brakoulias et al., 2008), as the latter did not effectively reduce delusions in some schizophrenia patients (for discussion also see Ross, Freeman, Dunn, & Garety, 2011). In another study, schizophrenia patients performed a computerized interactive training to treat jumping to conclusions biases (Waller et al., 2011). They found that a one-time training (approximately 90 min) ameliorated jumping to conclusions biases in the patients for at least up to 1 month. Further, Garety et al. (2017) suggested the use of a novel therapy that targets slow and fast modes of reasoning (known as SlowMo). It involves 8 sessions focusing on training to monitor thoughts and slow down jumping to conclusions and can ameliorate positive symptoms in schizophrenia patients.

Future directions

Based on the review of the previous studies administering reasoning tasks in schizophrenia and related disorders, there can be various avenues for future studies. For example, future studies should focus on developing techniques that aim to treat or remediate the reasoning deficits in schizophrenia and related disorders. While there have been some attempts to developing reasoning-based treatments as discussed earlier, it remains to be shown whether ameliorating reasoning deficits may help reduce delusions in schizophrenia patients. To our knowledge, only one study has investigated the relationship between inductive reasoning biases in the beads task and learning and reported that the jumping to conclusion biases are related to impaired learning from positive feedback (Averbeck et al., 2011). However, future studies should also investigate whether reasoning abilities are related impaired learning from negative feedback. If corrective feedback is related to schizophrenia patients' performance in reasoning tasks, this then suggests that reasoning deficits can be ameliorated by training.

One limitation of most prior studies is they assume reasoning deficits in schizophrenia are related to positive symptoms in the patients. However, most of these studies did not focus on any role played by negative symptoms and cognitive impairments. For instance, several studies have reported cognitive impairment in schizophrenia including attention (Bergman, O'Brien, Osgood, & Cornblatt, 1995; Moustafa et al., 2016; Sapir, Dobrusin, Ben-Bashat, & Henik, 2007), IQ (Kappelmann et al., 2019; van Os, Marsman, van Dam, & Simons, 2017), and working memory (Anticevic, Repovs, & Barch, 2013; Frydecka et al., 2014; Moustafa et al., 2016). These processes are also known to influence reasoning abilities (Howe, Rabinowitz, & Powell, 1998; Ren, Schweizer, & Xu, 2013). Accordingly, it is possible that reasoning deficits in schizophrenia could be related more to cognitive impairments rather than positive symptoms. Future research should address these symptoms.

References

Abi-Dargham, A., Mawlawi, O., Lombardo, I., Gil, R., Martinez, D., Huang, Y., ... Laruelle, M. (2002). Prefrontal dopamine D1 receptors and working memory in schizophrenia. *The Journal of Neuroscience*, *22*(9), 3708–3719. https://doi.org/10.1523/jneurosci.22-09-03708.2002.

American Psychiatric Association. (2013). *Diagnostic and statistical manual of mental disorders* (5th ed.). American Psychiatric Publishing. https://doi.org/10.1176/appi.books.9780890425596.

Anticevic, A., Repovs, G., & Barch, D. M. (2013). Working memory encoding and maintenance deficits in schizophrenia: Neural evidence for activation and deactivation abnormalities. *Schizophrenia Bulletin*, *39*(1), 168–178. https://doi.org/10.1093/schbul/sbr107.

Averbeck, B. B., Evans, S., Chouhan, V., Bristow, E., & Shergill, S. S. (2011). Probabilistic learning and inference in schizophrenia. *Schizophrenia Research*, *127*(1–3), 115–122. https://doi.org/10.1016/j.schres.2010.08.009.

Balzan, R. P., Delfabbro, P. H., Galletly, C. A., & Woodward, T. S. (2012). Over-adjustment or miscomprehension? A re-examination of the jumping to conclusions bias. *The Australian and New Zealand Journal of Psychiatry*, *46*(6), 532–540. https://doi.org/10.1177/0004867411435291.

Bergman, A., O'Brien, J., Osgood, G., & Cornblatt, B. (1995). Distractibility in schizophrenia. *Psychiatry Research*, *57*(2), 131–140. https://doi.org/10.1016/0165-1781(95)02590-s.

Brakoulias, V., Langdon, R., Sloss, G., Coltheart, M., Meares, R., & Harris, A. (2008). Delusions and reasoning: A study involving cognitive behavioural therapy. *Cognitive Neuropsychiatry*, *13*(2), 148–165. https://doi.org/10.1080/13546800801900587.

Colbert, S. M., & Peters, E. R. (2002). Need for closure and jumping-to-conclusions in delusion-prone individuals. *The Journal of Nervous and Mental Disease*, *190*(1), 27–31. https://doi.org/10.1097/00005053-200201000-00007.

Corcoran, R. (2000). Theory of mind in other clinical conditions: Is a selective 'theory of mind'deficit exclusive to autism? In S. Baron-Cohen, H. Tager-Flusberg, & D. Cohen (Eds.), *Understanding other minds: Perspectives from developmental cognitive neuroscience* (pp. 391–421). Oxford University Press.

Corcoran, R. (2003). Inductive reasoning and the understanding of intention in schizophrenia. *Cognitive Neuropsychiatry*, *8*(3), 223–235. https://doi.org/10.1080/13546800244000319.

Corcoran, R., & Frith, C. D. (2005). Thematic reasoning and theory of mind. Accounting for social inference difficulties in schizophrenia. *Evolutionary Psychology*, *3*(1), 1–19. https://doi.org/10.1177/147470490500300101.

Dudley, R. E., John, C. H., Young, A. W., & Over, D. E. (1997a). The effect of self-referent material on the reasoning of people with delusions. *The British Journal of Clinical Psychology*, *36*(4), 575–584. https://doi.org/10.1111/j.2044-8260.1997.tb01262.x.

Dudley, R. E., John, C. H., Young, A. W., & Over, D. E. (1997b). Normal and abnormal reasoning in people with delusions. *The British Journal of Clinical Psychology*, *36*(2), 243–258. https://doi.org/10.1111/j.2044-8260.1997.tb01410.x.

Dudley, R. E. J., & Over, D. E. (2003). People with delusions jump to conclusions: A theoretical account of research findings on the reasoning of people with delusions. *Clinical Psychology & Psychotherapy*, *10*(5), 263–274. https://doi.org/10.1002/cpp.376.

Dudley, R. E. J., Young, A. W., John, C. H., & Over, D. E. (1998). Conditional reasoning in people with delusions: Performance on the Wason selection task. *Cognitive Neuropsychiatry*, *3*(4), 241–258. https://doi.org/10.1080/135468098396071.

Esslinger, C., Braun, U., Schirmbeck, F., Santos, A., Meyer-Lindenberg, A., Zink, M., & Kirsch, P. (2013). Activation of midbrain and ventral striatal regions implicates salience processing during a modified beads task. *PLoS One*, *8*(3). https://doi.org/10.1371/journal.pone.0058536, e58536.

Evans, S. L., Averbeck, B. B., & Furl, N. (2015). Jumping to conclusions in schizophrenia. *Neuropsychiatric Disease and Treatment*, *11*, 1615–1624. https://doi.org/10.2147/ndt.S56870.

Fine, C., Gardner, M., Craigie, J., & Gold, I. (2007). Hopping, skipping or jumping to conclusions? Clarifying the role of the JTC bias in delusions. *Cognitive Neuropsychiatry*, *12*(1), 46–77. https://doi.org/10.1080/13546800600750597.

Fraser, J., Morrison, A., & Wells, A. (2006). Cognitive processes, reasoning biases and persecutory delusions: A comparative study. *Behavioural and Cognitive Psychotherapy*, *34*(4), 421–435. https://doi.org/10.1017/S1352465806002852.

Freeman, D., Garety, P. A., Fowler, D., Kuipers, E., Bebbington, P. E., & Dunn, G. (2004). Why do people with delusions fail to choose more realistic explanations for their experiences? An empirical investigation. *Journal of Consulting and Clinical Psychology*, *72*(4), 671–680. https://doi.org/10.1037/0022-006x.72.4.671.

Freeman, D., Pugh, K., & Garety, P. (2008). Jumping to conclusions and paranoid ideation in the general population. *Schizophrenia Research*, *102*(1–3), 254–260. https://doi.org/10.1016/j.schres.2008.03.020.

Frydecka, D., Eissa, A. M., Hewedi, D. H., Ali, M., Drapała, J., Misiak, B., … Moustafa, A. A. (2014). Impairments of working memory in schizophrenia and bipolar disorder: The effect of history of psychotic symptoms and different aspects of cognitive task demands. *Frontiers in Behavioral Neuroscience*, *8*. https://doi.org/10.3389/fnbeh.2014.00416, 416.

Garety, P. A., & Freeman, D. (1999). Cognitive approaches to delusions: A critical review of theories and evidence. *The British Journal of Clinical Psychology*, *38*(2), 113–154. https://doi.org/10.1348/014466599162700.

Garety, P. A., & Freeman, D. (2013). The past and future of delusions research: From the inexplicable to the treatable. *The British Journal of Psychiatry*, *203*(5), 327–333. https://doi.org/10.1192/bjp.bp.113.126953.

Garety, P. A., Freeman, D., Jolley, S., Dunn, G., Bebbington, P. E., Fowler, D. G., … Dudley, R. (2005). Reasoning, emotions, and delusional conviction in psychosis. *Journal of Abnormal Psychology*, *114*(3), 373–384. https://doi.org/10.1037/0021-843x.114.3.373.

Garety, P., Freeman, D., Jolley, S., Ross, K., Waller, H., & Dunn, G. (2011). Jumping to conclusions: The psychology of delusional reasoning. *Advances in Psychiatric Treatment*, *17*(5), 332–339. https://doi.org/10.1192/apt.bp.109.007104.

Garety, P. A., Hemsley, D. R., & Wessely, S. (1991). Reasoning in deluded schizophrenic and paranoid patients. Biases in performance on a probabilistic inference task. *The Journal of Nervous and Mental Disease*, *179*(4), 194–201. https://doi.org/10.1097/00005053-199104000-00003.

Garety, P. A., Ward, T., Freeman, D., Fowler, D., Emsley, R., Dunn, G., … Hardy, A. (2017). SlowMo, a digital therapy targeting reasoning in paranoia, versus treatment as usual in the treatment of people who fear harm from others: Study protocol for a randomised controlled trial. *Trials*, *18*(1), 510. https://doi.org/10.1186/s13063-017-2242-7.

Hayes, B. K., & Heit, E. (2018). Inductive reasoning 2.0. *WIREs Cognitive Science*, *9*(3), e1459. https://doi.org/10.1002/wcs.1459.

Howe, M. L., Rabinowitz, F. M., & Powell, T. L. (1998). Individual differences in working memory and reasoning-remembering relationships in solving class-inclusion problems. *Memory & Cognition*, *26*(5), 1089–1101. https://doi.org/10.3758/bf03201185.

Huq, S. F., Garety, P. A., & Hemsley, D. R. (1988). Probabilistic judgements in deluded and non-deluded subjects. *The Quarterly Journal of Experimental Psychology*, *40*(4), 801–812. https://doi.org/10.1080/14640748808402300.

Kappelmann, N., Khandaker, G. M., Dal, H., Stochl, J., Kosidou, K., Jones, P. B., … Karlsson, H. (2019). Systemic inflammation and intelligence in early adulthood and subsequent risk of schizophrenia and other non-affective psychoses: A longitudinal cohort and co-relative study. *Psychological Medicine*, *49*(2), 295–302. https://doi.org/10.1017/s0033291718000831.

Keefe, K. M., & Warman, D. M. (2011). Reasoning, delusion proneness and stress: An experimental investigation. *Clinical Psychology & Psychotherapy*, *18*(2), 138–147. https://doi.org/10.1002/cpp.683.

Langdon, R., Ward, P. B., & Coltheart, M. (2010). Reasoning anomalies associated with delusions in schizophrenia. *Schizophrenia Bulletin*, *36*(2), 321–330. https://doi.org/10.1093/schbul/sbn069.

Lunt, L., Bramham, J., Morris, R. G., Bullock, P. R., Selway, R. P., Xenitidis, K., & David, A. S. (2012). Prefrontal cortex dysfunction and 'Jumping to Conclusions': Bias or deficit? *Journal of Neuropsychology*, *6*(1), 65–78. https://doi.org/10.1111/j.1748-6653.2011.02005.x.

Menon, M., Pomarol-Clotet, E., McKenna, P. J., & McCarthy, R. A. (2006). Probabilistic reasoning in schizophrenia: A comparison of the performance of deluded and nondeluded schizophrenic patients and exploration of possible cognitive underpinnings. *Cognitive Neuropsychiatry*, *11*(6), 521–536. https://doi.org/10.1080/13546800544000046.

Moustafa, A. A., Garami, J. K., Mahlberg, J., Golembieski, J., Keri, S., Misiak, B., & Frydecka, D. (2016). Cognitive function in schizophrenia: Conflicting findings and future directions. *Reviews in the Neurosciences*, *27*(4), 435–448. https://doi.org/10.1515/revneuro-2015-0060.

Moustafa, A. A., & Gluck, M. A. (2011). Computational cognitive models of prefrontal-striatal-hippocampal interactions in Parkinson's disease and schizophrenia. *Neural Networks*, *24*(6), 575–591. https://doi.org/10.1016/j.neunet.2011.02.006.

Moustafa, A. A., Keri, S., Herzallah, M. M., Myers, C. E., & Gluck, M. A. (2010). A neural model of hippocampal-striatal interactions in associative learning and transfer generalization in various neurological and psychiatric patients. *Brain and Cognition*, *74*(2), 132–144. https://doi.org/10.1016/j.bandc.2010.07.013.

Moustafa, A. A., Misiak, B., & Frydecka, D. (2017). Computational models of schizophrenia. In A. A. Moustafa (Ed.), *Computational models of brain and behavior* Wiley-Blackwell.

Northrop, L. C. (1977). *The definition and measurement of verbal comprehension.* U.S. Civil Service Commission.

Peters, E. R., Thornton, P., Siksou, L., Linney, Y., & MacCabe, J. H. (2008). Specificity of the jump-to-conclusions bias in deluded patients. *The British Journal of Clinical Psychology, 47*(Pt 2), 239–244. https://doi.org/10.1348/014466507x255294.

Phillips, L. D., & Edwards, W. (1966). Conservatism in a simple probability inference task. *Journal of Experimental Psychology, 72*(3), 346–354. https://doi.org/10.1037/h0023653.

Rausch, F., Mier, D., Eifler, S., Fenske, S., Schirmbeck, F., Englisch, S., … Zink, M. (2015). Reduced activation in the ventral striatum during probabilistic decision-making in patients in an at-risk mental state. *Journal of Psychiatry & Neuroscience, 40*(3), 163–173. https://doi.org/10.1503/jpn.140191.

Ren, X., Schweizer, K., & Xu, F. (2013). The sources of the relationship between sustained attention and reasoning. *Intelligence, 41*, 51–58. https://doi.org/10.1016/j.intell.2012.10.006.

Ross, K., Freeman, D., Dunn, G., & Garety, P. (2011). A randomized experimental investigation of reasoning training for people with delusions. *Schizophrenia Bulletin, 37*(2), 324–333. https://doi.org/10.1093/schbul/sbn165.

Ross, R. M., McKay, R., Coltheart, M., & Langdon, R. (2015). Jumping to conclusions about the beads task? A meta-analysis of delusional ideation and data-gathering. *Schizophrenia Bulletin, 41*(5), 1183–1191. https://doi.org/10.1093/schbul/sbu187.

Sapir, A., Dobrusin, M., Ben-Bashat, G., & Henik, A. (2007). Neuroleptics reverse attentional effects in schizophrenia patients. *Neuropsychologia, 45*(14), 3263–3271. https://doi.org/10.1016/j.neuropsychologia.2007.06.007.

So, S. H., Garety, P. A., Peters, E. R., & Kapur, S. (2010). Do antipsychotics improve reasoning biases? A review. *Psychosomatic Medicine, 72*(7), 681–693. https://doi.org/10.1097/PSY.0b013e3181e7cca6.

Stuke, H., Stuke, H., Weilnhammer, V. A., & Schmack, K. (2017). Psychotic experiences and overhasty inferences are related to maladaptive learning. *PLoS Computational Biology, 13*(1), e1005328. https://doi.org/10.1371/journal.pcbi.1005328.

Toulmin, S. E. (1984). *Introduction to reasoning* (2nd ed.). Pearson.

van Os, J., Marsman, A., van Dam, D., & Simons, C. J. (2017). Evidence that the impact of childhood trauma on IQ is substantial in controls, moderate in siblings, and absent in patients with psychotic disorder. *Schizophrenia Bulletin, 43*(2), 316–324. https://doi.org/10.1093/schbul/sbw177.

Waller, H., Freeman, D., Jolley, S., Dunn, G., & Garety, P. (2011). Targeting reasoning biases in delusions: A pilot study of the Maudsley review training programme for individuals with persistent, high conviction delusions. *Journal of Behavior Therapy and Experimental Psychiatry, 42*(3), 414–421. https://doi.org/10.1016/j.jbtep.2011.03.001.

Warman, D. M., Lysaker, P. H., Martin, J. M., Davis, L., & Haudenschield, S. L. (2007). Jumping to conclusions and the continuum of delusional beliefs. *Behaviour Research and Therapy, 45*(6), 1255–1269. https://doi.org/10.1016/j.brat.2006.09.002.

Part Two

Recent topics in schizophrenia and related disorders

Religious delusions in psychotic patients: Prevalence, possible origin, and effects

5

Mahmoud H.I. El-Essawy[a], Alaa M.A. Soliman[a], Alejandro Morris[b], Victor Counted[b], Abeer M. Eissa[a], Ahmad Valikhani[c], and Ahmed A. Moustafa[b,d]
[a]Faculty of Medicine, Ain Shams University, Cairo, Egypt, [b]School of Psychology & Marcs Institute for Brain and Behaviour, Western Sydney University, Sydney, NSW, Australia, [c]Department of Clinical Psychology, School of Education and Psychology, Shiraz University, Shiraz, Iran, [d]Department of Human Anatomy and Physiology, the Faculty of Health Sciences, University of Johannesburg, South Africa

Chapter outline

Introduction

Religious delusions

Delusions are present in many severe neuropsychiatric disorders as they are experienced by over 70% of individuals who suffer psychotic episodes (McLean, Mattiske, & Balzan, 2017). Delusions are a fundamental feature of insanity, as stated by Lord Erskine (West & Walk, 1977) because they hard to change even when the patient is presented with

Cognitive and Behavioral Dysfunction in Schizophrenia. https://doi.org/10.1016/B978-0-12-820005-6.00001-3

evidence contrary to their beliefs. It is agreed upon that delusions have a significant effect on an individual's behavior and emotions, as seen in patients with schizophrenia (Paolini, Moretti, & Compton, 2016). Delusions are a core component of the diagnostic criteria used by psychiatrists to assess patients who have lost touch with reality (Maher, 1988). Nevertheless, as Spitzer notes, their nature is poorly understood, their etiology is unknown, and their nosological status remains problematic (Spitzer, 1990).

Recent conceptualizations of delusions characterize them as negative epistemic features, namely beliefs that are unwarranted, fixed, resistant to counterargument, and implausible (Lancellotta & Bortolotti, 2019). This view is supported by the Statistical Manual of Mental Disorders (American Psychiatric Association, 2013), which states that a delusion is a false belief based on an incorrect inference about an external reality that is firmly held despite evidence to the contrary. The APA description incorporates issues identified by Coltheart, Menzies, and Sutton (2010), namely that delusions are not described as false, but rather as "fixed beliefs that are not amenable to change in light of conflicting evidence".

Only recently have religious constructs in psychiatry started to be investigated using experimental studies in spite of religion being a subject of interest in psychiatry and psychosis for over 200 years (Bhavsar & Bhugra, 2008; Duñó, Oliva, Tobeña, Palao, & Labad, 2020; Mohr & Pfeifer, 2009). Atallah, El-Dosoky, Coker, Nabil, and El-Islam (2001) defined a religious delusion as any symptom containing religious references, such as holding special knowledge or power from God, being cursed by black magic, controlled by an evil spirit, identified or related with religious figures, and being punished by God, among others. Religious delusions are often classified as bizarre and are associated with higher levels of positive psychotic symptomology (Noort, Beekman, van Gool, & Braam, 2018).

Religious delusions exert a pervasive influence on patients' thoughts, affect, and behavior, and tend to co-occur with other delusions (Noort et al., 2018). They can be persecutory (often involving Satan), grandiose (messianic) or related to worries of condemnation (Clark & Harrison, 2012). Individuals who present such delusions tend to have higher rates of aggression and homicide (Waugh, 1986), as well as overall psychopathology. In addition, they exhibit a longer history of psychotic illness and worse global functioning (Raja, Azzoni, & Lubich, 2000). The misinterpretation of hallucinations as mystical experiences may reinforce their delusional system and cause an obstacle to recovery (Hanevik et al., 2017). In addition, individuals who suffer a psychotic disorder and experience religious delusions are more likely to interpret first rank symptoms as being common, and normal experiences (Lazarescu, Hurmuz, Draghici, & Blajovan, 2015), and therefore it is expected that they will not seek treatment, which could pose a problem for their long-term prognosis.

Religious delusions are held with greater conviction than other types of delusions (Appelbaum, Robbins, & Roth, 1999). Reaction to hypothetical contradiction is a measure of the severity of a delusion (Brett-Jones, Garety, & Hemsley, 1987). It can be used to evaluate the patient's responsiveness to evidence, contrary to the delusional idea, and can be used as a predictor of change. Low scores on this measure are indicative of a dismissal of relevant evidence, a factor likely to contribute to delusion maintenance.

In the current study, "religious delusions" are defined as all delusional symptoms with religious content. These can include altered religious behavior such as increased praying or reading of religious books, increased religiosity, increased reading of religious texts, altered practices/beliefs, insulting/cursing (God, religion, Church), joining religious groups, renouncing faith, growing hair, fasting, spending all one's time in the church or mosque, to delusional themes of a religious nature (e.g., believing oneself to be or be in relationship with a religious figure), on a religious mission (from God or Prophet) to save the world, special knowledge or power from God and so on as well as supernatural beliefs such as cursed by black magic (A'mal in Arabic), controlled by an evil spirit, possessed by an evil spirit (demon possession), punished by God, and/or is a sinner, persecution because of religion, or the evil eye were included (Atallah et al., 2001).

Attribution biases, religious delusions, and cognitive continuity

Attribution theory offers a potential mechanism for the movement along this continuum towards religious delusions (So, Tang, & Leung, 2015). It might begin as an adaptive religious belief whereby you attribute events to the figure of God as a means of belonging and self-actualization (McKay & Ross, 2020). However, as a result of suffering a mental illness such as schizophrenia, the religious thoughts become maladaptive and prejudicial for an individual's functioning in their social and work life. This is the point at which the severity of the delusions will be contingent on whether or not belief conviction strengthens community ties. If religiosity strengthens the individual's community ties, it will be harder to detect religious delusions within the context of a psychotic spectrum disorder (McCauley & Graham, 2020). Having a religious belief or having a religious delusional belief provides a framework by which people can make sense of negative life experiences. This is said to be helpful to people as it allows them something of a buffer against the depressing effects of uncontrollable life stresses (Park, Cohen, & Herb, 1990).

Recently, McCauley and Graham (2020) provided a scheme of three cognitive continuities that explains the interaction between religious cognition, normal cognition, and cognitions associated with mental disorders. Interestingly, it aims to explain the process by which normal and religious cognitions can become maladaptive cognitions in psychotic-spectrum disorders. It is suggested that glossolalia and tangled speech associated with mental disorders such as schizophrenia share similarities, and therefore future research should investigate the factors that facilitate the salient continuity between both forms of speech.

On the other hand, religious delusions have routinely been linked to poorer prognosis for people with psychotic disorders (Mohr et al., 2010). Mohr et al. suggested delusions with religious content may lead to a poorer therapeutic alliance. Deluded patients with religious content in their study had been hospitalized for a shorter time than other deluded patients and were more likely to experience a conflict between their religion and psychiatric treatment. The latter issue could be related to the fact that some patients may find hallucinations or delusions to be agreeable, in their function as coping mechanisms that help avoid the painful experience of reality (Jenner, Rutten, Beuckens, Boonstra, & Sytema, 2008). Beyond cognitive elements preventing insight, this could be the main factor explaining their reluctance to seek medical care. Thus, it is harder for clinicians to treat patients when their delusions have a religious content. In addition, when religious coping is taken into account, these patients are less likely to benefit from the support of their religious communities, and their religion is more often a burden than a support. This situation is likely to be challenging for both clinicians and religious clergy (Mohr et al., 2010). Many studies have confirmed that delusions with a religious content have been associated with a poorer prognosis and higher levels of psychosis (Appelbaum et al., 1999; Gawad et al., 2018; Siddle, Haddock, Tarrier, & Faragher, 2002; Thara & Eaton, 1996). Levels of disability, distress, and conviction have all been reported to be higher in people with religious delusions compared to other types of delusions (Appelbaum et al., 1999; Bhavsar & Bhugra, 2008; Cannon & Kramer, 2012; Huguelet et al., 2007; Mohr et al., 2011; Siddle et al., 2002). In a study, a total of 25,542 adult respondents across 18 countries from the WHO World Mental Health Surveys showed that there was a significant association between increased religiosity and reporting more types of psychotic experiences (Kovess-Masfety et al., 2018). On the other hand, the presence of religious delusions may influence the help-seeking pathways chosen through religious avenues.

Religious delusions are also associated with poor engagement, low satisfaction with services and with treatment, and longer duration of untreated psychosis (Gearing et al., 2011; Huang, Shang, Shieh, Lin, & Su, 2011; Mohr et al., 2010; Mohr & Huguelet, 2004; Moss, Fleck, & Strakowski, 2006). People with religious delusions appear, therefore, to be a particularly problematic group to treat effectively, and ought to be targeted for psychological therapies (Mohr et al., 2009; NICE, 2009). However, as the mechanisms underlying the treatment resistance are poorly understood, further study is required to establish what the particular foci of psychological intervention for people with religious delusions should be, and what issues are likely to arise in implementation.

Prevalence across cultures

Despite religious delusions being present in most major cultures, their prevalence varies greatly between countries and sociocultural contexts. In Western clinical settings, 47% of individuals with psychotic depression and 32% in patients with schizophrenia have reported suffering religious delusions (Noort et al., 2018). Other findings estimate between 25 and 39% of patients with schizophrenia and between 15% and 22% of those with bipolar disorder have religious delusions (Koenig, 2009). The range in prevalence seen in the literature might be due to intercultural differences as well as sociodemographic variables such as personal religiosity (Anderson-Schmidt et al., 2019).

There is high prevalence in the USA, specifically 25% (Appelbaum et al., 1999), with 21% in Austrian samples and lower in Pakistan with 4.6% (Saavedra, 2014). In one study with 270 schizophrenia individuals, 44% of Malay patients compared to 5% of Chinese patients reported having religious delusions (Azhar, Varma, & Hakim, 1995). Meanwhile, a South-African study found 42 out of 73 (70%) Xhosa individuals with schizophrenia reported having religious delusions (Connell et al., 2015). Wilson (1998) also reported religious delusions being culturally driven: a manifestation of psychotic illness rather than a cause of it. Longitudinal studies of large-scale changes in the content and/or structure of psychiatric symptoms are relatively rare. One study (Mitchell & Vierkant, 1989) looked at how delusional themes changed across time, according to the sub-cultural milieu. The delusional content of American patients in the 1930s reflected the material deprivation and personal powerlessness of that time, while in the 1980s, they reflected a more threatening and negative milieu, with visions of blood, snakes, and dead people.

Gender and social class may affect the rate of religious delusions as these are more prevalent in men compared to women and are found more in higher social classes compared with lower classes (Suhail, 2003). Moreover, a study conducted in Germany with a cohort of schizophrenia and schizoaffective individuals found that gender, age, school education, and marital status was significantly associated with religious delusions (Anderson-Schmidt et al., 2017). The prevalence of religious delusions varies widely not only within culture, gender, and social class, but also over time. For example, in Egypt, the rate of religious delusions rose from 5% to 21% during a 22-year period when patterns of religious emphasis in Egyptian society have changed (Atallah et al., 2001). Aside from cultural and political affiliation, the content of delusions is found the be highly influenced by religious background. Studies show that the risk of experiencing religious delusions among patients with schizophrenia or schizoaffective disorder is significantly higher in subjects with a strong religious activity compared to individuals without a religious denomination (Anderson-Schmidt et al., 2017).

Japanese individuals' delusional content was found to change over a 20-year period (1941–1961) (Asai, 1964). There was a decrease in emphasis on traditional figures such as the Emperor, and shift towards the radio, television, and the United States (Asai, 1964). Other studies found that current sociopolitical events and media influenced the presentation and phenomenology of psychiatric disorders (Axer, Corrigan, & Liberman, 1992; Bhugra & Gupta, 1996; Bohlken & Priebe, 1990; Grover, Davuluri, & Chakrabarti, 2014; Kim et al., 1993; Sher, 1997; Mishra, Das, & Goyal, 2018; Yorston, 1997). Kim et al. (1993) found that religious delusional themes were among those most sensitive to changes in the social/political climate. Societal and individual support of, or opposition to, religion was found to positively correlate with the overall frequency of religious delusions or symptoms within the population (Ahmed, 1978; Iyassu et al., 2014; Levenson, 1973; Lowe, 1954; Maslowski, 1988; Siddle et al., 2002. Klaf and Hamilton (1961) found that in the West, the prevalence of religious symptomatology during the 20th century dropped to approximately one-third of its level in the 19th century. This was assumed to be a function of the declining emphasis on religion and religious affiliation in Western culture.

In Egypt and the rest of the Arab world, religion and religious beliefs do not only hold an important place in the society at large, but traditionally provide the basis for explanations of emotional distress and dysfunctional behavior in general (El-Islam, 1978). On one hand, delusions and/or illness interpretations involving possession by "jinn" and other spirits derive from traditional beliefs in the devil and other supernatural agents (El-Islam, 1982). On the other hand, most emotional illnesses and distress are attributed to factors such as a "lack of faith" or improper religious practice. While more affluent and educated sectors of the Egyptian population may not necessarily adhere to traditional beliefs involving spirit possession or black magic, religion (particularly Islam) exerts a strong cultural influence and provides many of the symbols used to express emotional and social distress.

Symptoms involving "supernatural" themes have included over time delusions or hallucinations involving the "jinn", "black magic", and "spirit possession". These themes share a common "paranoid" ideation, and their suggestion of a negative outside influence on the body of the person. These themes are very common in Egyptian religious ideology and are often invoked as nonpathological explanations for misfortune or disease.

Since religious delusional explanations should be anticipated in any culture where religion is present, one might also expect that cultures high in religiosity will produce higher rates of religious delusions. This is in fact what has been established, with figures regarding the prevalence of religious delusions in schizophrenia varying from 7% in Japanese patients, 21% in Germans (Tateyama et al., 1993), and 80% in Afro-Caribbean populations (Kiev, 1963). Moreover, a South African Xhosa sample of schizophrenia individuals was tested on the content of their delusions. The majority (72.5%) reported that the cause of their mental illness was being bewitched by an outsider (Campbell et al., 2017). Similarly, a Zimbabwean sample of schizophrenia individuals believed their illness had been caused by spirits or witchcraft, which in turn influenced their symptomology explanation and help-seeking behavior (Chidarikire, Cross, Skinner, & Cleary, 2020). Such studies highlight the important role culture can play in the content of delusions.

There have been a number of well-publicized cases, in which patients exhibiting religious delusions have acted upon them with fatal consequences. Aside from the rare occurrence of these homicides, religious delusions are of clinical significance for two reasons. First, religiously deluded people have taken religious texts literally and attacked other people (Blackner & Wong, 1963; Field & Waldfogel, 1995; Kushner, 1967; Waugh, 1986). Second, religious delusions have been associated with poorer treatment outcomes (Doering et al., 1998; McCabe, Fowler, & Cadoret, 1972; Thara & Eaton, 1996). The reasons for such outcomes are unclear and the publications referenced rarely specify a proposed mechanism of action. Few scientific investigations have focused on religious delusions in schizophrenia populations (Cook, 2015; Gearing et al., 2011).

The content of delusions has been shown to vary between populations and over time (Al-Issa, 1995; Cook, 2015; Kent & Wahass, 1996; Ndetei & Vadher, 1984, 1985). Religious delusions were more prevalent in the past than currently. Nevertheless, even in a largely secular society, there are schizophrenia individuals who report having religious content in their delusions. Delusional ideas being on a continuum with normal beliefs (Harrow, Rattenbury, & Stoll, 1988) is supported by a number of sources, with researchers concluding that normal religious beliefs are held in many cases as overvalued ideas, somewhere between delusions and "normal beliefs" (Jackson, 1991; Jones & Watson, 1997; Peters, Day, McKenna, & Orbach, 1999; Strauss, 1991). It seems likely that many religiously deluded patients will have shifted along the continuum from the "normal" but overvalued religious ideas eventually to religious delusions.

Religion and psychiatry

Religion is a means by which we understand the world and assign meaning to our lives (Tseng, 2001). There are numerous religions even within the same society that directly or indirectly shape our lives and influence our thoughts and behavior.

In psychiatric patients, religiosity may impact psychopathology and treatment of the patient (Bartocci, 2006a, 2006b). It is therefore essential for clinicians to understand the nature of religion and distinguish it from religious delusions bearing in mind the socio-political context of the patient. The term spirituality in health care has expanded above and beyond its original meaning.

Spirituality and religiosity (or religion, religious, religiousness) are terms that have been used somewhat interchangeably. While some people see these terms as polar opposites, others view them as having overlapping dimensions. Hill et al. (2000) proposed a definitional criterion suggesting that religiosity ought to include "the subjective feelings, thoughts, and behaviors that arise from a search for the sacred" (p. 68). From his perspective, spirituality is a "central and essential function" of religiosity (Hill & Hood, 1999). Similarly, Zinnbauer et al. (1997) argue "religion in its broadband sense includes the personal and the institutional, the traditional and the progressive, the helpful and the harmful". It is this broadband sense of the term "religiosity" that will be used in the context of this study (Zinnbauer et al., 1997).

Until not long ago, religion and mental health care were closely aligned. Many of the first mental hospitals were located in monasteries and run by priests. The first form of psychiatric care in the United States was moral treatment, which involved the compassionate and humane treatment of people with mental illness—a revolutionary notion at a time when patients were often displayed and (or) housed in despicable conditions in the back wards of hospitals or prisons (Koenig, McCullough, & Larson, 2001).

Previous studies have demonstrated the connection between cultural variables, the social environment, and delusional and behavioral manifestations of psychiatric illness (Azhar et al., 1995; Bose, 1997; Draguns, 1995; Duñó et al., 2020; El-Fatatry, El-Kashlan, El-Garem, & Ghazi, 1980; Saavedra, 2014; Scott, 1967). The manifestations of illness experiences, whether they are ultimately considered "delusions," "flat affect" or any other of a number of "universal symptoms," are difficult, if not impossible, to interpret outside of the cultural and experiential context in which they occur.

Religion and religious beliefs (as well as spirituality) are increasingly recognized as important in the understanding of psychiatric disorders and in the clinical assessment and treatment of patients (Böhmer, 2016). Religious beliefs are associated with enhance well-being and a higher sense of empowerment which can give patients meaning to their illness (Pargament & Lomax, 2013). Therefore, faith can help better comprehend mental health, and can enrich psychiatry overall (Huguelet, Brandt, & Mohr, 2016; Huguelet, Brandt, & Mohr, 2016). In spite of religions being associated with emotional comfort, attachment, or self-regulation, theorists have also started to study the problematic aspects of religiousness, namely religious-based violence with oneself and with others (Pargament & Lomax, 2013). No single explanation will offer a complete understanding of a complex process such as religious violence within the context of psychosis-spectrum disorders. Nevertheless, it has been suggested that threats to ideals or ideologies can trigger command hallucinations and those "dangerous" commands increase the likelihood that an individual will engage in violent behavior (Patel, Barot, Vankar, & Pal, 2019). Chronic mental illnesses have been commonly perceived to be associated with higher risk of harmful behavior

(Patel et al., 2019), and recent findings indicate that high religiousness could be an added risk factor. In congruence with an increased interest in the role religion can play in psychiatry, neurobiological hypotheses have been postulated. One states the limbic system produces divergent affect and cognitions such as perceptions of overheated importance, self-reference, and noetic feelings (Ventriglio, Bonfitto, Ricci, Cuoco, & Bhavsar, 2018). A second one states dysfunctional mesolimbic activities generate altered perceptions of reality, including a distorted sense of time, autoscopy, and depersonalization (Ventriglio et al., 2018).

Delusional content

Childhood socialization and adverse early life experiences can influence the onset and content of delusions (Catone et al., 2016; Westermeyer, 1988). The conceptualization of delusions is an attempt to provide meaning to internal and external events. For example, there is a positive association between humiliating events (e.g., bullying) and developing persecutory delusions later in life (Catone et al., 2016). Furthermore, the concept of understandability provides a framework under which each delusion can be understandable if the psychopathological analysis is thorough enough (Broome, 2012). A Kuwaiti-based study found that the rates of delusional themes of a traditional nature did not vary with subsequent educational achievement (El-Islam & Malasi, 1985). That is, recently acquired, rational information did not replace cultural influences ingrained during childhood. Therefore, it is likely that exposure to religion and religious ideology at the societal level might find expression at the individual level in terms of themes acquired during early socialization, that is, possession beliefs and black magic.

Another content-specific theme that has varied across time periods is the reference to God. References to God, of course, may overlap with most, if not all of the other symptoms. Furthermore, this was the single most commonly reported theme in our study. This reference increased significantly in frequency right around the time of the initial surge in religious symptoms overall (around the late 1970s early 1980s), then peaked in the mid-1980s and early 1990s, returning to low levels thereafter. With some caution, these findings might be interpreted in the following manner: God is the ultimate symbol of religion and religiosity. In Muslim-majority countries, including Egypt, references to God are ubiquitous and form an integral part of everyday speech. With the increased emphasis on religion in the Egyptian society in the early 1980s, God would naturally have been a potent symbol of expression for this newfound (or "refound") awareness. In later time periods, when religious expression had become more commonplace, references to God might be expected to return to previous levels (as was found here). No other delusional theme or religious symbol showed significant changes in form or content across the time period of the study. This is not surprising in light of what we suggested previously about the effect of societal factors on the content of delusional and hallucinatory themes. Religious delusional themes included things such as "thinks he/she is God," "believes he/she possesses special powers from God," etc. There is no reason to think that any one of these themes would vary relative to the others according to societal factors; rather, we can conclude here that they are culturally common pathological symbols of religious expression that became uniformly more frequent in a more religiously "charged" environment.

When psychotic experiences are encountered, people seek causal explanations for these (Maher, 1988) and will inevitably draw upon their existing knowledge and belief systems. In a recent model of positive symptoms of psychosis (Garety, Kuipers, Fowler, Freeman, & Bebbington, 2001), biased appraisal is said to contribute to a tendency for anomalous experiences to "feel external," resulting in a cognitive style characterized by jumping to conclusions, external attritional bias and deficits in understanding social situations (Garety & Freeman, 1999).

Religious coping appeared to impact outcomes in a positive way, since it was associated with greater insight and compliance. Higher church attendance has been associated with good prognosis in patients with schizophrenia (Schofield, Hathaway, Hastings, & Bell, 1954). Furthermore, schizophrenia patients living in urban areas (as opposed to rural settings) were less likely to be re-hospitalized if their families encourage religious worship during their hospitalization (Chu & Klein, 1985). Overall, a lack of religious affiliation is associated with a greater risk of relapse and re-admission. A study conducted among a largely Hindu sample of 386 Indian outpatients with schizophrenia reported that a decrease in religious activities at baseline resulted in a more rapid deterioration over time (Verghese et al., 1989). Further, culturally acceptable religious beliefs are cited as an important coping strategy for many people with schizophrenia, and may contribute to lower symptom severity in both severe and enduring mental illnesses (Aukst-Margetic & Jakovljevic, 2008; Campion & Bhugra, 1997) and common mental disorders (Braam, Beekman, Deeg, Smit, & Tilburg, 1997; Maselko & Buka, 2008). In addition, religious involvement was found to be among the factors that predicted fewer suicide attempts (along with healthy family relationships and better health) in a Swedish sample of adolescents with psychotic-spectrum disorders (mostly schizophrenia) (Jarbin & Von Knorring, 2004).

Rationale of the study

The current study arose from a desire to establish the prevalence of religious delusions in a representative sample of inpatients suffering psychosis who had been admitted to El-Abbassia Mental Health Hospital (Cairo, Egypt). In addition, we wanted to assess the significance religious delusions play in the lives of these patients. These types of delusions are of clinical interest because they may have an impact upon the individual's health belief model (Kelly, Mamon, & Scott, 1987) and, thus, their adherence to treatment.

The prevalence of religious delusions in psychotic patients living in Egypt is not well documented at this point in time. Past research has suggested a fluctuating pattern within the Egyptian community, with a possible increase in numbers in the last years. The relationship between the emergence of religious delusions in patients and their social class or gender is not clear. There is insufficient data about the impact of religious delusions on the severity of psychotic episodes and their relation to the prognosis of the disorder. The relationship between religious delusions and religiosity is still obscure, and therefore more research is required.

Methods

Stage 1: Descriptive methods

Participants

A random sample of 500 inpatients from El-Abbassyia mental health hospital (Cairo, Egypt) were included in this study. The exclusion criteria were patients with evidence of mental retardation as well as subjects with any physical handicap. Our sample included both acute and chronic individuals. They were all given appropriate information about the study and its rationale. A written informed consent was obtained and socio-demographic data (age, sex, level of education, occupation, marital status) was collected from patients prior to commencing. The diagnosis of the selected patients was confirmed using ICD-10 symptom checklist for mental disorders. The ICD-10 Symptom Checklist for mental disorders (Janca, Ustun, van Drimmelen, Dittmann, & Isaac, 1994) is a semi-structured instrument intended for clinician's assessment of psychiatric symptoms and syndromes in the F0-F6 categories of the International Classification of Diseases, Tenth revision (ICD-10). The difference between routine clinical interview and the checklist-guided interview is that in the later chances for oversights are less and the variabilities that typically contribute to the unreliability of unstructured clinical examinations are minimized.

All patients were assessed for the presence of religious delusions depending on an operational definition from a previous Egyptian study in 2001 as Atallah and colleagues defined religious delusion as any symptom with religious content (Atallah et al., 2001). Further, patients were asked if they have any religious delusions in the past. This stage helped calculate the prevalence of religious delusions. The sample showed the following distribution of diagnosis according to ICD-10: 353 cases were diagnosed as schizophrenia (70.6%), 125 cases were diagnosed as bipolar affective disorder (25%) and 21 cases were diagnosed as schizoaffective (4.2%) and one case was diagnosed as mania with psychotic features (0.2%).

Stage 2: Group differences

A group of 80 patients with religious delusions (experimental group) and another group of 80 patients without religious delusions (control group) from the first stage were included in the second stage of our study. Patients with history of religious delusions (not active at the time of the study) are excluded from control group. As for diagnosis, the cases were composed of 40 individuals (50%) diagnosed as schizophrenia, 29 cases (36.3%) diagnosed as bipolar affective Disorder, 1 case (1.3%) diagnosed as mania with psychotic feature and 10 cases (12.5%) diagnosed as schizoaffective disorder. The Controls were composed of 50 cases (62.5%) diagnosed as schizophrenia, 27 cases (33.8%) diagnosed as bipolar affective disorder, 1 case (1.3%) diagnosed as mania with psychotic feature and 2 cases (2.5%) diagnosed as schizoaffective disorder. The difference between cases and controls regarding diagnosis using Chi square test was statistically insignificant. As for the number of previous episodes, the cases' mean number of previous episodes was 3.93 ± 2.8, while controls' mean number of previous episodes was 3.5 ± 1.8. The difference between cases and controls' number of previous episodes using Chi square test was statistically insignificant.

Both experimental and control groups were assessed for: (a) The social class of the patients using Fahmy and El-Sherbini's Social Classification Scale and Family Socio-Economic Status (SES); (b) The current psychopathology of the illness using Brief Psychiatric Rating Scale (BPRS), (c) The functionality of patients using Global Assessment of Functioning (GAF) Scale; (d) The religiosity of the patients using Religious Orientation Scale; (e) Assessing conviction, perception of others' views of belief, explanation of differing views, fixity of ideas, attempt to disprove ideas and insight of patients using Brown Assessment of Beliefs Scale (BABS); and (f) Violent behavior of the patients regarding physical aggression against objects, self or other people and intervention needed. Verbal aggression was considered mild violent behavior and was not considered further in our analyses.

The scales used in this study:

Fahmy and El-Sherbini's Social Classification Scale (Fahmy & El-Sherbini, 1988): This classification is based on 5 parameters: the father and mother's education, income, crowding index and sanitation. The aggregate score based on the five parameters can range between four classes: a score of 25–30 is considered high social class 1, a score of 20–25 is considered middle social class 2, a score of 15–20 is considered low social class 3, and a score of 14 or lower is considered very low social class 4.

Family Socio-Economic Status (SES): This scale includes 7 domains. Socioeconomic level is classified as very low, low, middle, and high levels depending on the quartiles of the score calculated.

Brief Psychiatric Rating Scale (BPRS-4): The BPRS has been originally developed by Overall and Gorham (1962). Our version was adapted by Ventura, Green, Shaner, and Liberman (1993). It has 24 items that can be rated from not present (given 1 point) to extremely severe (given 7 points), and the item is rated zero if not assessed. Rating is according to the presence of the symptom, frequency of occurrence, and the degree of impairment. The total score of each patient is compared to assess the degree of psychopathology.

Global Assessment of Functioning (GAF) Scale: A scale used for reporting the clinician's judgment of the individual's overall level of functioning. The scale is presented and described as Axis V of the internationally accepted Diagnostic and Statistical Manual of Mental Disorders, Fourth Edition Text Revision (DSM-IV-TR; American Psychiatric Association, 2000). The GAF Scale is to be rated with respect only to psychological, social, and occupational functioning, that is, not including impairment of functioning due to physical or environmental limitations. The score is rated from 100 (superior functioning, no symptoms) to 1 (persistent danger of severely hurting self or others).

Religious Orientation Scale (Al-Behairi & Demerdash, 1988): This scale was developed by Dr. Abd El-Rakeeb Al-Behairi and Dr. Adel Demerdash in 1988. It assesses intrinsic and the extrinsic religious orientation. The scale has been standardized on Egyptians with high inter-rater reliability and validity. The scale has two forms: form (A) for Muslims (34 questions) and form (B) for Christians (26 questions). Each question is given the 4-point (1 = strongly disagree to 4 = strongly agree) response format.

Brown Assessment of Beliefs Scale (BABS): The BABS is a seven-item, semi-structured interview which assesses delusionality of beliefs (obsession, concern, idea, worry, or delusion) during the past week in a wide range of psychiatric disorders. The BABS assesses the degree of delusional thinking related to a dominant belief dimensionally and also provides cut-off points to differentiate poor from good insight and delusional from nondelusional beliefs. BABS items measure the following components of delusionality: (1) conviction (how certain the patient is about the accuracy of the belief), (2) perception of others' views (the patient's ability to accurately assess the beliefs of others), (3) explanation of differing views (the patient's explanation for the difference between his/her and others' views of the belief), (4) fixity of beliefs (how unshakable the patient's conviction about the beliefs), (5) attempt to disprove beliefs (how actively and frequently the patient tries to disprove or reject his/her belief), (6) insight into the symptomatic nature of the belief (whether the patient recognizes that the belief has a psychiatric/psychological cause), (7) referential thinking (an additional item that assesses whether the patient has ideas of reference congruent with the content of the belief). Each item is rated from zero to four, with higher scores indicating poorer insight. The first six items are summed to reach a total score, ranging from 0 to 24 (referential thinking is not included in the total score). The BABS has good psychometric properties, including inter-rater reliability, test–retest reliability, and internal consistency. Also, BABS is sensitive to change and has a high correlation with other measures of delusionality suggesting that the Brown Assessment of Beliefs Scale is a valid measure of delusionality. (Eisen et al., 1998).

Statistical analysis

In stage 1, descriptive statistics are used to organize, summarize, and describe the measures of our sample. In stage 2, we conducted Chi-square tests to compare between the experimental and control groups. All data have been analyzed using Statistical Package for Social Sciences (SPSS) version 20.

Results

The first stage is descriptive and is designed to calculate the prevalence of religious delusions in the current sample. The second stage aimed at testing the relationship between prevalence of religious delusions in each social status, and the severity of the psychotic episode as indicated by the Brief Psychiatric Rating Scale (BPRS), the Global Assessment of Functioning (GAF) Scale which aids in assessing the patient's social, occupational and psychological functioning; BABS elements (conviction, perception of others' views of belief, explanation of differing views, fixity of ideas, attempt to disprove ideas and insight) in both experimental and control groups.

Stage 1: Descriptive analysis

The mean age of the sample was 46.32 ± 11.6 years, the youngest case was 21 and the eldest was 71 years old. The median was 47 and the mode was 55. The sample

Table 1 Prevalence of religious delusion across the sample.

Religious delusions		**Frequency**	**Percentage**
Valid	Present	191	38.2
	Not present	309	61.8
	Total	500	100

consisted of 328 males (65.6%) and 172 females (34.4%). The sample was distributed according to its marital status as 260 cases were single (52%), 105 were married (21%), 108 were divorced (21.6%), and 27 were widow (5.4%).

As for educational level, the sample included three illiterates (0.6%), 69 (13.8%) who were able to read and write were, 88 (17.6%) who were primary school educated, 99 (19.8%) who were preparatory educated, 170 (34%) who were cases with general and technical secondary education, and 71 (14.2%) who were the university graduates. As for occupation, the sample showed that 235 cases were not working (47%), 79 were manual worker (15.8%) and 68 cases were professional/clerk (13.6%) and 118 were on pension (23.6%).

The prevalence of religious delusion in the sample is shown in Table 1.

Stage 2: Group differences

Demographic differences

The cases' mean age was 44.28 ± 11.1 years while the controls' mean age was 45.14 ± 12.08 years. The difference between cases and controls regarding age in years using independent student's t-test was statistically insignificant ($p=9.6$).

As for gender, the cases were composed of 57 males (71.3%) and 23 females (28.7%); similarly, the controls were composed of 58 males (72.5%) and 22 females (27.5%). The difference between cases and controls regarding gender using Chi Square test was statistically insignificant ($p=0.8$). As for marital status, the cases were composed of 34 singles (42.5%), 23 married (28.7%), and 23 divorced (28.7%) similarly the controls were composed of 43 single (53.8%), 21 married (26.3%), and 16 divorced (20%). The difference between cases and controls regarding the marital status using Chi Square test was statistically insignificant ($p=0.3$).

As for educational level, the cases were composed of 6 individuals (7.5%) who can read and write, 11 cases (13.8%) who obtained primary education only, 13 cases (16.3%) who obtained preparatory education only, 19 cases (23.8%) who obtained secondary education only and 31 cases (38.8%) who obtained university education. The controls were composed of 3 cases (3.8%) can read and write, 15 cases (18.8%) finished primary education only, 15 cases (18.8%) finished preparatory education only, 26 cases (32.5%) finished secondary education only and 21 cases (26.3%) finished university education. The difference between cases and controls using Chi square test was statistically insignificant ($p=0.3$).

As for occupation, the cases were composed of 22 individuals (27.5%) not-working, 24 cases (30%) working as manual worker, 17 cases (21.3%) working as clerk or a professional, and 17 cases (21.3%) on pension. The controls were composed of 26 cases (32.5%) not-working, 15 cases (18.8%) working as manual worker, 11 cases (13.8%) working as clerk or a professional, and 28 cases (35%) on pension. The difference between cases and controls using Chi square test was statistically insignificant ($p=0.09$).

Variable differences

Table 2 shows the number of case patients and control group individuals who exhibited signs of violence towards their family, co-workers, staff, and other patients. The difference between cases and controls using Chi square was statistically insignificant.

The cases' mean Fahmy and El-Sherbini's scale was 22.18 ± 4.8, while the controls' mean Fahmy and El-Sherbini's scale was 21.96 ± 3.6. The cases' mean Family Socio-Economic Status was 46.1 ± 8.3, while the controls' Family Socio-Economic Status was 45.6 ± 6.11. The differences between cases and controls regarding Fahmy and El-Sherbini's scale and Family Socio-Economic Status using Chi square test was statistically insignificant (all p's > 0.05). The cases' mean GAF scale was 46.2 ± 11.7 while the controls' mean GAF scale was 56.7 ± 8.7. The difference between cases and controls regarding the GAF scale using Chi square test was highly significant ($p=0.001$). This indicates that a religious delusion in patients is related to poor functioning of patients in their society. The cases' mean BPRS was 77.66 ± 13.7 while the controls' mean BPRS was 60.29 ± 12.12. The difference between the cases and controls regarding BPRS using Chi square test was highly significant ($p=0.001$). This indicates that religious delusions in patients are related to the severity of their psychopathology.

Religious orientation

The total cases were 80 cases divided as 70 Muslim cases and 10 Christian cases while the total control was 80 cases divided as 69 Muslim cases and 11 Christian individuals.

Table 3 summarizes the levels of religious orientation within the Muslim cohort according to extrinsic and intrinsic orientation, as well as belonging to either case

Table 2 Differences between cases and controls regarding frequency of physical violence.

Violence against		Case	Control	χ^2	p
Family	Yes	45 (83.3%)	17 (77.3%)	0.3	0.5 NS
	No	9 (16.7%)	5 (22.7%)		
Co worker	Yes	9 (16.7%)	4 (18.2%)	0.02	0.8 NS
	No	45 (83.3%)	18 (81.8%)		
Staff	Yes	41 (75.9%)	14 (63.6%)	1.18	0.2 NS
	No	13 (24.1%)	8 (36.4%)		
Other patients	Yes	10 (18.5%)	1 (4.5%)	2.4	0.1 NS
	No	44 (81.5%)	21 (95.5%)		

NS, not significant.

Table 3 Differences between cases and controls regarding Religious Orientation Scale (Muslim).

Delusion		*N*	Mean	Std. deviation	T	*P*
Extrinsic	Case	70	52.37	6.029	−5.7	0.001
	Control	69	57.49	4.286		
Intrinsic	Case	70	53.53	12.898	−6.5	0.001
	Control	69	65.26	7.793		
Total	Case	70	105.9	13.003	−9.6	0.001
	Control	69	123.07	7.136		

group or control group. The difference between cases and controls using Chi square test was statistically significant for extrinsic, intrinsic, and total religious orientation scale (see Table 3).

Table 4 outlines the levels of religious orientation within the Christian cohort according to extrinsic and intrinsic orientation, and whether they belong to case group or control group. The difference between cases and controls using Chi square test was statistically significant for intrinsic and total orientation scales only (see Table 4). This indicates that a religious delusion in patients—whether Muslims or Christians—is related to distortion in their religious orientation.

Table 5 summarizes the level of differences between case group and control individuals on levels of conviction and insight concerning their beliefs. The difference between cases and controls using Chi square test was highly significant ($p < 0.001$).

Discussion

Our study found that 38.2% (191 cases) of inpatients had religious delusions. Furthermore, individuals in the case group showed significantly higher rates of belief conviction in their delusions compared to controls. Our results also indicate that in the Muslim cohort, individuals in the case group reported significantly less intrinsic

Table 4 Difference between cases and controls regarding Religious Orientation Scale (Christian).

Delusion		*N*	Mean	Std. deviation	T	*P*
Extrinsic	Case	10	46.2	1.989	−0.3	0.7 NS
	Control	11	46.82	4.976		
Intrinsic	Case	10	42	5.142	−3.6	0.001
	Control	11	48.82	2.96		
Total	Case	10	88.1	3.872	−3.9	0.001
	Control	11	95.64	4.864		

NS, not significant.

Table 5 Difference between cases and controls regarding all six dimensions of the Brown Assessment of Belief Scale.

		N	**Mean**	**Std. deviation**	**T**	***P***
Conviction	Case	80	4.73	0.551	6.7	0.001
	Control	80	4	0.779		
Perception of others' views of beliefs	Case	80	3.78	0.981	9.6	0.001
	Control	80	2.5	0.656		
Explanation of differing views	Case	80	4.51	0.746	14.8	0.001
	Control	80	3.11	0.39		
Fixity of ideas	Case	80	4.36	0.733	6.5	0.001
	Control	80	3.7	0.537		
Attempt to disprove ideas	Case	80	4.73	0.711	5.2	0.001
	Control	80	4.1	0.805		
Insight	Case	80	4.59	0.688	10.7	0.001
	Control	80	3.51	0.574		
Total Score	Case	80	20.68	3.415	12.6	0.001
	Control	80	14.9	2.259		

and extrinsic religious orientation. Similarly, the case group in the Christian cohort reported less intrinsic (but not extrinsic) religious orientation compared to controls. On the other hand, no significant differences were found in levels of aggression between the case group and controls.

The level of prevalence of religious delusions in this study is in line with previous meta-analyses (Amro et al., 2019; Cook, 2015) which indicate that between 20% and 60% of inpatients suffering a psychosis-spectrum disorder will report suffering delusions with religious content. Previous studies have found higher levels of delusional religiosity in Christian cohorts compared to Muslim and Buddhist groups (Grover et al., 2014), which in this study was not the case because firstly there were insufficient participants in the Christian group to make a significant comparison and secondly, this group reported less extrinsic religious orientation compared to the Muslim group which could explain a reduced tendency to report delusions of religious nature.

In our study, patients with religious delusions and the control group (who had delusions but without any religious content at time of study) were nearly equal in terms of gender, marital status, educational level achieved, occupations, and the different diagnoses involved in this study. There were no statistically significant differences between the numbers of cases' group and control group. This is consistent with other studies (Anderson-Schmidt et al., 2017; Raja et al., 2000). Furthermore, we found no difference in age of patients with or without religious delusions, as seen in other studies (Iyassu et al., 2014; Siddle et al., 2002). However, Atallah et al. found in his study that patients with religious symptoms tend to be younger (Atallah et al., 2001), while Raja found that patients with religious delusions were significantly older (Raja et al., 2000). These differences could be due to methodological differences or under-diagnosed, but do not reflect any clinical significance.

However, it has been reported that delusions of a religious theme are particularly common in male patients in their study in Turkey (Gecici et al., 2010) which can be explained by under-diagnosed female patients especially in rural areas where psychotic patients have a stigma for weak faith and a bad person. In one study, the number of previous episodes in both cases and control groups was about the same with no statistically significant difference. This was not expected or consistent with other United Kingdom studies' results that patients with religious delusions had mental health problems for significantly longer than those without religious delusions (Siddle et al., 2002). That is probably due to misdiagnosed episodes or missed religious symptoms in previously known patients due to cultural miss-understanding about difference between religious affiliation and religious delusions.

In our study, the frequency of physical violent episodes of patients within their immediate environment in case and control groups was nearly the same with no statistically significant difference. This is consistent with a study in United States that found no particular subgroup of delusions displaying threat or represents an important risk factor for violence in the general population and in several patient groups (Appelbaum, Robbins, & Monahan, 2000). Our results can be explained by the fact that number or frequency of episodic physical violence is more affected by agitation and psychomotor activity of patients than content of their delusions, especially if not confronted with opposite opinion. Confrontations is better expressed in perception of others' views of beliefs, and explanation of differing views, fixity of ideas of Brown Assessment of Belief Scale (BABS), while his reaction to that confrontation (based on his delusional content) can be expressed in attempt to disprove ideas of BABS.

There was no difference in the social class between patients with or without religious delusions in our study. This denotes that the presence of religious delusions in psychotic population is not related to their social class. This is consistent with other studies in Rome (Raja et al., 2000) that assessed Patients' social class according to an original scale including the following three items (rated 1–5): patient's employment, patient's residence, and family head's employment. Further, Stompe et al. (1999) investigated the content of delusions among Austrian and Pakistani patients with schizophrenia and found that neither in Pakistan nor in Austria any connection was established between contents of delusions and social status as well as level of education of patients with schizophrenia (Stompe et al., 1999). Only cultural factors seem to have a decisive influence on shaping the contents of delusions.

Our results show that the Global Assessment of Functioning (GAF) showed a highly significant poorer functioning in the religiously deluded patients than other psychotic patients. In congruence with previous studies performed in various countries such as Italy (Raja et al., 2000), United Kingdom (Siddle et al., 2002), which is a cross-sectional examination and description of religious delusions in 193 patients with schizophrenia, and Taiwan (Huang et al., 2011). The three studies indicated that religious delusions have more negative effect on the psychological, social, and occupational functioning of the patients. This poor functioning is explained by the greater effect of religion on patients' life and role in society.

The Brief Psychiatric Rating Scale (BPRS) was significantly higher in patients with religious delusions than other patients, indicating more severe symptoms of psychosis in religiously deluded patients. As expected, religious delusions may have a very serious impact on the severity of the psychosis, and it should not pass lightly. Further, Iyassu and colleagues found in a study in United Kingdom that religious delusions were associated with higher levels of positive symptoms, auditory hallucinations, and bizarre behavior. People with religious delusions also reported more internal evidence for their delusions (anomalous experiences or mood changes) and were very likely to have an accompanying grandiose delusion (Iyassu et al., 2014). Iyassu even proposed that these characteristics could plausibly underlie the persistence of religious delusions and their resistance to treatment. However, Iyassu used Scales for the assessment of positive/negative symptoms (SAPS/SANS) developed by Andreasen (1984). Raja et al. found that patients with religious delusions presented higher level of psychopathology and, in particular, severer psychotic positive symptoms (Raja et al., 2000), scoring higher using BPRS, SAPS, and SANS.

Further, other previous studies reported that schizophrenia patients with religious delusion/hallucination had more severe psychotic symptoms and lower functioning (Siddle et al., 2002) using the Hallucination Scale (AH) and the Delusion Scale (DS) from PSYRATS (Haddock, McCarron, Tarrier, & Faragher, 1999) to evaluate the dimensions and severity of these particular symptoms. Presumably, their baseline conditions were poorer, and their psychotic exacerbation was severer. These differences could be explained by association of religious delusion with severer psychopathological crises, possibly due to a more pervasive influence of religious delusion on patients' thought, affect, and behavior (Raja et al., 2000).

Our results of Religious Orientation Scale (ROS) in Muslims' patients, was significantly higher in the control group than in patients with religious delusions in all aspects: intrinsic, extrinsic, and total ROS. In Christian's patients, the results of ROS were significantly higher in control group than in religiously deluded patients in intrinsic and total religious orientation scale with no significant change in extrinsic scale. This is nearly the same as in Muslims' patients with the exception of extrinsic scale which may be due to methodological differences between different questions in the 2 forums of the test. Generally, ROS rates were higher in control group than religiously deluded patients denoting a more deterioration in the religiously deluded psychotic patients. This aligns with a significant association between increased religiosity and reporting more types of psychotic experiences (Kovess-Masfety et al., 2018). However, one study demonstrated that religiosity in general as well as personal importance of the faith are not directly related to the religious content of delusions in patients with schizophrenia, that is, religious delusions are not influenced by personal religiosity by asking all 295 patients with schizophrenia about their personal religiosity, asking "Are you a religious person?" and "Is your faith personally important for you?" (Rudalevičienė, Stompe, Narbekovas, Raškauskienė, & Bunevičius, 2008). Although no standardized test has been applied to patients, but simple questions demonstrated no apparent relation between religiosity and development of psychosis.

Siddle et al. (2002) assessed religiosity using the patients' own classification of whether they said they were religious or not when asked to make a forced choice. They found that no obvious and clear linear relationship between psychotic symptomatology in general and religiosity, though it was admitted that religiously deluded subjects were more religious on self-assessed degree of religiosity than the comparison group. This study reflects psychotic patients' own view of their religiosity, which is not accurate reflection of pre-psychosis religiosity. Even though, still no relation has been found between religiosity and development of psychosis, that is, personal religiosity is not necessary for the development of religious delusions. This only indicates that religious delusions are not proportional to the usual religious practices or to the intrinsic feeling of religion in patient's spiritual life. However, this is not an indication for religiously deluded patient's reaction upon his delusion, because the test only scale the usual daily religious practice already accepted in society.

In our data, the degree of delusionality in the religiously deluded patients was significantly higher than nonreligiously deluded patients using Brown Assessment of Belief Scale in the total score and all included dimensions (Conviction, Perception of others' views of beliefs, Explanation of differing views, Fixity of ideas, Attempt to disprove ideas, Insight). This is expected because religious delusions are proportionately considered one of the most likely delusions (after persecutory and body/mind control) to be chosen as having the greatest impact on subjects' lives (Appelbaum et al., 1999). Appelbaum interviewed 1136 actually hospitalized psychiatric patients, a total of 328 subjects (29%) were rated as definitely or possibly delusional. Their rating was done on dimensions of MacArthur-Maudsley Delusions Assessment Schedule (which included seven dimensions: conviction, negative affect, action, inaction, preoccupation, pervasiveness, and fluidity). Appelbaum et al. noted that patients with religious delusions scored significantly higher on ratings of conviction, insight, and pervasiveness, so they may be least susceptible to cognitive behavioral interventions (Appelbaum et al., 1999).

However, in a study in United Kingdom of 383 adult participants (only 87 of them are religiously deluded) with delusions and a schizophrenia spectrum Iyassu et al. (2014) found that no significant differences in delusional conviction or insight between religiously deluded patients and other deluded patients. For measuring conviction, they used PSYRATS Psychotic Symptoms Rating Scale (a semi-structured interviews designed to assess the subjective characteristics of hallucinations and delusions). The inter-rater reliability of the PSYRATS subscales was very good but that of the items was less consistent as concluded by Drake, Haddock, Tarrier, Bentall, and Lewis (2007).

Limitations and future work

First, our sample was collected randomly from inpatients in a single hospital, with a limited number of patients to study (80 religiously deluded vs. 80 non-religiously deluded). Second, our study was concerned with the study of delusional belief in psychotic patients (whether religiously deluded or non-religiously deluded). However, normal religious beliefs, and delusional religious belief in non-psychotic population are not accounted for. Third, the frequency of episodes of physical violence from patients (whether observed or reported) refers to patients' whole agitation and aggression, not to the patients' aggression in response to denial or refusal of their delusional thought content. Future work should address these limitations.

References

Ahmed, S. H. (1978). Cultural influences on delusion. *Psychiatria Clinica, 11*(1), 1–9.

Al-Behairi, A., & Demerdash, A. (1988). *Religious orientation scale (Arabic version).*

Al-Issa, I. (1995). The illusion of reality or the reality of illusion: Hallucinations and culture. *British Journal of Psychiatry, 166*, 368–373.

American Psychiatric Association. (2000). *Diagnostic and statistical manual of mental disorders, fourth edition, text revision (DSM-IV-TR).* Washington, DC: American Psychiatric Association.

American Psychiatric Association. (2013). *Diagnostic and Statistical Manual of Mental Disorders, Fourth Edition, Text Revision (DSM-5).* Washington, DC: American Psychiatric Association.

Amro, I., Ghuloum, S., Mahfoud, Z., Opler, M., Khan, A., Hammoudeh, S., … Al-Amin, G. (2019). Cross cultural adaptation of the Arabic positive and negative syndrome scale of schizophrenia: Qualitative analysis focus group. *Transcultural Psychiatry, 56*(5), 573–991. https://doi.org/10.1177/1363461519850345.

Anderson-Schmidt, H., Gade, K., Malzahn, D., Papiol, S., Budde, M., Heilbronner, U., … Schulze, T. G. (2019). The influence of religious activity and polygenic schizophrenia risk on religious delusions in schizophrenia. *Schizophrenia Research, 210*, 255–261. https://doi.org/10.1016/j.schres.2018.12.025.

Anderson-Schmidt, H., Gade, K., Malzahn, D., Papiol, S., Budde, M., Kalman, J., ... Falkai, P. (2017). Dissecting religious delusions in schizophrenia: The interplay of religious activity and polygenic burden. *European Neuropsychopharmacology, 27,* S457–S458.

Andreasen, N. C. (1984). *Scale for the assessment of negative symptoms (SANS).* Iowa City: The University of Iowa.

Appelbaum, P., Robbins, P., & Monahan, J. (2000). Violence and delusions: Data from the MacArthur violence risk assessment study. *American Journal of Psychiatry, 157,* 566–572.

Appelbaum, P., Robbins, P., & Roth, L. (1999). Dimensional approach to delusions: Comparison across types and diagnoses. *American Journal of Psychiatry, 156,* 1938–1943.

Asai, T. (1964). The content of delusions of schizophrenic patients in Japan: Comparisons between periods from 1941–1961. *Transcultural Psychiatric Research Review, 1,* 27–28.

Atallah, S., El-Dosoky, A., Coker, E., Nabil, K., & El-Islam, M. (2001). A 22 year retrospective analysis of the changing frequency and patterns of religious symptoms among inpatients with psychotic illness in Egypt. *Social Psychiatry and Psychiatric Epidemiology, 36*(8), 407–415.

Aukst-Margetic, B., & Jakovljevic, M. (2008). Religiosity and schizophrenia. *Psychiatria Danubina, 20,* 437–438.

Axer, H. A., Corrigan, P. W., & Liberman, R. P. (1992). Helping chronic psychiatric patients adjust to sociopolitical changes in Poland. *Psychiatry, 55,* 207–213.

Azhar, M., Varma, S., & Hakim, H. (1995). Phenomenological differences of delusions between schizophrenic patients of two cultures of Malaysia. *Singapore Medical Journal, 26,* 273–275.

Bartocci, G. (2006a). Recent advances in cultural and transcultural psychiatry. *Newsletter, 21*(1), 24–29.

Bartocci, G. (2006b). The influence of religion on psychiatric theories and practices. *World Cultural Psychiatry Research Review, 3*(4), 106–113.

Bhavsar, V., & Bhugra, D. (2008). Religious delusions: Finding meaning in psychosis. *Psychopathology, 41*(3), 165–172.

Bhugra, D., & Gupta, K. R. (1996). Psychiatric episodes precipitated by elections. *Journal of Nervous and Mental Disease, 184,* 129–130.

Blackner, K., & Wong, N. (1963). Four cases of autocastration. *Archives of General Psychiatry, 8,* 169–176.

Bohlken, J., & Priebe, S. (1990). Political change and the course of affective psychosis: Berlin 1989–1990. *Psychiatry Research, 37,* 1–4.

Böhmer, M. (2016). Does psychiatry need religion and spirituality in its treatment approach? Narcissism as an example. *South African Journal of Psychiatry, 22*(1), 563. https://doi.org/10.4102/sajpsychiatry.v22i1.563.

Bose, R. (1997). Psychiatry and the popular conception of possession among the Bangladeshis in London. *International Journal of Social Psychiatry, 43,* 1–15.

Braam, A. W., Beekman, A. T. F., Deeg, D. J. H., Smit, J. H., & Tilburg, W. V. (1997). Religiosity as a protective or prognostic factor of depression in later life; results from a community survey in the Netherlands. *Acta Psychiatrica Scandinavica, 96,* 199–205.

Brett-Jones, J., Garety, P. A., & Hemsley, D. (1987). Measuring delusional experiences: A method and its application. *British Journal of Clinical Psychology, 26,* 257–265.

Broome, M. R. (2012). *The Maudsley reader in phenomenological psychiatry.* Cambridge, New York: Cambridge University Press.

Campbell, M. M., Sibeko, G., Mall, S., Baldinger, A., Nagdee, M., Susser, E., & Stein, D. J. (2017). The content of delusions in a sample of South African Xhosa people with schizophrenia. *BMC Psychiatry, 17*(1), 41.

Campion, J., & Bhugra, D. (1997). Experience of religious healing in psychiatric patients in South India. *Social Psychiatry and Psychiatric Epidemiology*, *32*, 215–221.

Cannon, B. J., & Kramer, L. M. (2012). Delusion content across the 20th century in an American Psychiatric Hospital. *International Journal of Social Psychiatry*, *58*, 323–327.

Catone, G., Pisano, S., Broome, M., Lindau, J. F., Pascotto, A., & Gritti, A. (2016). Continuity between stressful experiences and delusion content in adolescents with psychotic disorders—A pilot study. *Scandinavian Journal of Child and Adolescent Psychiatry and Psychology*, *4*(1), 14–22. http://orcid.org/0000-0002-1769-4489.

Chidarikire, S., Cross, M., Skinner, I., & Cleary, M. (2020). An ethnographic study of schizophrenia in Zimbabwe: The role of culture, faith and religion. *Journal of Spirituality in Mental Health*, *22*(2), 173–194. https://doi.org/10.1080/19349637.2018.1531366.

Chu, C. C., & Klein, H. E. (1985). Psychosocial and environmental variables in outcome of black schizophrenics. *Journal of the National Medical Association*, *77*, 793–796.

Clark, S. M. L., & Harrison, D. A. (2012). How to care for patients who have delusions with religious content. *Current Psychiatry*, *11*(1), 47.

Coltheart, M., Menzies, P., & Sutton, J. (2010). Abductive inference and delusional belief. *Cognitive Neuropsychiatry*, *15*(1), 261–287.

Connell, A., Koen, L., Niehaus, D., Cloete, K. J., Jordaan, E., & Botha, U. (2015). Religious delusions in a Xhosa schizophrenia population. *Journal of Religion and Health*, *54*(5), 1555–1562.

Cook, C. C. H. (2015). Religious psychopathology: The prevalence of religious content of delusions and hallucinations in mental disorder. *The International Journal of Social Psychiatry*, *61*(4), 404–425.

Doering, S., Muller, E., Kopcke, W., Pietzcker, A., Gaebel, W., Linden, M., ... Schussler, G. (1998). Predictors of relapse and rehospitalization in schizophrenia and schizoaffective disorder. *Schizophrenia Bulletin*, *24*(1), 87–98.

Draguns, J. G. (1995). Cultural influences upon psychopathology: Clinical and practical implications. (Special issue) A psychosocial view of mental illness *Journal of Social Distress and Homeless*, *4*, 79–103.

Drake, R., Haddock, G., Tarrier, N., Bentall, R., & Lewis, S. (2007). The psychotic symptom rating scales (PSYRATS): Their usefulness and properties in first episode psychosis. *Schizophrenia Research*, *89*, 119–122.

Duñó, R., Oliva, J. C., Tobeña, A., Palao, D., & Labad, J. (2020). Religiosity and psychotic ideation in stable schizophrenia: A roles for empathic perspective-taking. *Behavioral Science*, *10*(2), 53. https://doi.org/10.3390/bs10020053.

Eisen, J. L., Phillips, K., Baer, L., Beer, D., Atala, K., & Rasmussen, S. (1998). The brown assessment of beliefs scale: Reliability and validity. *American Journal of Psychiatry*, *155*, 102–108.

El-Fatatry, M., El-Kashlan, K., El-Garem, O., & Ghazi, A. M. (1980). Psychiatric patients of Egyptian culture in Alexandria. *International Journal of Social Psychiatry*, *26*, 69–71.

El-Islam, M. F. (1978). Transcultural aspects of psychiatric patients in Qatar. *Comparative Medicine East and West*, *6*, 33–36.

El-Islam, M. F. (1982). Arabic cultural psychiatry. *Transcultural Psychiatric Research Review*, *19*, 5–24.

El-Islam, M. F., & Malasi, T. H. (1985). Delusions and education. *Journal of Operational Psychiatry*, *16*, 2–4.

Fahmy, S. I., & El-Sherbini, A. F. (1988). Determining simple parameters for social classification for health researchers. *The Bulletin of the High Institute of Public Health Journal*, *10*, 95–108.

Field, H. L., & Waldfogel, S. (1995). Severe ocular self-injury. *General Hospital Psychiatry, 17*(3), 224–227.

Garety, P. A., & Freeman, D. (1999). Cognitive approaches to delusions: A critical review of theories and evidence. *British Journal of Clinical Psychology, 38*(2), 113–154.

Garety, P. A., Kuipers, E., Fowler, D., Freeman, D., & Bebbington, P. E. (2001). A cognitive model of the positive symptoms of psychosis. *Psychological Medicine, 31*, 189–195.

Gawad, N. A., Desai, P., Ali, T., Lewis, K. K., Polo, R., Engstrom, A., … Pigott, T. (2018). Religious activity, psychotic features, and suicidality in 688 acute psychiatric inpatients. *Journal of Psychiatric Practice, 24*(4), 253–260.

Gearing, R. E., Alonzo, D., Smolak, A., McHugh, K., Harmon, S., & Baldwin, S. (2011). Association of religion with delusions and hallucinations in the context of schizophrenia: Implications for engagement and adherence. *Schizophrenia Research, 126*, 150–163.

Gecici, O., Kuloglu, M., Guler, O., Ozbulut, O., Kurt, E., Onen, S., … Albayrak, Y. (2010). Phenomenology of delusions and hallucinations in patient with schizophrenia. *Bulletin of Clinical Psychopharmacology, 20*, 204–212.

Grover, S., Davuluri, T., & Chakrabarti, S. (2014). Religion, spirituality, and schizophrenia: A review. *Indian Journal of Psychological Medicine, 36*(2), 119–124.

Haddock, G., McCarron, J., Tarrier, N., & Faragher, E. B. (1999). Scales to measure dimensions of hallucinations and delusions: The psychotic symptom rating scales (PSYRATS). *Psychological Medicine, 29*, 879–889.

Hanevik, H., Hestad, K. A., Lien, L., Joa, I., Larsen, T. K., & Danbolt, L. J. (2017). Religiousness in first-episode psychosis. *Archive for the Psychology of Religion, 39*(2), 139–164.

Harrow, M., Rattenbury, F., & Stoll, F. (1988). Schizophrenic delusions: An analysis of their persistence, of related premorbid ideas, and of three major dimensions. In F. Oltmanns, & B. A. Maher (Eds.), *Delusional beliefs* (pp. 185–211). New York: John Wiley.

Hill, P. C., & Hood, R. (1999). *Measures of religiosity*. Birmingham, AL: Religious Education Press.

Hill, P. C., Pargament, K. I., Hood, R. W., McCullough, M. E., Swyers, J. P., Larson, D. B., & Zinnbauer, B. J. (2000). Conceptualizing religion and spirituality: Points of commonality, points od departure. *Journal for the Theory of Social Behavior, 30*(1), 51–77.

Huang, C. L.-C., Shang, C.-Y., Shieh, M.-S., Lin, H.-N., & Su, J. (2011). The interactions between religion, religiosity, religious delusion/hallucination, and treatment-seeking behavior among schizophrenic patients in Taiwan. *Psychiatry Research, 187*, 347–353.

Huguelet, P., Brandt, P., & Mohr, S. (2016). The assessment of spirituality and religiousness in patients with psychosis. *L'Encéphale, 42*(3), 219–225. https://doi.org/10.1016/j.encep.2015.12.005.

Huguelet, P., Mohr, S., Jung, V., Gillieron, C., Brandt, P., & Borras, L. (2007). Effect of religion on suicide attempts in outpatients with schizophrenia or schizo-affective disorders compared with inpatients with non-psychotic disorders. *European Psychiatry, 22*, 188–194.

Iyassu, R., Jolley, S., Bebbington, P., Dunn, G., Emsley, R., Freeman, D., … Garety, P. (2014). Psychological characteristics of religious delusions. *Social Psychiatry and Psychiatric Epidemiology, 49*, 1051–1061.

Jackson, M. C. (1991–2007). A study of the relationship between psychotic and spiritual experience. Unpublished D. Phil Thesis, University of Oxford. Chung, M. C In M. C. Chung, K. W. M. Fulford, & G. Graham (Eds.), *Reconceiving schizophrenia*. Oxford: Oxford University Press.

Janca, A., Ustun, T. B., van Drimmelen, J., Dittmann, V., & Isaac, M. (1994). *ICD-10 symptom checklist for mental disorders (version 1.1). Geneva, division of mental health*. World Health Organization.

Jarbin, H., & Von Knorring, A. L. (2004). Suicide and suicide attempts in adolescent-on-set psychotic disorders. *Nordic Journal of Psychiatry*, *58*, 115–123.

Jenner, J. A., Rutten, S., Beuckens, J., Boonstra, N., & Sytema, S. (2008). Positive and useful auditory vocal hallucinations: Prevalence, characteristics, attributions, and implications for treatment. *Acta Psychiatrica Scandinavica*, *118*(3), 238–245.

Jones, E., & Watson, J. P. (1997). Delusion, the overvalued idea and religious beliefs: A comparative analysis of their characteristics. *British Journal of Psychiatry*, *170*, 381–386.

Kelly, G. R., Mamon, J. A., & Scott, J. E. (1987). Utility of the health belief model in examining compliance among psychiatric outpatients. *Social Science and Medicine*, *25*, 1205–1211.

Kent, G., & Wahass, S. (1996). The content and characteristics of auditory hallucinations in Saudi Arabia and the UK: A cross-cultural comparison. *Acta Psychiatrica Scandinavica*, *94*, 433–437.

Kiev, A. (1963). Beliefs and delusions of West Indian immigrants to London. *British Journal of Psychiatry*, *109*, 356–363.

Kim, K. I., Li, D., Jiang, Z., Cui, X., Lin, L., Kang, J. J., … Kim, C. K. (1993). Schizophrenic delusions among Koreans, Korean-Chinese and Chinese: A transcultural study. *International Journal of Social Psychiatry*, *39*, 190–199.

Klaf, F. S., & Hamilton, J. G. (1961). Schizophrenia: A hundred years ago and today. *The Journal of Mental Science*, *107*, 819–827.

Koenig, H. G. (2009). Research on religion, spirituality, and mental health: A review. *The Canadian Journal of Psychiatry*, *54*(5), 283–291.

Koenig, H. G., McCullough, M. E., & Larson, D. B. (2001). A history of religion, science and medicine. In H. G. Koenig, M. E. McCullough, & D. B. Larson (Eds.), *Handbook of religion and health* (pp. 24–49). New York, NY: Oxford University Press.

Kovess-Masfety, V., Saha, S., Lim, C. C. W., Aguilar-Gaxiola, S., Al-Hamzawi, A., Alonso, J., … Florescu, S. (2018). Psychotic experiences and religiosity: Data from the WHO World Mental Health Surveys. *Acta Psychiatrica Scandinavica*, *137*(4), 306–315.

Kushner, A. W. (1967). Two cases of auto-castration due to religious delusions. *British Journal of Medical Psychology*, *40*, 293–298.

Lancellotta, E., & Bortolotti, L. (2019). Are clinical delusions adaptive? *Wiley Interdisciplinary Reviews: Cognitive Science*, *10*(5), e1502. https://doi.org/10.1002/wcs.1502.

Lazarescu, M., Hurmuz, M., Draghici, A. M., & Blajovan, J. (2015). Schneider's first rank symptoms in relation to religious delusion. *European Psychiatry*, *30*, 1580.

Levenson, P. (1973). Religious delusions in counter-culture patients. *American Journal of Psychiatry*, *130*, 1265–1269.

Lowe, W. L. (1954). Group beliefs and socio-cultural factors in religious delusions. *The Journal of Social Psychology*, *40*, 267–274.

Maher, B. A. (1988). Anomalous experience and delusional thinking: The logic of explanations. In T. F. Oltmann, & B. A. Maher (Eds.), *Delusional beliefs* (pp. 15–33). New York: Wiley.

Maselko, J., & Buka, S. (2008). Religious activity and lifetime prevalence of psychiatric disorder. *Social Psychiatry and Psychiatric Epidemiology*, *43*, 18–21.

Maslowski, J. (1988). Cross-cultural study of productive phenomenology of schizophrenia. *Psychiatria Polska*, *22*, 193–197.

McCabe, M. S., Fowler, R. C., & Cadoret, R. J. (1972). Symptom differences in schizophrenia with good and poor prognosis. *American Journal of Psychiatry*, *128*(10), 59–63.

McCauley, R. N., & Graham, G. (2020). *Hearing voices and other matters of the mind: What mental abnormalities can teach us about religions*. Oxford University Press.

McKay, R. T., & Ross, R. M. (2020). Religion and delusion. *Current Opinion in Psychology*, *40*, 160–166.

McLean, B. F., Mattiske, J. K., & Balzan, R. P. (2017). Association of the jumping to conclusions and evidence integration biases with delusions in psychosis: A detailed meta-analysis. *Schizophrenia Bulletin*, *43*(2), 344–354. https://doi.org/10.1093/schbul/sbw056.

Mishra, A., Das, B., & Goyal, N. (2018). Religiosity and religious delusions in schizophrenia—An observational study in a Hindu population. *Asian Journal of Psychiatry*, *32*, 35–39.

Mitchell, J., & Vierkant, A. D. (1989). Delusions and hallucinations as a reflection of the subcultural milieu among psychotic patients of the 1930s and 1980s. *Journal of Psychology*, *123*, 269–274.

Mohr, S., Borras, L., Betrisey, C., Pierre-Yves, B., Gilliéron, C., & Huguelet, P. (2010). Delusions with religious content in patients with psychosis: How they interact with spiritual coping. *Psychiatry*, *73*(2), 158–172.

Mohr, S., Borras, L., Rieben, I., Betrisey, C., Gillieron, C., Brandt, P. Y., … Huguelet, P. (2009). Evolution of spirituality and religiousness in chronic schizophrenia or schizo-affective disorders: A 3-year follow up study. *Social Psychiatry and Psychiatric Epidemiology*, *45*, 1095–1103.

Mohr, S., & Huguelet, P. (2004). The relationship between schizophrenia and religion and its implications for care. *Swiss Medical Weekly*, *134*(25–26), 369–376.

Mohr, S., Perroud, N., Gillieron, C., Brandt, P., Rieben, I., Borras, L., & Huguelet, P. (2011). Spirituality and religiousness as predictive factors of outcome in schizophrenia and schizo-affective disorders. *Psychiatry Research*, *186*, 177–182.

Mohr, S., & Pfeifer, S. (2009). Delusions and hallucinations with religious content. In P. Huguelet, & G. Koenig (Eds.), *Religion and spirituality in psychiatry* (p. 81). Cambridge University Press.

Moss, Q., Fleck, D. E., & Strakowski, S. M. (2006). The influence of religious affiliation on time to first treatment and hospitalization. *Schizophrenia Research*, *84*, 421–426.

Ndetei, D. M., & Vadher, A. (1984). Frequency and clinical significance of delusions across cultures. *Acta Psychiatrica Scandinavica*, *70*(1), 73–76.

Ndetei, D. M., & Vadher, A. (1985). Cross cultural study of religious phenomenology in psychiatric in-patients. *Acta Psychiatrica Scandinavica*, *72*, 59–62.

NICE. (2009). *Core interventions in the treatment and management of schizophrenia in primary and secondary care (update) (cg82)*. London: National Institute for Health and Clinical Excellence.

Noort, A., Beekman, A. T. F., van Gool, A. R., & Braam, A. W. (2018). Religious delusions in older adults: Diagnoses, combinations and delusional characteristics. *International Journal of Geriatric Psychiatry*, *33*(12), 1680–1687. https://doi.org/10.1002/gps.4973.

Overall, J. E., & Gorham, D. R. (1962). The brief psychiatric rating scale. *Psychological Reports*, *10*, 790–812.

Paolini, E., Moretti, P., & Compton, M. T. (2016). Delusions in first-episode psychosis: Principal component analysis of twelve types of delusions and demographic and clinical correlates of resulting domains. *Psychiatry Research*, *243*, 5–13.

Pargament, K. I., & Lomax, J. W. (2013). Understanding and addressing religion among people with mental illness. *World Psychiatry*, *12*(1), 26–32. https://doi.org/10.1002/wps.20005.

Park, C., Cohen, L. H., & Herb, L. (1990). Intrinsic religiousness and religious coping as life stress moderators for Catholics versus Protestants. *Journal of Personality and Social Psychology*, *59*, 562–574.

Patel, A., Barot, C. K., Vankar, G., & Pal, S. (2019). Acting on delusions in patients suffering from schizophrenia. *Archives of Psychiatry and Psychotherapy*, *4*, 52–61. https://doi.org/10.12740/APP/109009.

Peters, E., Day, S., McKenna, J., & Orbach, G. (1999). Delusional ideation in religious and psychotic populations. *British Journal of Clinical Psychology*, *38*(Issue 1), 83–96.

Raja, M., Azzoni, A., & Lubich, L. (2000). Religious delusion: An observational study of religious delusion in a population of 313 acute psychiatric inpatients. *Schweiz Archives of Neurology Psychiatry and Psychotherapy*, *151*, 22–29.

Rudalevičienė, P., Stompe, T., Narbekovas, A., Raškauskienė, N., & Bunevičius, R. (2008). Are religious delusions related to religiosity in schizophrenia? *Medicina (Kaunas, Lithuania)*, *44*(7), 529–535.

Saavedra, J. (2014). Function and meaning in religious delusions: A theoretical discussion from a case study. *Mental Health, Religion and Culture*, *17*(1), 39–51. https://doi.org/10.1080/13674676.2012.745493.

Schofield, W., Hathaway, S. R., Hastings, D. W., & Bell, D. M. (1954). Prognostic factors in schizophrenia. *Journal of Consulting Psychology*, *18*, 155–166.

Scott, E. H. M. (1967). A study of the contents of delusions and hallucinations in 100 African female psychotics. *South African Medicine Journal*, *4*, 853–858.

Sher, L. (1997). The influence of sociopolitical events on the content of delusions. *The Israel Journal of Psychiatry and Related Sciences*, *34*, 165.

Siddle, R., Haddock, G., Tarrier, N., & Faragher, E. B. (2002). Religious delusions in patients admitted to hospital with schizophrenia. *Social Psychiatry and Psychiatric Epidemiology*, *37*, 130–138.

So, S. H., Tang, V., & Leung, P. W. (2015). Dimensions of delusions and attribution biases along the continuum of psychosis. *PLoS One*, *10*(12), e0144558.

Spitzer, M. (1990). On defining delusions. *Comprehensive Psychiatry*, *31*, 377–397.

Stompe, T., Friedman, A., Ortwein, G., Strobi, R., Chaudhry, H. R., Najam, N., & Chaudhry, M. R. (1999). Comparisons of delusions among schizophrenics in Austria and Pakistan. *Psychopathology*, *32*, 225–234.

Strauss, J. S. (1991). The person with delusions. *British Journal of Psychiatry*, *159*(Suppl 14), 57–61.

Suhail, K. (2003). Phenomenology of delusions in pakistani patients: Effect of gender and social class. *Psychopathology*, *36*, 195–199.

Tateyama, J., Asai, M., Kamisada, M., Hashimoto, M., Bartels, M., & Heimann, H. (1993). Comparison of schizophrenic delusions between Japan and Germany. *Psychopathology*, *26*(3–4), 151–158.

Thara, R., & Eaton, W. W. (1996). Outcome of schizophrenia: The Madras longitudinal study. *Australian and New Zealand Journal of Psychiatry*, *30*, 516–522.

Tseng, W. S. (2001). *Handbook of cultural psychiatry*. San Diego, London, Boston, New York, Sydney, Tokyo, Toronto: Academic Press. 2001.

Ventriglio, A., Bonfitto, I., Ricci, F., Cuoco, F., & Bhavsar, V. (2018). Delusion, possession and religion. *Nordic Journal of Psychiatry*, *72*(sup1), s13–s15. https://doi.org/10.1080/08039488.2018.1525639.

Ventura, M. A., Green, M. F., Shaner, A., & Liberman, R. P. (1993). Training and quality assurance with the Brief Psychiatric Rating Scale: "The drift buster". *International Journal of Methods in Psychiatric Research*, *3*, 221–224.

Verghese, A., John, J. K., Rajkumar, S., Richard, J., Sethi, B. B., & Trivedi, J. K. (1989). Factors associated with the course and outcome of schizophrenia in India: Results of a two-year multicentre follow-up study. *British Journal of Psychiatry*, *154*, 499–503.

Waugh, A. C. (1986). Autocastration and biblical delusions in schizophrenia. *British Journal of Psychiatry*, *149*(5), 656–659.

West, D., & Walk, A. (1977). *Daniel McNaughton: His trial and the aftermath*. Ashford: Headley Brothers Ltd.

Westermeyer, J. (1988). Some cross-cultural aspects of delusions. In T. F. Oltmanns, & B. A. Maher (Eds.), *Delusional beliefs* (pp. 230–258). New York: John Wiley.

Wilson, W. P. (1998). Religion and psychoses. In H. G. Koenig (Ed.), *Handbook of religion and mental health* (pp. 161–173). San Diego, CA: Academic Press.

Yorston, G. (1997). Depressive delusions and general election. *British Journal of Psychiatry, 171*, 585.

Zinnbauer, B. J., Pargament, K. I., Cole, B., Rye, M. S., Butter, E. M., Belavich, T. G., ... Kadar, J. L. (1997). Religion and spirituality: Unfuzzying the fuzzy. *Journal for the Scientific Study of Religion, 36*(4), 549–564.

Urbanicity and familial liability interact and influence auditory verbal hallucinations in first-episode schizophrenia patients

6

Alejandro Morris[a], *Ahmed A. Moustafa*[a,b], *Kristina Ulm*[c], *Dorota Frydecka*[d], *Patryk Piotrowski*[d], *and Błażej Misiak*[e]
[a]School of Psychology & Marcs Institute for Brain and Behaviour, Western Sydney University, Sydney, NSW, Australia, [b]Department of Human Anatomy and Physiology, the Faculty of Health Sciences, University of Johannesburg, South Africa, [c]Faculty of Built Environment, University of New South Wales, Sydney, NSW, Australia, [d]Department of Psychiatry, Wroclaw Medical University, Wroclaw, Poland, [e]Department of Genetics, Wroclaw Medical University, Wroclaw, Poland

Chapter outline

Introduction

More than half of the global population is living in urban areas, which are growing at a higher pace than rural areas (The United Nations, 2018). At the same time, living in urban environments is associated with increased mental health rates, including childhood psychiatric disorders, adult depression, and neurotic disorders (Engemann et al., 2019). Consequently, understanding the impact of living in an urban environment on mental health is crucial for the prevention and treatment of mental health disorders in large parts of the population.

Research has found that individuals living in urban environments are at a higher risk of developing psychosis spectrum disorders compared to individuals living in rural settings (Vassos, Pedersen, Murray, Collier, & Lewis, 2012). Evidence shows that urban upbringing contributes to the development of schizophrenia spectrum disorders, after controlling for drug use and minority group affiliation (Krabbendam & van Os, 2005). One large-scale

Cognitive and Behavioral Dysfunction in Schizophrenia. https://doi.org/10.1016/B978-0-12-820005-6.00008-6

study also found that an increase in urbancity is associated with an increase in symptom severity and risk to develop schizophrenia (Luo, Pang, Guo, Zhang, & Zheng, 2020). Epidemiological studies have sought to understand the association between urbanicity and schizophrenia. Urbanicity can be defined as "the impact of living in urban areas at a given time" (Vlahov & Galea, 2002) and is most commonly measured as population size of a place of residence or population density (van Os, Hanssen, Bak, Bijl, & Vollebergh, 2003; Vassos et al., 2012). Despite urbanicity being viewed as a proxy for risk-increasing factors, there is evidence indicating it can provide protective factors such as readily available psychiatric care, resource access and better nutrition (He et al., 2018). Nevertheless, the connection between urbanicity and the prevalence of schizophrenia remains constant irrespective of outcome measure (schizophrenia or broad psychosis), the method used to measure urban environment (population size of place of residence or population density), and time of exposure (birth and upbringing or onset of illness) (Vassos et al., 2012). Although there are multiple studies demonstrating the link between higher population density and higher risk of schizophrenia (van Os et al., 2003; Vassos et al., 2012), there is also evidence that other urban environmental factors affect schizophrenia rates (Essock, 2017; Fan et al., 2018; van Os, Kenis, & Rutten, 2010). Urban risk factors that could explain this relationship can be socio-environmental, such as low socioeconomic status, social fragmentation, belonging to migrant/ethnic minorities (Jongsma et al., 2018; Kirkbride et al., 2017; Schofield et al., 2017) or part of the physical environment, such as toxins or auditory pollution (DeVylder et al., 2018; March et al., 2008). Research on socio-environmental factors indicates links between higher psychosis rates in neighborhoods with high proportions of households disadvantaged in terms of employment, education, health, and/or living environment (Essock, 2017). There is evidence that psychotic disorders are associated with indicators of social maladjustment such as single parent family or residential instability (van Os et al., 2010; van Os, Driessen, Gunther, & Delespaul, 2000). If individual social maladjustment factors differ significantly from the neighborhood environment, they will exacerbate the risk of psychotic disorders (van Os et al., 2000). In sum, it is acknowledged that although it is difficult to distinguish between environmental and individual risk factors that interact with each other and are associated with living in urban settings (Silva & Steffen, 2019), there is a significant body of research confirming the link between urbanicity and schizophrenia that requires further investigation.

To fully understand the rural–urban differences in schizophrenia risk, familial factors ought to be considered as variables that increase susceptibility to developing schizophrenia as urban environments do not increase risk of psychosis by default (Fett, Lemmers-Jansen, & Krabbendam, 2019). Despite the link between schizophrenia and urbanicity, little is known regarding the effect personal risk factors can have on this association, specifically familial liability to psychosis. Two studies revealed that family history of psychosis used as a proxy measure of genetic liability might be a missing element linking urbanicity and schizophrenia risk (van Os et al., 2003; van Os, Pedersen, & Mortensen, 2004). The environmental influences associated with growing up in an urban setting can interact with familial liability to psychosis and moderate the expression of schizophrenia symptomology. Moreover, further research implemented poor social and cognitive abilities as markers of genetic liability and were found to interact with levels of urbanicity on the expression of schizophrenia

(Weiser et al., 2007). However, the validity of the genetic markers is uncertain as familial mental illness history was not considered, nor was it specified the degree to which each component within social and cognitive dysfunction contributed to higher genetic vulnerability. To address previous shortcomings, recent work identified familial liability as the phenotypic correlation of psychotic symptoms between related individuals (Grech & van Os, 2017). Higher familial liability led to increased positive symptoms of schizophrenia for those individuals who had been raised in an urban environment as opposed to a non-urban setting. Grech and van Os (2017) revealed that the effect of family history on schizophrenia symptomology might be moderated by higher levels of urbanicity. However, the interaction of genetic liability, as measured by a polygenic risk score, and urbanicity is unclear as higher schizophrenia rates were found in both low and high urban areas (Gasse et al., 2019; Paksarian et al., 2018; Wimberley et al., 2016), after accounting for genetic liability. One possible explanation for lower rates of psychotic symptomology in urban areas compared to less urbanized areas is that former research (Paksarian et al., 2018) lacked direct measures on parents' genetic information or personality characteristics that would enable direct assessment of hypothesized mechanisms of gene–environment correlation. In spite of previous research, little is known about symptomatic manifestation of psychosis with respect to levels of urbanicity and familial liability. Smeets and colleagues (Smeets, Lataster, Viechtbauer, & Delespaul, 2015) revealed that familial psychosis, but not urban upbringing, was associated with the risk of delusions and hallucinations. Nonetheless, the influence of the interaction between familial liability and the level of urbanicity on symptomatic manifestation of psychosis has not been tested so far. In this study, we aim to investigate whether proxy genetic risk (defined as positive family history of schizophrenia in first- and second-degree relatives) and the level of urbanicity interact and influence the expression of auditory verbal hallucinations (AVH) in first-episode schizophrenia (FES) patients.

Method

We recruited 112 FES patients (59 males aged 25.00 ± 4.80 years and 53 females aged 29.24 ± 6.63 years). A diagnosis of schizophrenia was based on ICD-10 and DSM-IV criteria. The Operational Criteria for Psychotic Illness (OPCRIT) checklist was used to validate a diagnosis (McGuffin, Farmer, & Harvey, 1991). Lifetime occurrence of AVH was also assessed using OPCRIT, which recognizes following categories of AVH: thought echo, third person auditory hallucinations, running commentary voices, abusive/accusatory/persecutory voices and other (nonaffective) auditory hallucinations. Hallucinatory behavior on the day of recruitment was evaluated using the P3 item of the Positive and Negative Syndrome Scale (PANSS) (Kay, Fiszbein, & Opler, 1987). Patients were treated with the following antipsychotics: amisulpride (2 patients), haloperidol (20 patients), olanzapine (49 patients), quetiapine (1 patient), and risperidone (19 patients). There were 21 antipsychotic-naïve patients. The average treatment duration and chlorpromazine equivalent were 5.98 ± 4.41 days and 157.65 ± 117.85 mg/day, respectively. All patients were Caucasians, and the majority came from the same geographic area—Lower Silesia (Poland). Four patients came from other Polish regions. They did not migrate abroad for a considerable time period. Current place of residence and place of birth were recorded for all patients. Two levels of urbanicity were defined for place of birth and current place of residence: (1) low urbanicity—population density below 2000 people/km^2 and (2) high urbanicity—population density at least 2000 people/km^2. Analysis of covariance (ANCOVA) was used to test the effects of current place of residence together with family history of schizophrenia on total number of AVH categories and the PANSS P3 item score after co-varying for education, duration of untreated psychosis (DUP) and chlorpromazine equivalent. The study was approved by the Wroclaw Medical University Ethics Committee and all subjects gave an informed consent for participation.

Results

There was a significant effect of the interaction between family history of schizophrenia and current place of residence on total number of AVH categories ($F=4.41$, $p=0.038$) and the PANSS P3 item score ($F=4.21$, $p=0.042$) (Fig. 1). After excluding the patients who changed place of residence since birth date in terms of the level of urbanicity (34 patients), this effect remained significant with respect to total number of AVH categories ($F=5.23$, $p=0.025$) and PANSS P3 item score ($F=4.26$, $p=0.043$). The effects of chlorpromazine equivalent and DUP were not significant.

Discussion

In this preliminary study, results indicate urban living and familial liability interacted and influenced the number of AVH categories and the severity of hallucinations in FES patients. There was a main effect for patients who had a family history of

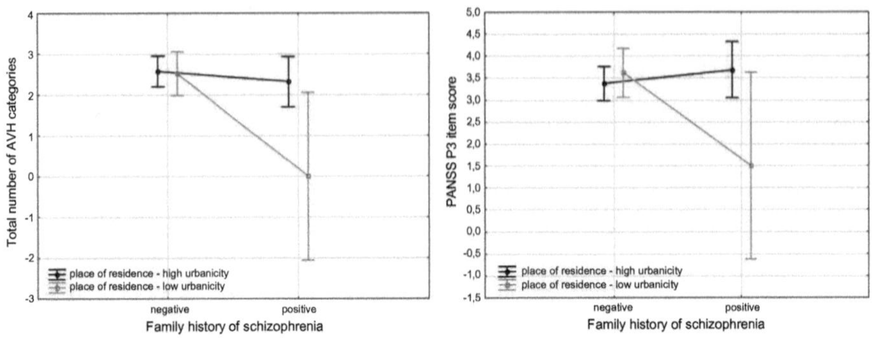

Fig. 1 The effect of interaction between family history of schizophrenia and the level of urbanicity on total number of AVH categories and PANSS P3 item score (hallucinatory behavior). Error bars represent 95%CI.

schizophrenia and lived in low urbanicity areas as they showed significantly less AVH symptomology and lower scores on behavioral hallucinations (PANSS) compared to individuals who lived in the same environment but had no family history. Furthermore, there was a significant interaction between urbanicity and family history on levels of AVH and PANSS as the decrease in psychotic symptomology from negative family history to positive family history was greater for those in low urbanicity areas than in high urbanicity areas. Finally, no main effect was found for individuals residing in high urbanicity areas as their psychosis phenotype did not change significantly as a function of family history of schizophrenia, indicating that the association between high urbanicity and schizophrenia risk was not confounded by genetic liability. Given that three categories of AVH assessed in this study (thought echo, running commentary voices and third person auditory hallucinations) are Schneiderian first-rank hallucinations, our results might be also perceived as a proxy support for studies showing that the interaction between low levels of urbanicity and family history of psychosis influence schizophrenia risk (van Os et al., 2003, 2004).

A significant interaction was found whereby the difference between negative family history and positive family history of schizophrenia was dictated by whether participants were in the high or low urbanicity environments. These findings depart from previous research (Paksarian et al., 2018) in that it tests whether urbanicity moderates the relationship between genetic liability to psychosis and positive symptomology. Urban upbringing may affect brain regions involved in stress processing including dorsolateral prefrontal cortex and perigenual anterior cingulate cortex (Haddad et al., 2015; Lederbogen et al., 2011), which can in turn increase the likelihood of developing schizophrenia. In addition, current city living has been associated with increased amygdala activity (Lederbogen et al., 2011), the brain region involved in the development of AVH (Escarti et al., 2010). Individual differences in stress reactivity are also dependent on corticotropin-releasing hormone (CRH) and the locus coeruleus-norepinephrine (LCN) (Boyce & Ellis, 2005) which are highly active in high stimuli environments and can result in hyper-vigilance and behavioral avoidance in schizophrenia patients. The findings would suggest individuals in high urbanicity develop a weaker neurosensory "gating" (Aron & Aron, 1997) system that does not allow them to attenuate auditory stimuli nor engage in prepulse inhibition, two intrinsic mechanisms that contribute to positive symptoms in schizophrenia. Improving sensory gating and regulation of stress responses has been associated with protective environments such as low urbanicity (Paksarian et al., 2018) as they are less exposed to auditory pollution and develop better auditory filters. This could explain the effect levels of urbanicity had on the relationship between genetic liability and positive symptomology. Further research should elucidate with more precision the particular characteristics of the current urban environment, as it has been shown that it can increase or decrease positive and negative symptoms according to the country of residence (Fett et al., 2019).

Genetic liability, as measured in the current study, does not appear to moderate the association between high urbanicity levels and schizophrenia symptomology (congruent with Paksarian et al., 2018). Previous research suggested that higher polygenic scores are associated with higher risk of schizophrenia (Agerbo et al., 2015), which the current findings support partially as behavioral hallucinations increased non-significantly when individuals had a history of schizophrenia in their family. Negative schematic beliefs and negative affect could have mediated the effects of urbanicity on hallucinatory behavior as paranoia can build upon negative beliefs about the self (Freeman et al., 2014). Meanwhile, AVH levels decreased (albeit not significantly). The high-risk environment triggered similar levels of auditory and behavioral hallucinations irrespective of genetic history when, based on previous research (Vassos et al., 2012), it was expected schizophrenia scores would increase concomitantly with high urbanicity. This leads to the possibility that that there are biopsychosocial factors that are protective against high reactivity to stressful situations in patients with schizophrenia. Phenomenological studies (Riches et al., 2018) of AVH suggest higher IQ is a protective factor against AVH in individuals who have a history of schizophrenia in their family. It was not the case that it reduced symptomology, but rather a more balanced emotional appraisal and greater control over AVH symptoms was found. Secondly, greater neighborhood cohesion characterized by trust between neighbors and shared values was predictive of a reduced psychotic experience (Riches et al., 2018; van Os et al., 2000). This might be indicative that intra and interpersonal factors mediate in the stabilization of auditory hallucinations for individuals in high-risk environments who have a genetic liability to developing schizophrenia.

The current findings indicate a significant decline in AVH and behavioral hallucinations when individuals live in low urbanicity areas and have a family history of schizophrenia. These findings might be counterintuitive as one would expect lower levels of psychotic symptoms in low urban areas and no family history (Fett et al., 2019). There appears to be incongruity between epidemiological heritability estimates based on previous studies (van Os et al., 2003, 2004) and the proportion of phenotypic expression of schizophrenia in subjects with a family history of psychosis. This may be a case of epigenetics regulating genomic activities such as cognition of AVH through covalent modifications of DNA and histones (Labrie, Pai, & Petronis, 2012). Positive environmental factors may impact epigenetic regulation of familial psychosis as families in tame visual and auditory environments learn the ability to manage positive symptoms through avoiding auditory pollution and maintaining familial cohesion (Daxinger & Whitelaw, 2012). Meanwhile, families without past history do not inherit epigenetic regulation of psychotic symptoms, thereby exhibiting higher levels of AVH and behavioral hallucinations. More research is needed to understand the protective properties of epigenetic regulation in schizophrenia under favorable conditions such as low urbanicity. Nonetheless, the current research suggests that having a history of schizophrenia increases resilience towards positive symptoms in low-risk environments.

Epigenetic factors might explain the adaptive function positive environments can have on the expression of schizophrenia. However, the underlying cognitive processes that facilitate a significant decrease in schizophrenia symptomology in low-urban areas, as found in the current study, is not yet explained. The Differential Susceptibility Hypothesis (DSH) (Belsky, 2005; Boyce & Ellis, 2005) posits that we ought to consider the developmental pathway of psychopathology by observing not only negative (Diathesis-Stress Model; Walker & Diforio, 1997), but also positive environments and their effect on symptomology. Long-term exposure (Fox & Beevers, 2016) to low-risk environments reduces negative attentional bias as potentially threatening stimuli (such as noise pollution or toxins) are less present, thereby reducing the frequency of stress reactivity and increasing sensitivity to protective stimuli such as low-frequency noise environments. Similarly, healthy environments foster adaptive voice hearers as they confront less stressful stimuli and thereby possess greater feeling of control over their experiences through the use of problem solving and distraction (Larøi, 2012). Inhibitory control and appraisal of content of AVH are suggested as possible cognitive and emotional mechanisms that aid in the control of hallucinations (Fett et al., 2019). Such protective mechanisms would be learnt and fostered in families who have a pre-disposition to psychosis and live in low-risk environments that contain less visual and auditory threats. In turn, this would result in better coping of positive symptoms in first-episode schizophrenia patients, as found in the current study. Despite the current explanations, further research is required to understand how epigenetic factors can foster protective mechanisms in families with a history of psychosis, and how this relationship can be moderated by urban and non-urban environments (DSH model).

Some important limitations should be addressed in studies replicating our findings: low sample size, cross-sectional study design and the lack of more detailed assessment of urbanicity. Indeed, we did not collect the data indicating a time point, when the patients changed place of residence. However, the exclusion of this group of patients did not change considerably our results. Importantly, one study has shown that even short exposition to city stress in a busy urban area (and not actually living there) may increase the level of hallucinations in patients with current persecutory delusions (Freeman et al., 2014). In addition, Freeman et al. (2014) found that some of the patients have reported a fear of going outside. Future research should investigate how urban environment also exacerbate psychotic symptoms, and how these relate to family history of schizophrenia.

While there is an ongoing quest to understand the GxE interaction effect on the expression of schizophrenia symptoms, new therapeutic approaches are being developed to enhance patients' wellbeing in urban areas. Current proposals do not yet integrate the role genetic liability can play in moderating the effect urbanicity has on patients with schizophrenia symptomology. This is due mainly to a lack of consensus on the degree to which genetic liability is responsible for the variance found in schizophrenia symptomology as a function of living in urban and nonurban environments. Notwithstanding, in order to achieve an effective treatment, an understanding of how patients with schizophrenia experience stress in an urban environment is required. Urban remediation (Baumann et al., 2020; Södeström, 2019; Södeström et al., 2016; Södeström, Södeström, Codeluppi, Empsom, & Conus, 2017) posits that schizophrenia patients have three sources of possible stress: the built environment, the social interactions occurring within that environment, and the mobility of the subject within its environment. Within a concept where schizophrenia is a multifactorial disorder (Baumann et al., 2020), there are indicators that higher demographic density is associated with lower rates of treatment resistant schizophrenia, which suggests urban psychosis may be a form of psychosis more responsive to treatment (Wimberley et al., 2016). To this end, urban remediation suggests three steps in reducing stress in patients with first-episode schizophrenia. First, creating adapted housing in which the individual feels secure in order to create a safe from which to explore a city. Second, increase contact with restorative places such as green places, areas of positive social interaction (Nanda, Eisen, Zadeh, & Owen, 2011), public places with art and engaging in activities that avoid overcrowded and noisy places. Third, planning and regulating trajectories in the city in order decrease potential crowded areas and thereby render urban environments more predictable. These three steps would assist patients with auditory hallucinations to be less prone to paranoiac ideation and protect against active social withdrawal (Baumann et al., 2020). Furthermore, urban remediation posits that strengthening cognitive resources such as spatial navigation (route planning), selective attention, as well as providing go-along therapy (i.e., patient accompanied by a person of their choice) are strategies that increase urban self-efficacy in first-episode schizophrenia patients. Increased metacognition is also promoted as it is argued to facilitate re-examination of cognitive problems experienced by the person and promotes more awareness and better understanding of these deficits (Tsapekos, Taylor, & Cella, 2017). Despite the potential benefits of urban remediation, more research is required to establish its efficacy in different urban environments.

Neurourbanism (Adli et al., 2017) aims to bring neuroscience conceptually and methodologically out of the lab and focus on fieldwork that can yield insights into how to envisage the urban milieu as a nexus of possible sites of recovery for first-episode patients with psychotic disorders. The conceptual framework draws upon the geographies of mental health- experiencing the city as a relation between social interaction, built environment and mobility. Compared to urban remediation, neurourbanism emphasizes a mixed-method approach that includes video-recorded go-along video-elicitation interviews, focus groups with care workers and surveys with large groups of first-episode schizophrenia patients. This new perspective aims to create an inter-disciplinary approach that incorporates neurobiological and social research in order to characterize the urban stressors and their modulators, as well as identifying high-risk populations. This new framework is still developing as an academic discipline and therefore, further case-studies are required to explore the validity of this biopsychological approach in the context of psychosis-spectrum disorders. Taken together, the proposed urban remediation therapies provide first-episode schizophrenia patients with metacognitve competencies to navigate urban settings, albeit further research is required across different mental health conditions in order to establish their reliability as efficacious treatments.

Acknowledgments

B.M. conducted the experiments, performed the literature search, and analyzed the data.
All authors performed the literature search, and wrote the paper, and all authors contributed to the final version of the manuscript.

References

Adli, M., Berger, M., Brakemeier, E. L., Engel, L., Fingerhut, J., Gomez-Carrillo, A., ... Stollman, J. (2017). Neurourbanism: Towards a new discipline. *The Lancet Psychiatry*, *4*(3), 183–185.

Agerbo, E., Sullivan, P. F., Vihjalmsson, B. J., Pederson, C. B., Mors, O., Borgium, A. D., ... Mortensen, P. B. (2015). Polygenic risk score, parental socioeconomic status, family history of psychiatric disorders, and the risk for schizophrenia: A Danish population-based study and meta-analysis. *JAMA Psychiatry*, *72*(7), 635–641.

Aron, E. N., & Aron, A. (1997). Sensory-processing sensitivity and its relation to introversion and emotionality. *Journal of Personality and Social Psychology*, *73*, 345–368.

Baumann, P. S., Södeström, O., Empson, L. A., Södeström, D., Codeluppi, Z., Golay, P., ... Conus, P. (2020). Urban remediation: A new recovery-oriented strategy to manage urban stress after first-episode psychosis. *Social Psychiatry and Psychiatric Epidemiology*, *55*, 273–283.

Belsky, J. (2005). Differential susceptibility to rearing influences: An evolutionary hypothesis and some evidence. In B. Ellis, & D. Bjorklund (Eds.), *Origins of the social mind: Evolutionary psychology and child development* (pp. 139–163). New York: Guilford.

Boyce, W. T., & Ellis, B. J. (2005). Biological sensitivity to context: I. An evolutionary-developmental theory of the origins and functions of stress reactivity. *Development and Psychopathology*, *17*, 271–301.

Daxinger, L., & Whitelaw, E. (2012). Understanding transgenerational epigenetic inheritance via the gametes in mammals. *Nature Reviews. Genetics*, *13*(3), 153–162.

DeVylder, J. E., Kelleher, I., Lalane, M., Oh, H., Link, B. G., & Koyanagi, A. (2018). Association of urbanicity with psychosis in low- and middle-income countries. *JAMA Psychiatry*, *75*(7), 678–686.

Escarti, M. J., de la Iglesia-Vaya, M., Marti-Bonmati, L., Robles, M., Carbonell, J., Lull, J. J., ... Sanjuan, J. (2010). Increased amygdala and parahippocampal gyrus activation in schizophrenic patients with auditory hallucinations: An fMRI study using independent component analysis. *Schizophrenia Research*, *117*(1), 31–41.

Essock, S. M. (2017). When social and environmental adversity causes schizophrenia. *American Journal of Psychiatry*, *174*(2), 89–90.

Fan, C. C., McGrath, J. J., Appadurai, V., Buil, A., Gandal, M. J., Schork, A. J., ... Pedersen, C. B. (2018). Spatial fine-mapping for gene-by-environment effects identifies risk hot spots for schizophrenia. *Nature Communications*, *9*, 5296.

Fett, A. K., Lemmers-Jansen, I. M. J., & Krabbendam, L. (2019). Psychosis and urbanicity: A review of the recent literature from epidemiology to neurourbanism. *Current Opinion in Psychiatry*, *32*(3), 232–241.

Fox, E., & Beevers, C. G. (2016). Differential sensitivity to the environment: Contribution of cognitive biases and genes to psychological wellbeing. *Molecular Psychiatry*, *12*, 1657–1662.

Freeman, D., Emsley, R., Dunn, G., Fowler, D., Bebbington, P., Kuipers, E., ... Garety, P. (2014). The stress of the street for patients with persecutory delusions: A test of the symptomatic and psychological effects of going outside into a busy urban area. *Schizophrenia Bulletin*, *41*(4), 971–979.

Gasse, C., Wimberley, T., Wang, Y., Mors, O., Borglum, A., Als, T. D., ... Horsdal, H. T. (2019). Schizophrenia polygenic risk scores, urbanicity and treatment-resistant schizophrenia. *Schizophrenia Research*, *212*, 79–85.

Grech, A., & van Os, J. (2017). Evidence that the urban environment moderates the level of familial clustering of positive psychotic symptoms. *Schizophrenia Bulletin*, *43*(2), 325–331.

Haddad, L., Schafer, A., Streit, F., Lederbogen, F., Grimm, O., Wust, S., … Meyer-Lindenberg, A. (2015). Brain structure correlates of urban upbringing, an environmental risk factor for schizophrenia. *Schizophrenia Bulletin*, *41*(1), 115–122.

He, P., Chen, G., Guo, C., Wen, X., Song, X., & Zheng, X. (2018). Long-term effect of prenatal exposure to malnutrition on risk of schizophrenia in adulthood: Evidence from the Chinese famine of 1959-1961. *European Psychiatry: The Journal of the Association of European Psychiatrists*, *51*, 42–47.

Jongsma, H. E., Gayer-Anderson, C., Lasalvia, A., Quattrone, D., Mulè, A., Szöke, A., … Kirkbride, J. B. (2018). Treated incidence of psychotic disorders in the multinational EU-GEI study. *JAMA Psychiatry*, *75*(1), 36–46.

Kay, S. R., Fiszbein, A., & Opler, L. A. (1987). The positive and negative syndrome scale (PANSS) for schizophrenia. *Schizophrenia Bulletin*, *13*(2), 261–276.

Kirkbride, J. B., Hameed, Y., Ioannidis, K., Ankireddypalli, G., Crane, C. M., Nasir, M., … Jones, P. B. (2017). Ethnic minority status, age-at-immigration and psychosis risk in rural environments: Evidence from the SEPEA study. *Schizophrenia Bulletin*, *43*(6), 1251–1261.

Krabbendam, L., & van Os, J. (2005). Schizophrenia and urbanicity: A major environmental influence-conditional on genetic risk. *Schizophrenia Bulletin*, *31*(4), 795–799.

Labrie, V., Pai, S., & Petronis, A. (2012). Epigenetics of major psychosis: Progress, problems, and perspectives. *Trends in Genetics*, *28*(9), 427–435.

Larøi, F. (2012). How do auditory verbal hallucinations in patients differ fomr those in non-patients? *Frontiers in Human Neuroscience*, *6*, 25.

Lederbogen, F., Kirsch, P., Haddad, L., Streit, F., Tost, H., Schuch, P., … Meyer-Lindenberg, A. (2011). City living and urban upbringing affect neural social stress processing in humans. *Nature*, *474*(7352), 498–501.

Luo, Y., Pang, L., Guo, C., Zhang, L., & Zheng, X. (2020). Association of urbanicity with schizophrenia and related mortality in China: Association de l'urbanicite avec la schizophrenie et la mortalite qui y est reliee en Chine. *Canadian Journal of Psychiatry*. https://doi.org/10.1177/0706743720954059.

March, D., Hatch, S. L., Morgan, C., Kirkbride, J. B., Bresnahan, M., Fearon, P., & Susser, E. (2008). Psychosis and place. *Epidemiologic Reviews*, *30*, 84–100.

McGuffin, P., Farmer, A., & Harvey, I. (1991). A polydiagnostic application of operational criteria in studies of psychotic illness. Development and reliability of the OPCRIT system. *Archives of General Psychiatry*, *48*(8), 764–770.

Nanda, U., Eisen, S., Zadeh, R. S., & Owen, D. (2011). Effect of visual art on patient anxiety and agitation in a mental health facility and implications for the business case. *Journal of Psychiatric and Mental Health Nursing*, *18*(5), 386–393.

Paksarian, D., Trabjerg, B. B., Merikangas, K. R., Mors, O., Borglum, A. D., Haugaard, D. M., … Agerbo, E. (2018). The role of genetic liability in the association of urbanicity at birth and during upbringing with schizphrenia in Denmark. *Psychological Medicine*, *48*(2), 305–315.

Engemann, K., Pedersen, C. B., Arge, L., Tsirogiannis, C., Mortensen, P. B., & Svenning, J. C. (2019). Residential green space in childhood is associated with lower risk of psychiatric disorders from adolescence into adulthood. *Proceedings of the National Academy of Sciences of the United States of America*, *116*(11), 5188–5193.

Riches, S., Arseneault, L., Bagher-Niakan, R., Alsultan, M., Crush, E., & Fisher, H. L. (2018). Protective factors for early psychotic phenomena among children of mothers with psychosis. *Frontiers in Psychology*, *9*, 750.

Schofield, P., Thygesen, M., Das-Munshi, J., Becares, L., Cantor-Graae, E., Pedersen, C., & Agerbo, E. (2017). Ethnic density, urbanicity and psychosis risk for migrant groups—A population cohort. *Schizophrenia Research*, *190*, 82–87.

Silva, C. E. J. A., & Steffen, R. E. (2019). Urban environment and psychiatry disorders: A review of the neuroscience and biology. *Metabolism, Clinical and Experimental*, *100*, 153940.

Smeets, F., Lataster, T., Viechtbauer, W., & Delespaul, P. (2015). Evidence that environmental and genetic risks for psychotic disorder may operate by impacting on connections between core symptoms of perceptual alteration and delusional ideation. *Schizophrenia Bulletin*, *41*(3), 687–697.

Södeström, O. (2019). Precarious encounters with urban life: The city/psychosis nexus beyond epidemiology and social constructivism. *Geoforum*, *101*, 80–89.

Södeström, O., Empsom, L. A., Codeluppi, Z., Södeström, D., Baumann, P. S., & Conus, P. (2016). Unpacking 'the City': An experience-based approach to the role of urban living in psychosis. *Health & Place*, *42*, 104–110.

Södeström, O., Södeström, D., Codeluppi, Z., Empsom, L. A., & Conus, P. (2017). Emplacing recovery: How persons diagnosed with psychosis handle stress in cities. *Psychosis: Psychological, Social and Integrative Approaches*, *9*(4), 322–329.

The United Nations. (2018). *Department of Economic and Social Affairs web site*. May 16 https://www.un.org/development/desa/en/news/population/2018-revision-of-world-urbanization-prospects.html.

Tsapekos, D., Taylor, R., & Cella, M. (2017). Feasibility and acceptability of brief cognitive remediation targeting metacognition in acute inpatients with psychosis: A case series. *Neuropsychological Rehabilitation*, *29*(3), 361–375.

van Os, J., Driessen, G., Gunther, N., & Delespaul, P. (2000). Neighbourhood variation in incidence of schizophrenia. Evidence for person-environment interaction. *The British Journal of Psychiatry: the Journal of Mental Science*, *176*, 243–248.

van Os, J., Hanssen, M., Bak, M., Bijl, R. V., & Vollebergh, W. (2003). Do urbanicity and familial liability coparticipate in causing psychosis? *The American Journal of Psychiatry*, *160*(3), 477–482.

van Os, J., Kenis, G., & Rutten, B. P. (2010). The environment and schizophrenia. *Nature*, *468*(7321), 203–212.

van Os, J., Pedersen, C. B., & Mortensen, P. B. (2004). Confirmation of synergy between urbanicity and familial liability in the causation of psychosis. *The American Journal of Psychiatry*, *161*(12), 2312–2314.

Vassos, E., Pedersen, C. B., Murray, R. M., Collier, D. A., & Lewis, C. M. (2012). Meta-analysis of the association of urbanicity with schizophrenia. *Schizophrenia Bulletin*, *38*(6), 1118–1123.

Vlahov, D., & Galea, S. (2002). Urbanization, urbanicity, and health. *Journal of Urban Health: Bulletin of the New York Academy of Medicine*, *79*(4 Suppl 1), S1–S12.

Walker, E. F., & Diforio, D. (1997). Schizophrenia: A neural diathesis-stress model. *Psychological Review*, *104*(4), 667–685.

Weiser, M., van Os, J., Reichenberg, A., Rabinowitz, J., Nahon, D., Kravitz, E., … Davidson, M. (2007). Social and cognitive functioning, urbanicity and risk of schizophrenia. *The British Journal of Psychiatry: the Journal of Mental Science*, *191*, 320–324.

Wimberley, T., Pedersen, C. B., MacCabe, J. H., Stovring, H., Astrup, A., Sorensen, H. J., … Gasse, C. (2016). Inverse association between urbanicity and treatment resistance in schizophrenia. *Schizophrenia Research*, *174*, 150–155.

Sexual dysfunctions in male schizophrenia patients

7

Ahmed A. Moustafa[a,b], *Belinda Favaloro*[c], *Doaa H. Hewedi*[d], *Nagla N. El Mahallawy*[d], *and Hossam ElKhatib*[e]
[a]School of Psychology & Marcs Institute for Brain and Behaviour, Western Sydney University, Sydney, NSW, Australia, [b]Department of Human Anatomy and Physiology, the Faculty of Health Sciences, University of Johannesburg, South Africa, [c]School of Psychology, University of Western Sydney, Sydney, NSW, Australia, [d]Institute of Psychiatry, Faculty of Medicine, Ain Shams University, Cairo, Egypt, [e]Misr International University, Cairo, Egypt

Chapter outline

Introduction

Sexual dysfunction is prevalent in patients with mental illnesses, especially in patients with schizophrenia (Zhao et al., 2020). Epidemiological and clinical studies show that many patients with schizophrenia suffer from impairments in sexual functioning, with erectile dysfunction being prevalent in men and loss of libido the most frequent in women (Dumontaud et al., 2020). Psychiatric patients between 35 and 64 years old often have higher rates of sexual dysfunction than patients between 18 and 34 years old. Illness severity, depressive symptomology and antipsychotics have been identified as risk factors for the development of sexual dysfunction in schizophrenia (Dumontaud et al., 2020).

Most antipsychotic drugs used to treat schizophrenia have adverse sexual side effects, but it is difficult to identify if the impairment in the patients' sexual functioning can be attributed to their clinical diagnosis or to pharmacological treatments. Patients with schizophrenia often have underlying hormonal disturbances that may contribute to sexual disturbances that occur (Kelly & Conley, 2004). The age of onset of schizophrenia typically occurs around the reproductive period, which is when the secretion of luteinizing hormones increase. Luteinizing hormones are produced and released

Cognitive and Behavioral Dysfunction in Schizophrenia. https://doi.org/10.1016/B978-0-12-820005-6.00002-5

in the anterior pituitary gland and are important for ensuring a healthy reproductive system. These hormones have a role in controlling the function of ovaries in females and testicles in males. Lower levels of luteinizing hormones, including estrogen for females and testosterone for males, have been reported in schizophrenia patients when compared to healthy normal controls (Oades & Schepker, 1994; Van Cauter et al., 1991). There is a significant inverse correlation between negative symptomology and levels of testosterone in schizophrenia patients (Brzezinski-Sinai & Brzezinski, 2020), and lower levels of testosterone is linked to increased risk of sexual dysfunction among males (Kruljac et al., 2020). Lower estrogen levels have been correlated with sexual dysfunction in females (Kelly & Conley, 2004). Therefore, an association between reproductive hormone levels and sexual functioning may be a contributing factor to rates of sexual dysfunction in psychiatric patients.

The negative symptoms of schizophrenia, such as lack of interest and anhedonia, may also contribute to limiting the capacity for interpersonal and sexual relationships. Male patients with schizophrenia appear to have more negative symptoms than female patients (Wei, Chen, Ma, Xiu, & Zhang, 2020); this may be associated with an inverse correlation between negative symptomology and testosterone levels. Huang et al. (2019) identified an association between negative symptoms and sexual dysfunction in Chinese patients with schizophrenia, and a study from Europe found that negative symptoms of schizophrenia predicted decreased libido (Malik et al., 2011). Despite there being some evidence for an association between schizophrenia and sexual dysfunction, there are still inconsistencies in the research and results have been attributed to other factors, such as the effect of antipsychotics (Brzezinski-Sinai & Brzezinski, 2020). In addition, although some sexual dysfunction may be present due to the psychopathology, psychotropic medications used for treatment of schizophrenia tend to exacerbate these sexual dysfunctions (Zemishlany & Weizman, 2008).

Antipsychotics are the first line of treatment for the symptoms of schizophrenia, and they ameliorate positive, and to a lower extent negative symptoms of schizophrenia by acting on the dopamine receptor system (Lodha & Sousa, 2020). Many studies have reported an association between antipsychotic medications and problems with libido, arousal, and orgasm in patients with schizophrenia (Zemishlany & Weizman, 2008). Sexual dysfunction as a side effect associated with the use of psychotropic treatments, that is, treatment-emergent sexual dysfunction, is an important issue that needs attention in clinical treatment. Schizophrenia patients undergoing pharmacological treatment showed significantly more sexual dysfunctions than those who are unmedicated (Bains & Shah, 2012). Current research suggests that adverse sexual effects are frequent with prescribed psychotropic drugs, specifically erectile dysfunction in men with antipsychotics (Kelly & Conley, 2004). Erectile dysfunction is an arousal-related disorder defined as a consistent or recurrent inability of a man to attain and/or maintain penile erection sufficient for sexual activity. Diminished libido and decreased orgasm quality are also commonly reported in both men and women (Kelly & Conley, 2004). Some of the possible mechanisms underlying sexual dysfunction during antipsychotic therapy may involve lack of sexual interest due to sedation and weight gain, extrapyramidal side effects, tardive dyskinesia that may reduce mobility or elevated prolactin levels (Kelly & Conley, 2004).

It is believed that sexual dysfunction from psychotropic treatment is due to hyperprolactinemia resulting from the blockage of dopaminergic D2 receptors in the pituitary tuberoinfundibular pathway (Zhang et al., 2018). Hyperprolactinemia is increased levels of prolactin, which is a hormone produced by the pituitary gland in the brain. Many commonly used antipsychotics, including risperidone, amisulpride, and paliperidone may result in hyperprolactinemia. Antipsychotic medications such as quetiapine and aripiprazole are known to cause less sexual dysfunction due to having a smaller effect on prolactin (Zhang et al., 2018). A Cochrane review of randomized controlled trials involving schizophrenia patients with sexual dysfunction found sildenafil had beneficial effects in improving sexual dysfunction compared with placebo, and also use of olanzapine or quetiapine as treatment may have a positive impact on sexual functioning (Montejo, Montejo, & Baldwin, 2018). Therefore, antipsychotic medications may be interacting with specific sex hormones to contribute to sexual dysfunction; however, these mechanisms require further investigation (Zhang et al., 2018).

Understanding the association between psychotropic medication and sexual dysfunction in schizophrenia is crucial as it appears to impact treatment adherence of schizophrenia patients. Whilst this type of treatment is effective in up to 80% of schizophrenia patients, approximately 50% of patients do not adhere to their treatment. Various studies have shown that nonadherence rates can range from 37% to 74%, which then results in increased hospitalizations and resource usage (Goldstone, 2020). Nonadherence to antipsychotic treatment in schizophrenia is likely to result in an increase in the frequency of relapse, longer hospital admissions and increased symptoms severity, which can often lead to more utilization of health care resources (Dilla, Ciudad, & Alvarez, 2013). Sexual side effects may be a contributing factor to treatment noncompliance. Among patients with schizophrenia, 42% of men and 15% of women stopped taking their antipsychotic medication due to sexual dysfunction (Rosenberg, Bleiberg, Koscis, & Gross, 2003). Many young patients with schizophrenia drop out of pharmacological treatment due to the onset of sexual dysfunction, especially problems with erectile functioning, orgasm, and loss of desire (Montejo et al., 2018). Several studies have shown that schizophrenia patients are more concerned with the sexual side effects of antipsychotic medications than any other side effect. The National Schizophrenia Fellowship confirmed this increased concern with sexual side effects, through a survey of over 2000 mental health service users, which portrayed that a large proportion of the survey respondents had experienced side effects from their antipsychotic medication and that these sexual side effects were deemed to be the most troublesome (Smith & Henderson, 2000). Here, we argue that the investigation and management of these side effects is required as a part of treating psychiatric illnesses.

Sexual dysfunction in schizophrenia also tends to be under-reported, possibly due to shame, cultural difficulties or lack of questioning by health providers. The lack of adequate discussion about sexual functioning in standard clinical practice is rather common, affecting 50%–73% of those with sexual dysfunction (Montejo et al., 2010). Not only is enquiring into sexual problems with clients often avoided, but failure to inform patients of the possible sexual side effects is common due to shame and incompetence, especially in some conservative cultures (Souaiby, Kazour, Zoghbi, Bou Khalil, & Richa, 2019). Importantly, communication with a practicing clinician or psychiatrist is positively correlated with treatment adherence (Goldstone, 2020). Prior research highlights the need to examine, understand, and communicate on sexual dysfunction in schizophrenia patients, in order to increase clinician competence and hopefully reduce the shame around discussing sexual dysfunction in schizophrenia patients.

Research on antipsychotics and sexual dysfunction in schizophrenia is still limited and it is unclear whether systematic differences occurring through the measurement process have impacted rates of sexual dysfunction associated with specific drugs. Variability in rates of sexual dysfunction among schizophrenia patients may be affected by how sexual dysfunction is measured; subjective reports may result in more clinical variability (Waldinger, Zwinderman, Schweitzer, & Olivier, 2004). It can be difficult to attribute sexual dysfunctions in schizophrenia patients to the drugs themselves or to differences in methods of inquiry and difference patient samples (e.g., inclusion/exclusion of patients with mild sexual disorders, demographics) (Lodha & Sousa, 2020). Further systematic enquiries are needed to determine the incidence and severity of sexual dysfunction induced by various psychotropic treatments, including antipsychotics (Baggaley, 2008).

In addition, other factors such as substance use, negative or depressive symptoms and comorbidity with physical illness, may also contribute to sexual dysfunction and other related disorders in schizophrenia patients (for discussion, see Moustafa et al., 2017; Moustafa, Weickert, & Frydecka, 2016; Moustafa et al., 2016). The complexity of sexual dysfunction in schizophrenia emphasizes the need for further research to be done in this area, in order to improve clinical practice. Treatment-emergent sexual dysfunction may reduce the quality of an individual's life, impact relationship satisfaction and impact their adherence to treatment (Souaiby et al., 2019). Improved sexual functioning in patients with schizophrenia is associated with improvements in overall quality of life (Fanta, Haile, Abebaw, Assefa, & Hibdye, 2018). Since there are many contributing factors to sexual dysfunction, a biopsychosocial model of sexual dysfunction provides a compelling argument for combination treatment that integrates psychosocial interventions and pharmaceuticals. Although more research is needed, it seems probable that combination therapy will be the treatment of choice for sexual dysfunction, as new pharmaceuticals are developed for problems with desire, arousal, and orgasm in men (Lee, Surridge, Morales, & Heaton, 2000).

The relationship between sexual functioning and psychotropic medication requires further investigation. This is an important topic for clinical treatment as compared to many side effects of antipsychotic treatment, sexual side effects are reportedly the most distressing and impact schizophrenia patients' adherence to treatment. Treatment compliance results in improved outcomes and increased quality of life (Goldstone, 2020). The aim of this study is to address the association between sexual dysfunction and different types of psychotropic treatments for schizophrenia, in order to improve treatment outcome in clinical practice.

Methods

Participants

This is a cross-sectional study conducted at the General Psychiatric Clinic—Institute of Psychiatry at Ain Shams University, Cairo, Egypt, on male patients between ages 18 and 60 years old diagnosed with schizophrenia-related disorders. This age range was selected to avoid the effect of aging on sexual function. Participants recruited were those that attended the general psychiatric clinic seeking mental health services between December 2010 and June 2013. Those who were excluded from the study included males outside the aforementioned age group, females, geriatric, and child patients.

Procedure

Participants were told the rationale of the study, confidentiality and informed of their rights, including the right to withdraw from the study at any time without consequences. A pilot study was conducted on 80 cases to obtain preliminary data that assisted in assessing the applicability and reliability of the Sexual Behavior Questionnaire (SBQ). This was to inform any necessary modifications required for the measure to suit our participant demographics.

All patients were administered a psychiatric interview using the Psychiatric Sheet of the Institute of Psychiatry, Faculty of Medicine, Ain Shams University, with particular interest on sexual history, marital history, religious history, diagnosis, and current treatment received by patients (drugs, Electro-Convulsive Therapy, among other treatments). They were also administered the ICD-10 Symptom Checklist for Mental Disorders (Janca & Hiller, 1996) to assess symptoms according to ICD-10 classification. In addition to these, the male version of the Sexual Behavior Questionnaire (Macdonald et al., 2003) translated to Arabic was applied. The Sexual Behavior Questionnaire is a self-reported gender specific questionnaire designed to assess sexual dysfunction. The male version contains 11 questions, which cover four areas of sexual functioning: desire, arousal, performance, and satisfaction.

For patients who were married, marital satisfaction was assessed by using the Arabic version of the Marital Satisfaction Inventory, which is modified from Marital Satisfaction Inventory (MSI; Snyder, 1981). Married patients who were susceptible to having erectile dysfunction, identified by answering either number 1 or 2 on the Sexual Behavior Questionnaire, were subjected to the International Index of Erectile Function (IIEF-15) Arabic version (Alzohiery, 2011).

The wives of the married patients were given the Arabic version of the Marital Satisfaction Inventory as well as the Woman Abuse Scale (WAS), which was modified from the Woman Abuse Scale. Qualitative data were described using frequency and percentage while quantitative data was described using mean and standard deviation. A Chi-square test (Chi 2) was used to compare categorical variables and a Pearson Correlation was used to compare continuous variables.

Results

Of the 214 patients, 53.8% falling within the range of 18–28 years old and 38.5% falling between 29 and 38 years old. Fifty-two of the patients were on typical antipsychotics, 64 were on atypical antipsychotics, 93 were on mixed treatments in the form of antipsychotics, mood stabilizers, and/or antidepressants, and 5 patients were on other forms of treatments such as hypnotics and anti-epileptics. Many of the patients were smokers (61.1%). The most common level of education was high school level and 50.5% of the patients were employed, mainly in the technical sector. Totally, 175 of the patients had single relationship status while 39 patients were married, only 19 of the 39 married patients agreed to complete the Arabic version of the Marital Satisfaction Inventory.

Statistical analyses showed significant differences between patients suffering from schizophrenia and their experience of orgasm ($p=0.04$), sexual satisfaction ($p=0.05$), sexual enjoyment ($p=0.005$), ability to maintain an erection ($p=0.006$), and erection ($p=0.01$) measured by the Sexual Behavior Questionnaire. There was a significant negative correlation between sexual enjoyment and age of patients ($p=0.04$, $r=-0.76$). Sexual excitement and delayed ejaculation had significant correlations with smoking ($p=0.05$, $r=-0.73$; $p=0.01$, $r=0.69$, respectively). Table 1 provides further details of these results. When examining the association between treatment and

Table 1 Comparison of Sexual Behavior Questionnaire items in psychotic patients (***n***=214) and their experience of sexual functioning.

Item	Dysfunction		No Dysfunction		χ2 test (*p*-value)
	No.	%	No.	%	
Orgasm	96	44.9	118	55.1	0.04
Sexual satisfaction	77	36	137	64	0.05
Premature ejaculation	70	32.7	144	67.3	>0.05
Sexual desire frequency	70	32.7	144	67.3	>0.05
Sexual enjoyment	154	71.9	60	28.1	0.005
Sexual excitement	57	26.6	157	73.4	>0.05
Delayed ejaculation	20	9.3	194	90.7	>0.05
Ability to maintain erection	27	12.6	187	87.4	0.006
Erection	189	88.3	25	11.7	0.01
Sexual intercourse	155	72.4	59	27.6	>0.05
Masturbation	84	39.3	130	60.7	>0.05

Table 2 Results of Sexual Behavior Questionnaire in schizophrenia patients in relation to drug treatment type. "Others" represent anti-epileptic drugs.

	Satisfied	Dissatisfied	Total	*p*-value	Sig
Typical antipsychotic	31	**21**	**52**	0.05	Sig
Atypical antipsychotic	44	20	64	0.1	NS
Sedatives hypnotics	1	1	2	0.23	NS
SSRI	0	1	1	0.41	NS
Others	1	1	2	0.07	NS
Mixed	60	**33**	**93**	0.002	Sig
Total	137	77	214		

satisfaction of sexual life, only those who were receiving mixed treatment and those on typical antipsychotics, showed a significant association with dissatisfaction in their sexual life. These results are represented in Table 2.

Results investigating sexual dysfunction in married males who completed the MSI, showed that patients were significantly dissatisfied with their sexual life in their marriage, with 50% of them being dissatisfied due to side effects of medication ($p=0.05$). A total of 16 out of 19 wives answered both questionnaires provided, 2 wives refused to participate and 1 did not come with her husband in his follow-up sessions. Table 3 shows significant differences between the patients physically ($p=0.03$), sexually ($p=0.02$), and psychologically ($p=0.005$) abusing their wives. Analyses of the responses from the Women Abuse Scale in relation to drug treatment showed significant differences between the 31% and 33% ($n=4$) of patients who received mixed treatment are being physically and sexually abusing their wives, respectively. 40% ($n=6$) of the same group are psychologically abusing their wives ($p=0.05$).

Positive correlations were found between mixed drug treatment and mild erectile dysfunction ($p=0.0005$, $r=0.87$), and sudden onset of erectile function ($p=0.01$, $r=0.081$). A positive correlation was also found between receiving typical antipsychotic and mild erectile dysfunctions ($p=0.05$, $r=0.77$). Correlations between receiving typical antipsychotics and sudden onset of erectile function, and between receiving

Table 3 Number of patients abusing their wives and the different types of abuse occurring.

No abuse		Abuse		Total	*p* value
Physical abuse					
3	18.8%	13	81.2%	16	0.03
Sexual abuse					
4	25%	12	75%	16	0.02
Psychological abuse					
1	6.3%	15	93.7%	16	0.005

Table 4 Comparison of erectile function in the International Index of Erectile Function (IIEF).

Erectile function						
No dysfunction		**Mild dysfunction**		**Moderate dysfunction**		**Fisher's exact test (*p*-value)**
No.	**%**	**No.**	**%**	**No.**	**%**	
2	8%	**15**	**60%**	8	32%	0.05
Onset of erectile dysfunction						
Sudden onset		**Gradual onset**		**No dysfunction**		**Fisher's exact test (*p*-value)**
No.	**%**	**No.**	**%**	**No.**	**%**	
14	**56%**	8	32%	3	12%	0.02
Situation under which erectile dysfunction occur						
With partner only		**Under all circumstances**		**No dysfunction**		**Fisher's exact test (*p*-value)**
No.	**%**	**No.**	**%**	**No.**	**%**	
12	48%	8	32%	5	20%	0.04
Morning erection						
Absent			**Present**			**Fisher's exact test (*p*-value)**
No.	**%**		**No.**	**%**		
4	16.0%		**21**	**84.0%**		0.05

atypical antipsychotics and mild erectile dysfunctions and sudden onset of erectile function were not significant.

Table 4 shows significant differences found in patients with mild erectile dysfunction, sudden onset of erectile dysfunction, erectile dysfunction, with their partner only and presence of morning erection ($p=0.05$, 0.02, 0.04, and 0.05, respectively). Table 5 portrays significant differences between different types of erectile dysfunction and sexual dissatisfaction. As well as a significant association between erectile dysfunction and dissatisfaction with the time spent with their wives. Finally, a statistical significance was also found between patients with mild erectile dysfunction and their dissatisfaction with their financial issues ($p=0.04$).

Discussion

In the present study, most patients fell within the age range of 18–28 (51.8%) or between 29 and 38 years old (40.5%). This highlights the common age range of psychiatric illness presentations in Egypt. Our patients with schizophrenia reported problems with the experience of orgasm, sexual satisfaction, sexual enjoyment, and ability to maintain or achieve an erection. These problems were similarly reported as the most

Table 5 Correlation of sexual dissatisfaction and erectile function.

Erection	Condition	Sexual dissatisfaction		Total	Fisher's exact test (*p*-value)
		Satisfied	Dissatisfied		
		N	N		
Erectile function (IIEF)	No dysfunction	1	1	2	0.05
	Mild dysfunction	2	**13**	15	
	Moderate dysfunction	3	5	8	
	Severe dysfunction	0	0	0	
Onset of erectile dysfunction	Sudden onset	2	**12**	14	0.05
	Gradual onset	2	6	8	
	No dysfunction	1	2	3	
Situation under which erectile dysfunction occur	With partner only	2	**10**	12	0.05
	Under all circumstances	3	5	8	
	No dysfunction	2	3	5	
Morning erection	Absent	3	1	4	0.05
	Present	2	**19**	21	

frequent concerns in previous studies (Dumontaud et al., 2020). The negative correlation found between sexual enjoyment and age suggests that as people get older their sexual enjoyment decreased. This may be due to effects of aging on sexual functioning, which appear to be negatively correlated. Many studies show a negative association between age and sexual dysfunction in patients with schizophrenia (Huang et al., 2019).

There are higher rates of sexual dysfunction found in individuals with schizophrenia being treated with medication (Bains & Shah, 2012), and specifically with typical antipsychotics (Souaiby et al., 2019). Our results show a significant association between sexual functioning and side effects of drug treatment, specifically between receiving typical antipsychotics and mixed medications. Patients receiving mixed treatment were having a combination of antipsychotics, mood stabilizers and/or antidepressants. There is evidence to suggest sexual dysfunction is also associated with antidepressants and mood stabilizers (García-Blanco et al., 2020; Montejo et al., 2018). We were unable to assess whether the side effects from the mixed medications group can be attributed to one particular drug, which should be investigated in future research. The association between sexual dysfunction and antipsychotics may be due to hyperprolactinemia, as patients who have increased serum prolactin levels were most likely to have sexual dysfunction (Zhang et al., 2018). Common antipsychotics such as amisulpride, paliperidone and risperidone are associated with higher rates of sexual dysfunction compared to clozapine, olanzapine, aripiprazole, and quetiapine (Bhowmick, Darji, Parikh, & Shah, 2020). Aripiprazole and quetiapine have a minimal effect on prolactin, and these have shown to have the least amount of sexual side effects. In addition, adding aripiprazole to another antipsychotic can reduce the side effects of sexual dysfunction. This seems to occur because aripiprazole acts as a partial dopamine agonist, therefore, when it is added to a typical antipsychotic, it binds to D2 receptors more robustly and acts as a dopamine agonist (Bhowmick et al., 2020). Our present study did not measure prolactin levels of clients, but we did see increased rates of sexual dysfunction with typical antipsychotics, some of which, as previously mentioned, tend to have greater effects on prolactin levels (Bhowmick et al., 2020).

Both novel and conventional antipsychotics are associated with significant sexual side effects and the presence of sexual side effects may affect compliance and adherence to pharmacological treatment. In some specific clinical populations, these specific side effects turn out to be the most distressing and promote increased drop-out rates and poor adherence to treatment. Nevertheless, sexual dysfunction is often underestimated or not investigated in the treatment course of psychiatric disorders with psychotropic medications (De Hert, Detraux, & Peuskens, 2014). Many people also do not spontaneously report sexual dysfunction to their clinicians, and this has been shown through clinical trials relying on individuals reporting sexual dysfunctions in comparison to individuals being directly questioned about it (Kelly & Conley, 2004). In our study, almost half of the patient sample reported being sexually dissatisfied due to the side effects of their medication. This shows patients' insight into the effect the medication has on their sexual functioning; therefore, it comes as no surprise that distress associated with treatment side effects can impact compliance and adherence to treatment.

Other factors identified in our patient sample that may contribute to sexual dysfunction include financial stressors, and stressors associated with having morning erections yet being unable to perform full functioning. Our results showed significant differences were found between patients with mild erectile dysfunction and their dissatisfaction with their financial state. Psychosocial factors such as stress, anxiety, and depression are highly correlated with sexual dysfunction. Dumontaud et al. (2020) found that depressive symptoms of schizophrenia were associated with increased risk of sexual dysfunction, therefore treating these symptoms may be an important part of treating sexual dysfunction. These factors need to be considered when treating sexual dysfunction in schizophrenia. Further research may be required to distinguish what proportion of sexual dysfunction is psychogenic and what is due to pharmacological treatment side effects.

Many of our patients in the current study were found to be light smokers (61.1%), which is not uncommon in a sample of mentally ill patients as smoking has been found to alleviate symptoms of mental illness. Research suggests that individuals with mental health problems are more likely to engage in smoking, and other substance use behaviors, possibly for symptom alleviation. For example, nicotine improves the symptoms of attention deficit hyperactivity disorder in adults and stimulates the release of neurotransmitters that may be involved in counteracting depression. In addition, nicotine helps alleviate some of the negative symptoms of schizophrenia (Patkar et al., 2002). Smoking may also help alleviate some side effects associated with antipsychotic medication, such as the side effects of haloperidol treatment in individuals diagnosed with schizophrenia (Levin et al., 1996). Despite its help with symptom relief, smoking may increase the risk of developing mental health problems. For example, an association was found between smoking during pregnancy and increased risk of attention deficit hyperactivity disorder (Milberger, Biederman, Faraone, & Jones, 1998). In addition, smoking can affect hormonal balances and sexual libido, as well as have impacts on sexual functioning (Harte & Meston, 2008). Our results showed significant correlations between sexual excitement and delayed ejaculation, with smoking. The direction of this correlation is still unknown and should be investigated further.

A large portion of the patients in our study reported decreased sexual enjoyment, which can impact the quality of their relationships. This response to sexual dysfunction is not uncommon (Souaiby et al., 2019) and can impact the relationship in negative ways. Our results also highlighted significant abuse occurring within relationships. Poor marriage quality is associated with lower sexual satisfaction (Aggarwal, Grover, & Chakrabarti, 2019), which may explain why many of our patients reported more dissatisfaction with their sexual lives. Marital distress and conflict can result in further mental illness occurring within family members and unhealthy developmental attachments with children (Akhtar & Farooq, 2013). This may pose a limitation of this study, as it is unknown whether the marital distress and conflict in this study is a result of sexual dissatisfaction or whether it is a contributor to sexual dissatisfaction. The association does highlight the importance of exploring relationship satisfaction and safety of caregivers throughout treatment of psychiatric disorders.

Overall, it is evident that there is an association between sexual dysfunction and typical antipsychotics. Although some sexual dysfunction may be present due to the psychopathology, and possibly other psychogenic factors, psychotropic medications used for treatment tend to exacerbate these dysfunctions (Zemishlany & Weizman, 2008).

Conclusion

This study shows significant correlations between sexual dysfunction and receiving typical antipsychotic and mixed medications. It is crucially important to highlight this data during clinical practice. Growing awareness of sexual dysfunctions in schizophrenia and the adverse effects of psychotropic drugs have led to attempts to use adjuvants or substitute treatments to resolve sexual dysfunction. Sexual dysfunction in schizophrenia should be carefully diagnosed and treated; it should be clearly discussed with schizophrenia patients in order to preserve an adequate quality of life, promote greater adherence to treatment, and promote good remission and recovery.

References

Aggarwal, S., Grover, S., & Chakrabarti, S. (2019). A comparative study evaluating the marital and sexual functioning in patients with schizophrenia and depressive disorders. *Asian Journal of Psychiatry*, *39*, 128–134.

Akhtar, Z., & Farooq, M. S. (2013). *Marital conflicts can lead to major depression.*

Alzohiery, A. M. (2011). *Reliability and validity of Arabic version of international index of erectile function-15 in Egyptian population.* Thesis submitted in partial fulfillment of Msc degree in andrology, sexology and sexually transmitted diseases.

Baggaley, M. (2008). Sexual dysfunction in schizophrenia: Focus on recent evidence. *Human Psychopharmacology: Clinical and Experimental*, *23*(3), 201–209.

Bains, S., & Shah, A. A. (2012). Sexual side effects of antipsychotic drugs. *Advances in Pharmacoepidemiology and Drug Safety*, *1*, 109.

Bhowmick, S. S., Darji, V. M., Parikh, N. C., & Shah, N. D. (2020). Risperidone-induced sexual dysfunction reverted with aripiprazole: Experience from two cases. *Annals of Indian Psychiatry*, *4*(1), 81.

Brzezinski-Sinai, N. A., & Brzezinski, A. (2020). Schizophrenia and sex hormones: What is the link? *Frontiers in Psychiatry*, *11*.

De Hert, M., Detraux, J., & Peuskens, J. (2014). Second-generation and newly approved antipsychotics, serum prolactin levels and sexual dysfunctions: A critical literature review. *Expert Opinion on Drug Safety*, *13*(5), 605–624.

Dilla, T., Ciudad, A., & Alvarez, M. (2013). Systematic review of the economic aspects of non-adherence to antipsychotic medication in patients with schizophrenia. *Patient Preference and Adherence*, *7*, 275.

Dumontaud, M., Korchia, T., Khouani, J., Lancon, C., Auquier, P., Boyer, L., & Fond, G. (2020). Sexual dysfunctions in schizophrenia: Beyond antipsychotics. A systematic review. *Progress in Neuro-Psychopharmacology and Biological Psychiatry*, *98*. https://doi.org/10.1016/j.pnpbp.2019.109804.

Fanta, T., Haile, K., Abebaw, D., Assefa, D., & Hibdye, G. (2018). Assessment of sexual dysfunction and associated factors among patients with schizophrenia in Ethiopia, 2017. *BMC Psychiatry*, *18*(1), 158.

García-Blanco, A., García-Portilla, M. P., de la Fuente-Tomás, L., Batalla, M., Sánchez-Autet, M., Arranz, B., … Sierra, P. (2020). Sexual dysfunction and mood stabilizers in long-term stable patients with bipolar disorder. *The Journal of Sexual Medicine*, *17*(5), 930–940.

Goldstone, L. W. (2020). Unmet medical needs and other challenges in the treatment of patients with schizophrenia. *The American Journal of Managed Care*, *26*(3), S48–S54.

Harte, C. B., & Meston, C. M. (2008). Acute effects of nicotine on physiological and subjective sexual arousal in nonsmoking men: A randomized, double-blind, placebo-controlled trial. *The Journal of Sexual Medicine*, *5*(1), 110–121.

Huang, Y. H., Hou, C. L., Ng, C. H., Chen, X., Wang, Q. W., Huang, Z. H., & Jia, F. J. (2019). Sexual dysfunction in Chinese rural patients with schizophrenia. *BMC Psychiatry*, *19*(1), 218.

Janca, A., & Hiller, W. (1996). ICD-10 checklists—A tool for clinicians' use of the ICD-10 classification of mental and behavioral disorders. *Comprehensive Psychiatry*, *37*(3), 180–187.

Kelly, D. L., & Conley, R. R. (2004). Sexuality and schizophrenia: A review. *Schizophrenia Bulletin*, *30*(4), 767–779.

Kruljac, M., Finnbogadottir, H., Bobjer, J., Giraldi, A., Fugl-Meyer, K., & Giwercman, A. (2020). Symptoms of sexual dysfunction among men from infertile couples: Prevalence and association with testosterone deficiency. *Andrology*, *8*(1), 160–165.

Lee, J. C., Surridge, D., Morales, A., & Heaton, J. P. W. (2000). The prevalence and influence of significant psychiatric abnormalities in men undergoing comprehensive management of organic erectile dysfunction. *International Journal of Impotence Research*, *12*(1), 47–51.

Levin, E. D., et al. (1996). Nicotine-haloperidol interactions and cognitive performance in schizophrenics. *Neuropsychopharmacology*, *15*(5), 429–436. https://doi.org/10.1016/s0893-133x(96)00018-8.

Lodha, P., & Sousa, A. D. (2020). Female sexual dysfunction and schizophrenia: A clinical review. *Journal of Psychosexual Health*, *2*(1), 44–55.

Macdonald, S., Halliday, J., MacEwan, T., Sharkey, V., Farrington, S., Wall, S., & McCreadie, R. G. (2003). Nithsdale schizophrenia surveys 24: Sexual dysfunction: Case–control study. *The British Journal of Psychiatry*, *182*(1), 50–56.

Malik, P., Kemmler, G., Hummer, M., Riecher-Roessler, A., Kahn, R. S., Fleischhacker, W. W., & EUFEST Study Group. (2011). Sexual dysfunction in first-episode schizophrenia patients: Results from European first episode schizophrenia trial. *Journal of Clinical Psychopharmacology*, *31*(3), 274–280.

Milberger, S., Biederman, J., Faraone, S. V., & Jones, J. (1998). Further evidence of an association between maternal smoking during pregnancy and attention deficit hyperactivity disorder: Findings from a high-risk sample of siblings. *Journal of Clinical Child Psychology*, *27*(3), 352–358.

Montejo, Á. L., Majadas, S., Rico-Villademoros, F., LLorca, G., De La Gándara, J., Franco, M., … Spanish Working Group for the Study of Psychotropic-Related Sexual Dysfunction. (2010). Frequency of sexual dysfunction in patients with a psychotic disorder receiving antipsychotics. *The Journal of Sexual Medicine*, *7*(10), 3404–3413.

Montejo, A. L., Montejo, L., & Baldwin, D. S. (2018). The impact of severe mental disorders and psychotropic medications on sexual health and its implications for clinical management. *World Psychiatry*, *17*(1), 3–11.

Moustafa, A. A., Garami, J. K., Mahlberg, J., Golembieski, J., Keri, S., Misiak, B., & Frydecka, D. (2016). Neural and cognitive function in schizophrenia: Conflicting findings and future directions. *Reviews in the Neurosciences*, *27*(4), 435–448.

Moustafa, A. A., Salama, M., Peak, R., Tindle, R., Salem, A., Keri, S., … Mohamed, W. (2017). Interactions between Cannabis and schizophrenia in humans and rodents. *Reviews in the Neurosciences*, *28*(7), 811–823.

Moustafa, A., Weickert, T. W., & Frydecka, D. (2016). Schizophrenia: Human and animal studies. *Frontiers in Behavioral Neuroscience*. https://doi.org/10.3389/fnbeh.2016.00076.

Oades, R. D., & Schepker, R. (1994). Serum gonadal steroid hormones in young schizophrenic patients. *Psychoneuroendocrinology*, *19*(4), 373–385.

Patkar, A. A., Gopalakrishnan, R., Lundy, A., Leone, F. T., Certa, K. M., & Weinstein, S. P. (2002). Relationship between tobacco smoking and positive and negative symptoms in schizophrenia. *The Journal of Nervous and Mental Disease*, *190*(9), 604–610.

Rosenberg, K. P., Bleiberg, K. L., Koscis, J., & Gross, C. (2003). A survey of sexual side effects among severely mentally ill patients taking psychotropic medications: Impact on compliance. *Journal of Sex & Marital Therapy*, *29*(4), 289–296. https://doi.org/10.1080/00926230390195524.

Smith, S., & Henderson, M. (2000). What you don't know won't hurt you: Information given to patients about the side-effects of antipsychotic drugs. *Psychiatric Bulletin*, *24*(5), 172–174.

Snyder, D. K. (1981). *Marrital satisfaction inventory (MSI)—Manual*. Los Angeles, CA: Western Psychological Services.

Souaiby, L., Kazour, F., Zoghbi, M., Bou Khalil, R., & Richa, S. (2019). Sexual dysfunction in patients with schizophrenia and schizoaffective disorder and its association with adherence to antipsychotic medication. *Journal of Mental Health*, 1–8.

Van Cauter, E., Linkowski, P., Kerkhofs, M., Hubain, P., L'Hermite-Balériaux, M., Leclercq, R., … Mendlewicz, J. (1991). Circadian and sleep-related endocrine rhythms in schizophrenia. *Archives of General Psychiatry*, *48*(4), 348–356.

Waldinger, M. D., Zwinderman, A. H., Schweitzer, D. H., & Olivier, B. (2004). Relevance of methodological design for the interpretation of efficacy of drug treatment of premature ejaculation: A systematic review and meta-analysis. *International Journal of Impotence Research*, *16*(4), 369–381.

Wei, C. W., Chen, Y. Q., Ma, M., Xiu, M. H., & Zhang, X. Y. (2020). Sex differences in the association of body mass index with symptoms and cognitive deficits in Chinese patients with chronic schizophrenia. *Translational Psychiatry*, *10*(1), 1–8.

Zemishlany, Z., & Weizman, A. (2008). The impact of mental illness on sexual dysfunction. In *Vol. 29. Sexual dysfunction* (pp. 89–106). Karger Publishers.

Zhang, Y., Tang, Z., Ruan, Y., Huang, C., Wu, J., Lu, Z., … Wang, T. T. (2018). Prolactin and thyroid stimulating hormone (TSH) levels and sexual dysfunction in patients with schizophrenia treated with conventional antipsychotic medication: A cross-sectional study. *Medical Science Monitor: International Medical Journal of Experimental and Clinical Research*, *24*, 9136.

Zhao, S., Wang, X., Qiang, X., Wang, H., He, J., Shen, M., … Kang, R. (2020). Is there an association between schizophrenia and sexual dysfunction in both sexes? A systematic review and meta-analysis. *The Journal of Sexual Medicine*, *17*(8), 1476–1488.

Case studies of the treatment of schizophrenia patients

8

Pronab Ganguly[a], *Ahmed A. Moustafa*[b,c], *Eid Abo Hamza*[d,e], *and Ahmed A. Helal*[d]
[a]Flourish, Australia, [b]School of Psychology & Marcs Institute for Brain and Behaviour, Western Sydney University, Sydney, NSW, Australia, [c]Department of Human Anatomy and Physiology, the Faculty of Health Sciences, University of Johannesburg, South Africa, [d]Faculty of Education, Department of Mental Health, Tanta University, Egypt, [e]College of Graduate Studies, Arabian Gulf University, Bahrain

Chapter outline

Introduction

Case studies are detailed qualitative studies where few participants are investigated in detail. Data from case studies can be gathered by documentation, interviews, archival records, and direct observation of study participants. Interviewing is a well-established technique for data collection in case study (Alpi & Evans, 2019; Crowe et al., 2011). There are various case studies in the treatment options of the schizophrenia patients, as we discuss below in detail.

Schizophrenia is a brain disorder that determines how a person interacts, thinks, and perceives reality (Coyle, 2017; Hernaus et al., 2019; Keshavan, Nasrallah, & Tandon, 2011; Richter et al., 2019). The symptoms of schizophrenia relate to delusions, hallucinations, disorganized speech, and diminished emotional expression (Ruppin, Reggia, & Horn, 1996; Shenton et al., 1992; Szeszko et al., 2008). Although controversial, the root cause of these symptoms has been linked to excess of dopaminergic signaling mostly in subcortical structures including the basal ganglia and hippocampus (American Psychiatric Association, 2013; Berry, Abohamza, & Moustafa, 2019; Moustafa et al., 2016; Moustafa, Weickert, & Frydecka, 2016; (Moustafa, Keri, Herzallah, Myers, & Gluck, 2010; Pankow, Knobel, Voss, & Heinz, 2012; Schott et al., 2015; Siekmeier & van Maanen, 2014; Tamminga, Stan, & Wagner, 2010; Yoon, Minzenberg, Raouf, D'Esposito, & Carter, 2013). Schizophrenia is among the top 10 common brain disorders in the world (Mathers & Loncar, 2006), as

Cognitive and Behavioral Dysfunction in Schizophrenia. https://doi.org/10.1016/B978-0-12-820005-6.00005-0

about 1% of the general population suffer from schizophrenia (Simeone, Ward, Rotella, Collins, & Windisch, 2015). Schizophrenia usually appears in the late teens or early adulthood (Gogtay, Vyas, Testa, Wood, & Pantelis, 2011; Harrop & Trower, 2001). However, schizophrenia may also manifest in middle ages (Folsom et al., 2006; Kirkbride, Fearon, & Morgan, 2006). Generally, the early onset of schizophrenia is often accompanied with severe positive and negative symptoms (Galletly et al., 2016; Larson, Walker, & Compton, 2010). Schizophrenia is found to be more severe and more common in men than in women (Aleman, Kahn, & Selten, 2003; McGrath, Saha, Chant, & Welham, 2008; Ochoa, Usall, Cobo, Labad, & Kulkarni, 2012; Sommer, Tiihonen, van Mourik, Tanskanen, & Taipale, 2020). Schizophrenia is a chronic disorder that can be managed effectively with due care and management (i.e., non-pharmacological treatment), in addition to antipsychotics medications (Canas et al., 2013; Lauriello & Perkins, 2019). However, the likelihood of recovery is larger, when schizophrenia is diagnosed and treated early on (Galletly et al., 2016). With medications and non-pharmacological therapy, many schizophrenia patients can live independently and have a fulfilling lifestyle.

The long-term burden for supporting patients with schizophrenia is much more than any other mental disorders (Neil, Carr, & Mihalopoulos, 2014). The ongoing cost of supporting schizophrenia amounts to 1%–3% of the national health care cost in most of the Western nations as well as many other countries. This cost is almost 20% of the direct expenses of all types of mental health costs (Galletly et al., 2016). The aim of supporting schizophrenia patients is not only to reduce or manage schizophrenia symptoms, but also to enhance the quality of life of schizophrenia patients, by having successful jobs, relationships among others (Edinoff et al., 2020; Lim & Lee, 2018). There are various case studies on managing different symptoms and quality of life associated with schizophrenia patients (Deardorff & Burton, 2012; Teixeira, Venancio, & Araujo, 2013).

Types of case studies

In research methodology, there may be single-case or multiple-cases depending on the research question (Lobo, Moeyaert, Baraldi Cunha, & Babik, 2017). The single-case design can be adopted where there are no other cases available for replication. For instance, a case study on the effects of twin tower collapse, or the effects of tsunami, can be conducted using a single-case methodology, where events occur one time only. However, a single-case design may fail to draw a generalizable conclusion. One way to augment this drawback is by supporting the study with other auxiliary methods to confirm the validity of the process. In multiple-case studies a number of real-life scenarios are analyzed. Thus, in multiple studies a pattern matching, that is, finding similarities or dissimilarities among all cases, can be conducted (Campbell, 1975). This increases the level of confidence in the correctness of the method. Case studies must be designed so as to address the need of the research questions. It should follow a proper procedure and should be systematically recorded when conducted by interviews (Tellis, 1997).

There are two types of case studies: exploratory and explanatory (Yin, 1984). First, exploratory case studies are supposed to explore any event which serves as a point of interest for the research. A pilot study is an example of an exploratory case study (McDonough & McDonough, 1997; Yin, 1984) and validates the procedure that will be used for subsequent studies. Explanatory case studies investigate the information both at a surface and deep level in order to explain the event. Interpretive and evaluative case studies are other types of case studies (McDonough & McDonough, 1997). In interpretive case studies, data are analyzed by development of conceptual categories, supporting or challenging the hypothesis made regarding them. For evaluative case studies, the research goes a bit deeper by adding judgment to the event.

As defined by Stake (1995), there are three categories of case studies mainly the intrinsic, the instrumental and the collective. In intrinsic case studies, the case is investigated for its own sake. In instrumental case studies, a small group of subjects are investigated to examine a definite type of pattern of behavior, for example, to see how college students prepare for examination. In a collective case study, data are collected from several sources. In intrinsic case studies, specific problems of an individual case are solved whereas instrumental and collective case studies target generalization of analysis to a larger population. Case studies offer a number of advantages. First, investigation of information is conducted within the context of its use (Yin, 1984), that is, the problem is defined in its boundary and investigation is carried out relating to various issues linked to that boundary. Second, multiple case studies allow for both quantitative and qualitative analyses of the information. Multiple case studies allow for comparison and pattern matching. This analysis gives rise to meaningful interpretation. Third, the detailed qualitative interpretation in case studies help investigate the data in real-life environment as well as help comprehend the complex real-life situations that may not be possible through experimental or survey research. Case studies can be a realistic alternative to quantitative studies when a large sample population is difficult to obtain. It should be noted that case studies are sometimes criticized for a lack of rigor and the tendency for a biased interpretation of the information, although this is debatable.

Data collection in case studies

Data in case studies can be gathered by documentation, interview, archival records, direct observation, participant observation, and physical artifact. Interviews are well-established technique for data collection in case studies (Yin, 2017). In a case study (Ertem & Duman, 2016), the achievement of treatment collaboration, that is, how a patient adheres to treatment regime, was investigated through motivational interviews. The clinician practices motivational interviewing with general principles in mind: express empathy through reflective listening, develop discrepancy between clients' goals or values and their current behavior, avoid argument and direct confrontation. In the Ertem and Duman (2016) case study, motivational interview interventions are carried out through individual-centered counseling, cognitive-behavioral therapy, social-cognitive theory, the health belief model and the trans-theoretical model. In six motivational interviews, open-ended and reflective questions were asked, and empathy was established with the patient. Each interview was structured in accordance with the principles of motivational interviews. In this context, The Morisky Medication Adherence Scale and a questionnaire were used to assess medication adherence in the patients. The motivational interviews method can be used to improve continued treatment effectiveness, to increase patient awareness about the disease and benefits of treatment, and to increase patients' self-efficacy. In a case study interview, the questions should be fluid rather than rigid. Throughout the interview process, investigation should be followed in an unbiased manner. Thus, during the interview, while maintaining line of enquiry, friendly and nonthreatening questions should be asked. There are three types of interview techniques for case studies (Yin, 2017). In the first type of interview, commonly the questions are open ended where the respondents can be asked about their opinions. Even the respondents can be asked about their insight which might provide further basis of questioning. A second type of interview, called focused interview (Merton, Fiske, & Kendall, 1990; Zaidah, 2007), is conducted for a shorter period of time, around 1 h. The interview questions are still predominantly open ended, and the interview assume conversational nature. However, the set of questions are derived from the case study objective. A third type of interview is more structured in nature and consists of survey type questions.

Methods

In our study, the eligibility criteria for selection of studies are their effectiveness in addressing issues related to case studies in management of schizophrenia. The studies we considered are those which help manage symptoms of schizophrenia. Our search strategy included the following key words: schizophrenia, treatments, case study, medication, management, quality of life, and holistic. Many of these searches were conducted in combination. For example, we searched case studies that include all of these key words: schizophrenia, social relationship, and therapy (or treatment). We carefully examined articles to make sure the goal of the study is addressing the treatment of some symptoms of schizophrenia. Studies that did not address this topic were excluded. Throughout this review, we provide assessment of the validity of the findings. We have searched studies in Pubmed and Google Scholar. Out of 115 articles initially identified for the proposed review, 65 were removed for duplication. Again, out of 50 studies, 15 articles were excluded for nonrelevant design criteria, 10 articles were excluded for not meeting participant criteria, 10 articles were excluded for mode of intervention, and 5 articles were excluded for psychosocial reasons. Finally, 11 studies were included for review.

Case studies on schizophrenia

The case study methodology supports exploration and comprehension of complex issues. It can be deployed as a sound research methodology for holistic and deep investigation. It is recognized as a research tool in many social science studies such as education (Gulsecen & Kubat, 2006), sociology (Grassel & Schirmer, 2006) and community-based problems (Johnson, 2006) as well as management of schizophrenia (Omoaregba, James, & Eze, 2009). Quantitative methods are limited in providing holistic and in-depth explanations of the complex social and behavioral science; case studies research can address this limitation. By case study methodology, it is possible to go above and beyond the quantitative statistical results and comprehend the behavioral as well as psychosocial factors. Case studies can assist in comprehending both the process and outcome of an issue through total investigation and analysis of the cases (Tellis, 1997). Literature survey identifies the use of the case studies in various fields such as sociology (Grassel & Schirmer, 2006), law (Lovell, 2006), and medicine (Taylor & Berridge, 2006).

There are several case studies in management of schizophrenia patients. In a case study by Deardorff and Burton (2012), issues regarding treatment of refractory patients with schizophrenia (i.e., patients who do not respond to medications) were investigated and treatment options in patients were recommended. In this case study, the investigation was carried out on the treatment of a patient with schizophrenia who had stabbed a cab driver. A 31-year-old African American female patient was brought to the emergency room of a hospital in USA escorted by police after stabbing a cab driver with a pencil. The patient had auditory hallucinations and paranoid delusions starting at the age 14 with a diagnosis of major depression with psychotic features. The issues investigated in this study included the pharmacokinetics of fluphenazine decanoate, strategies to manage clozapine-associated agranulocytosis, and approaches to addressing hyperprolactinemia (i.e., having higher than normal levels of prolactin). This case study highlighted multiple strategies that can be considered when managing treatment refractory patients in which alternative options for therapy are not readily available. This case study discussed a few clinical aspects to be considered when working with treatment refractory patients with schizophrenia and outlined some unique types of treatment in forensic clients.

In the case study by Omoaregba et al. (2009), investigation was conducted for culturally relevant treatment options for minority psychiatric patients. The study focused on schizophrenia spectrum disorders affecting four women in a Nigerian family of Ibo tribal origin who responded marginally to pharmacological interventions and required insight-oriented psychotherapy and family therapy in resolving psychosocial problems. For these patients, cultural beliefs are supposed to play an important role in disease presentation, treatment, and result. This case study highlighted that limitations in contemporary treatment approaches require the development of culturally appropriate psychotherapeutic interventions. It also highlights how cultural beliefs hamper and influence management of schizophrenia patients.

In a case study by Bradshaw (1998), 3-year cognitive behavior therapy (CBT) of a female schizophrenia patient was investigated and resulted in large improvements in psychosocial functioning and attainment of treatment goals. This case study describes the application of techniques of CBT in the long-term outpatient care of a young woman with schizophrenia. The study emphasized the application of cognitive-behavioral strategies to the needs of schizophrenia patient and presents data regarding clinical outcomes. Reduction in symptomatology and hospitalizations frequency was also found in this case. This led evidence to the efficacy of CBT in schizophrenia patient. In this case study the model highlighted the use of CBT with persons with schizophrenia from the focus on brief treatment of delusions and hallucinations to the multiple problems experienced by clients over the course of recovery from the disorder.

In a case study by Kozlowski-Gibson Maria (2016), the issues of a court case for a schizophrenia patient seeking medical follow-up and anosognosia were explored. The objective of this case study was to identify the issues associated with a court case seeking medical follow-up and treatment for a family member with schizophrenia and anosognosia. This study examined the difference between clinical and medical-legal evaluation of the patient. The study established linkage of the law to the real-life experience resulting from the procedures for its implementation. It concluded that the application of the Therapeutic Jurisprudence principles to the high number of schizophrenia cases with anosognosia, the abandonment of the mentally ill, and family crisis require healthcare providers and the Judiciary for an improvement in the action of the process of guardianship.

In a case study by Lysaker, Buck, and Ringer (2007), metacognitive capacity, delusions, and insight were assessed for a schizophrenia patient using the psychotherapy transcripts for a period of 32 months. It is assumed that psychotherapy might help patients with schizophrenia to improve their capacity for metacognition, that is, their ability to think about their own thinking and the thinking of others. Correlational analyses revealed that metacognitive capacity increased as symptoms and lack of insight decreased. The result of this study concluded that metacognitive capacities increased before symptoms changed and that awareness of the patient's own thoughts emerged before awareness of others' thoughts. Progress seemed to be initially volatile, with early gains sustained only after approximately one and half years.

In a case study by Davis and Lysaker (2005), a schizophrenia patient was treated over a 6-month period using the Indianapolis Vocational Intervention Protocol (IVIP). While a lot of attention has been placed on how CBT can address symptoms in schizophrenia spectrum disorders, much less is known about how it might be applied to aim psychosocial dysfunction such as social isolation, withdrawal from the community, relationship problems, among other social issues. The IVIP provided a paid job and simultaneous group and individual CBT. Therapeutic strategies involved focus on enhancing metacognition and identifying and restructuring dysfunctional beliefs about self and work. Improvements were found in metacognitive capacity as well as reduction is found in dysfunctional beliefs. Work behaviors were found to improve and symptoms of emotional disorder were decreased.

In a case study by Teixeira et al. (2013), face validity and clinical utility were found in terms of epidemiology, symptom profile, and identified pathophysiology in the diagnosis of late-onset schizophrenia. In this case study a 66-year-old woman with no psychiatric background up until 2010 was investigated when she was admitted to the hospital due to symptoms, which she has been developing since 2008. The symptoms included mystical and persecutory delusions and visual and auditory hallucinations (she believed she was persecuted by little witches who insulted her and invaded her home). This resulted in behavioral disturbance with intense aggressiveness and anguish. The neuropsychological diagnosis did not detect any cognitive impairment. She was treated with high doses of an antipsychotic and discharged being medicated with injectable antipsychotic and followed in compulsory treatment.

In a case study by Jara et al. (2012), investigation was carried out to find out relationship between smoking and exacerbation of positive and negative symptoms of schizophrenia. This case study indicated that some ingredients of cigarette smoke (mainly polycyclic aromatic hydrocarbons) have an accelerating effect on the metabolism of several antipsychotics (i.e., clozapine, olanzapine, members of the phenotiazine group, and haloperidol). This study also suggested that nicotinic receptor agonists (such as nicotine) may have a therapeutic role in the treatment of cognitive impairments (i.e., disturbances in attention and in verbal, visual, and working memories) in schizophrenia, and in turn, abstinence from tobacco can lead to deterioration of cognitive and psychomotor performance in this patient's symptoms. This study concluded that exacerbations of positive symptoms may be related to decreased effectiveness of certain antipsychotics in result of an accelerated metabolism induced by cigarette smoking. It was also observed that Nicotine may reduce some negative symptoms of schizophrenia, including cognitive impairment.

In a case study by Gaebel (2017), the objective was to collect evidence-based information and provide a concise overview of what is needed to overcome the treatment gap in schizophrenia. In this case study with the use of a combined approach of systematic review and health economics assessment was done for the socioeconomic impact of medical interventions (or the lack of thereof) for schizophrenia. This case study analysis outlines socioeconomic impact and health improvements of best practices in interventions for schizophrenia in comparison with the cost burden of nontreatment.

In a case study by Ertem and Duman (2016), the features of treatment collaboration were investigated through motivational interviews. The clinician practices motivational interviewing (MI) with general principles in mind: express empathy through reflective listening, develop discrepancy between clients' goals or values and their current behavior, avoid argument, and direct confrontation. In this case study, motivational interview interventions are carried out through individual-centered counseling, cognitive-behavioral therapy, social-cognitive theory, the health belief model and the trans-theoretical model. In six motivational interviews, open-ended and reflective questions were asked, and empathy was established with the patient. Each interview was structured in accordance with the principles of motivational interview. It was observed that motivational interview can be used for effective treatment and to increase the patient awareness of the disorder.

In a case study by Lysaker and Buck (2006), challenges for the treatment associated with inclinations to "fix" the client, the client's own deficits and symptoms, and discomfort within the therapeutic relationship were investigated. In this study the requirements and challenges of psychotherapy that could facilitate recovery are investigated. It explored the difficulties related to treatment of a person with schizophrenia for over 19 months Techniques to address these difficulties are presented in this study.

Table 1 summarizes various case studies associated with schizophrenia patients and their implications:

Table 1 Prior cases studies on the management of schizophrenia.

Case study by	Summary
Deardorff and Burton (2012)	Treatment of refractory patients, that is, patients who show resistance to treatment. Investigation was carried out to identify treatment options for patients where alternative options for therapy are not readily available
Omoaregba et al. (2009)	Culturally relevant treatment options for minority patients with psychiatric disorders. Investigation was carried out to identify how cultural beliefs hamper and influence the management of schizophrenia patients.
Bradshaw (1998)	Cognitive behavior therapy (CBT) of a female schizophrenia patient. In this study, it was pointed out how CBT addresses the multiple problems experienced by clients over the course of recovery from the disorder
Maria (2016)	Identification of the issues associated with a court case seeking medical follow-up and treatment for a family member with schizophrenia and anosognosia. This study identified the issues related to improvement in the action of the process of guardianship of a schizophrenia patient
Lysaker et al. (2007)	Psychotherapy transcripts for a schizophrenia patient. This study identified the issues related to the ability of the patient to think about their own thinking and the thinking of others about them
Davis and Lysaker (2005)	Investigation of Indianapolis Vocational Intervention Protocol (IVIP).This study identified how work behaviors can be improved and symptoms of emotional disorder were decreased for a schizophrenia patient
Teixeira et al. (2013)	Pathophysiology in the diagnosis of late-onset schizophrenia. This study identified the various antipsychotic treatment options for a late-onset schizophrenia patient
Jara et al. (2012)	Relationship between smoking and exacerbation of positive and negative symptoms of schizophrenia. This study observed that nicotine may reduce some negative symptoms of schizophrenia, including cognitive impairment.
Gaebel (2017)	Treatment gap in schizophrenia. This study outlines the socioeconomic impact and health improvements of best practices required for interventions in schizophrenia patient
Ertem and Duman (2016)	Treatment collaboration through motivational interviews. This study outlined how motivational interviewing can be used for effective treatment and to increase the patient awareness of the disorder
Lysaker and Buck (2006)	Difficulties related to treatment of a person with schizophrenia. In this study the discomfort within the therapeutic relationship between the clinician and patient was investigated

Discussion

The above-mentioned case studies investigate various aspects of the management of schizophrenia patients. The case study by (Deardorff & Burton, 2012) investigates treatment options for schizophrenia patients. The implication of this study was to explore the strengths and weaknesses of different mechanisms and treatments available to schizophrenia patients. The case study by Omoaregba et al. (2009) highlights how cultural beliefs hamper and influence the management of schizophrenia patients. The implication of this study is to explore culturally relevant treatment options for minority psychiatric patients, as this may affect treatment success. A case study by (Bradshaw, 1998) investigates the strengths and weaknesses of Cognitive Behavior Therapy for a schizophrenia patient. The case study by Kozlowski-Gibson Maria (2016) investigates legal aspects related to the management of schizophrenia patients. This study explores the legal ramifications of some treatments for schizophrenia patients. They explain various legal issues related to the treatment of schizophrenia patients. The case study by Lysaker et al. (2007) addresses psychotherapy transcripts for a schizophrenia patient. This study identified the issues related to the ability of the patient to think about their own thinking and the thinking of others about them. The case study by Davis and Lysaker (2005) investigates the effect of psychosocial factors on the quality of life of schizophrenia patient. It analyses the effects of various related psychosocial factors such as employment, education, and training on the quality of life of schizophrenia patient. The case study by Teixeira et al. (2013) explored the pathopsychological issues associated with late onset of a schizophrenia patient. This study investigates the pros and cons of the treatment-related issues and provides some pointers on how to address them. The case study by Jara et al. (2012) investigates the effects of smoking on the lifestyle of schizophrenia patients. This study explores various effects smoking induces on the wellbeing of the schizophrenia patients. The case study by Gaebel (2017) outlines the socio-economic impact and health improvements of best practices required for interventions in schizophrenia patients. The case study by Ertem and Duman (2016) explores treatment adherence of a schizophrenia patient using motivational interviewing. It was found that these kinds of interviews improve the treatment adherence of the patience. The case study by Lysaker and Buck (2006) investigates the issues and difficulties associated with treating a schizophrenia patient. This study explores the issues related to the treatment difficulty of a schizophrenia patient.

The above-mentioned case studies investigate the impact of various individual issues on the quality of life of schizophrenia patient. The issues associated with the management of schizophrenia patients can broadly be classified into three categories: drug intervention, different kinds of psychiatric therapies, and management of psychosocial factors. Future research should use a holistic approach where all the above-mentioned factors related to management of schizophrenia patient should be investigated simultaneously. The holistic intervention includes pharmacological and nonpharmacological intervention, diet, and complimentary medication, cognitive behavior therapy, yoga therapy, mindfulness, and other psychosocial factors (Ganguly, Soliman, & Moustafa, 2018). The psychosocial factors include proper and secured accommodation, education, training, employment, financial management, recreation, and hobbies among others.

With the help of proper medication management and effective therapy, the symptoms of schizophrenia can be improved (Galletly et al., 2016). With effective adjustment of secured accommodation, education, training, employment, recreation and hobbies, the quality of life of the schizophrenia patients can also be improved (Ganguly et al., 2018). We have investigated how drug intervention, psychotherapies and adjustment of psychosocial factors influence the treatment of schizophrenia patient in our study (Ganguly et al., 2018). Future work should focus on conducting interview-based qualitative case studies with schizophrenia patients using a holistic management approach.

References

Aleman, A., Kahn, R. S., & Selten, J. P. (2003). Sex differences in the risk of schizophrenia: Evidence from meta-analysis. *Archives of General Psychiatry*, *60*, 565–571.

Alpi, K. M., & Evans, J. J. (2019). Distinguishing case study as a research method from case reports as a publication type. *Journal of the Medical Library Association*, *107*(1), 1–5. https://doi.org/10.5195/jmla.2019.615.

American Psychiatric Association. (2013). *Diagnostic and statistical manual of mental disorders* (5th ed.). Arlington, VA: American Psychiatric Publishing.

Berry, T., Abohamza, E., & Moustafa, A. A. (2019). Treatment resistant schizophrenia: Focus on the transsulfuration pathway. *Reviews in the Neurosciences*, *31*(2), 219–232.

Bradshaw, W. (1998). Cognitive-behavioral treatment of schizophrenia: A case study. *Journal of Cognitive Psychotherapy: An International Journal*, *12*(1), 13–25.

Campbell, D. (1975). Degrees of freedom and the case study. *Comparative Political Studies*, *8*, 178–185.

Canas, F., Alptekin, K., Azorin, J. M., Dubois, V., Emsley, R., Garcia, A. G., … Roca, M. (2013). Improving treatment adherence in your patients with schizophrenia: The STAY initiative. *Clinical Drug Investigation*, *33*(2), 97–107. https://doi.org/10.1007/s40261-012-0047-8.

Coyle, J. T. (2017). Schizophrenia: Basic and clinical. *Advances in Neurobiology*, *15*, 255–280.

Crowe, S., Cresswell, K., Robertson, A., Huby, G., Avery, A., & Sheikh, A. (2011). The case study approach. *BMC Medical Research Methodology*, *11*, 100. https://doi.org/10.1186/1471-2288-11-100.

Davis, L. W., & Lysaker, P. H. (2005). Cognitive behavioral therapy and functional and metacognitive outcomes in schizophrenia: A single case study. *Cognitive and Behavioral Practice*, *12*(4), 468–478. Autumn 2005.

Deardorff, G., & Burton, S. A. (2012). Case based clinical pearls: A schizophrenic case study. *Mental Health Clinician*, *18*, 191–195.

Edinoff, A., Ruoff, M. T., Ghaffar, Y. T., Rezayev, A., Jani, D., Kaye, A. M., … Urits, I. (2020). Cariprazine to treat schizophrenia and bipolar disorder in adults. *Psychopharmacology Bulletin*, *50*(4), 83–117.

Ertem, M., & Duman, Z. C. (2016). Motivational interviewing in a patient with schizophrenia to achieve treatment collaboration: A case study. *Psychiatric Nursing*, *30*(2016), 50–54.

Folsom, D. P., Lebowitz, B. D., Lindamer, L. A., Palmer, B. W., Patterson, T. L., & Jeste, D. V. (2006). Schizophrenia in late life: Emerging issues. *Dialogues in Clinical Neuroscience*, *8*(1), 45–52.

Gaebel, W. (2017). Closing the treatment gap: The EPA case study of schizophrenia. *European Psychiatry*, *41*, S4.

Galletly, C., Castle, D., Dark, F., Humberstone, V., Jablensky, A., Killackey, A., ... Tran, N. (2016). Royal Australian and new Zealand College of Psychiatrists clinical practice guidelines for the management of schizophrenia and related disorders. *The Australian and New Zealand Journal of Psychiatry*, *50*(5), 410–472.

Ganguly, P., Soliman, A., & Moustafa, A. A. (2018). Holistic management of schizophrenia symptoms using pharmacological and non-pharmacological treatment. *Frontiers in Public Health*, *6*, 166.

Gogtay, N., Vyas, N. S., Testa, R., Wood, S. J., & Pantelis, C. (2011). Age of onset of schizophrenia: Perspectives from structural neuroimaging studies. *Schizophrenia Bulletin*, *37*(3), 504–513. https://doi.org/10.1093/schbul/sbr030.

Grassel, E., & Schirmer, B. (2006). The use of volunteers to support family careers of dementia patients: Results of a prospective longitudinal study investigating expectations towards and experience with training and professional support. *Zeitschrift Fur Gerontologie Und Geriatrie*, *39*(3), 217–226.

Gulsecen, S., & Kubat, A. (2006). Teaching ICT to teacher candidates using PBL: A qualitative and quantitative evaluation. *Educational Technology & Society*, *9*(2), 96–106.

Harrop, C., & Trower, P. (2001). Why does schizophrenia develop at late adolescence? *Clinical Psychology Review*, *21*(2), 241–265. https://doi.org/10.1016/s0272-7358(99)00047-1.

Hernaus, D., Frank, M. J., Brown, E. C., Brown, J. K., Gold, J. M., & Waltz, J. A. (2019). Impaired expected value computations in schizophrenia are associated with a reduced ability to integrate reward probability and magnitude of recent outcomes. *Biological Psychiatry: Cognitive Neuroscience and Neuroimaging*, *4*(3), 280–290. https://doi.org/10.1016/j.bpsc.2018.11.011.

Jara, J., Costa, C., Paixao, L., Coutinho, R., Fernandes, I., & Bento, A. (2012). Smoking and schizophrenia—Case study. *European Psychiatry*, *27*(1).

Johnson, M. P. (2006). Decision models for the location of community corrections centers. *Environment and Planning. B, Planning & Design*, *33*(3), 393–412.

Keshavan, M. S., Nasrallah, H. A., & Tandon, R. (2011). Schizophrenia, "just the facts" 6. Moving ahead with the schizophrenia concept: from the elephant to the mouse. *Schizophrenia Research*, *127*(1–3), 3–13. https://doi.org/10.1016/j.schres.2011.01.011.

Kirkbride, J. B., Fearon, P., & Morgan, C. (2006). Heterogeneity in incidence rates of schizophrenia and other psychotic syndromes: Findings from the 3-center AeSOP study. *Archives of General Psychiatry*, *63*, 250–258.

Larson, M. K., Walker, E. F., & Compton, M. T. (2010). Early signs, diagnosis and therapeutics of the prodromal phase of schizophrenia and related psychotic disorders. *Expert Review of Neurotherapeutics*, *10*(8), 1347–1359. https://doi.org/10.1586/ern.10.93.

Lauriello, J., & Perkins, D. O. (2019). Enhancing the treatment of patients with schizophrenia through continuous care. *The Journal of Clinical Psychiatry*, *80*(1). https://doi.org/10.4088/JCP.al18010ah2c.

Lim, M. W. Z., & Lee, J. (2018). Determinants of health-related quality of life in schizophrenia: Beyond the medical model. *Frontiers in Psychiatry*, *9*, 712. https://doi.org/10.3389/fpsyt.2018.00712.

Lobo, M. A., Moeyaert, M., Baraldi Cunha, A., & Babik, I. (2017). Single-case design, analysis, and quality assessment for intervention research. *Journal of Neurologic Physical Therapy*, *41*(3), 187–197. https://doi.org/10.1097/NPT.0000000000000187.

Lovell, G. I. (2006). Justice excused: The deployment of law in everyday political encounters. *Law and Society Review*, *40*(2), 283–324.

Lysaker, H. P., & Buck, D. (2006). Narrative enrichment in the psychotherapy for persons with schizophrenia: A single case study. *Mental Health Nursing*, *27*(3).

Lysaker, P. H., Buck, K. D., & Ringer, J. (2007). The recovery of metacognitive capacity in schizophrenia across 32 months of individual psychotherapy: A case study. *Psychotherapy Research*, *17*(6), 713–720.

Maria, K.-G. (2016). The struggle for schizophrenia treatment: A case study. *International Journal of Law and Psychiatry*, *49*(A), 124–129.

Mathers, C. D., & Loncar, D. (2006). Projections of global mortality and burden of disease from 2002 to 2030. *PLoS Medicine*, *3*, e442.

McDonough, J., & McDonough, S. (1997). *Research methods for English language teachers*. London: Arnold.

McGrath, J. L., Saha, S., Chant, D., & Welham, J. (2008). Schizophrenia: A concise overview of incidence, prevalence, and mortality. *Epidemiologic Reviews*, *30*, 67–76.

Merton, R., Fiske, M., & Kendall, L. P. (1990). *The focused interview: A manual of problems and procedures*. Free Press.

Moustafa, A. A., Garami, J. K., Mahlberg, J., Golembieski, J., Keri, S., Misiak, B., & Frydecka, D. (2016). Neural and cognitive function in schizophrenia: Conflicting findings and future directions. *Reviews in the Neurosciences*, *27*(4), 435–448.

Moustafa, A. A., Keri, S., Herzallah, M. M., Myers, C. E., & Gluck, M. A. (2010). A neural model of hippocampal-striatal interactions in associative learning and transfer generalization in various neurological and psychiatric patients. *Brain and Cognition*, *74*(2), 132–144.

Moustafa, A., Weickert, T. W., & Frydecka, D. (2016). Schizophrenia: Human and animal studies. *Frontiers in Behavioral Neuroscience*.

Neil, A. L., Carr, V. J., & Mihalopoulos, C. (2014). What difference a decade? The costs of psychosis in Australia in 2000 and 2010: Comparative results from the first and second Australian national surveys of psychosis. *Australian and New Zealand Journal of Psychiatry*, *48*, 237–248.

Ochoa, S., Usall, J., Cobo, J., Labad, X., & Kulkarni, J. (2012). Gender differences in schizophrenia and first-episode psychosis: A comprehensive literature review. *Schizophrenia Research and Treatment*, *2012*, 916198. https://doi.org/10.1155/2012/916198.

Omoaregba, J. O., James, B. O., & Eze, G. O. (2009). Schizophrenia spectrum disorders in a Nigerian family: 4 case reports. *Cases Journal*, *2*, 14.

Pankow, A., Knobel, A., Voss, M., & Heinz, A. (2012). Neurobiological correlates of delusion: Beyond the salience attribution hypothesis. *Neuropsychobiology*, *66*(1), 33–43. https://doi.org/10.1159/000337132.

Richter, J., Hesse, K., Eberle, M. C., Eckstein, K. N., Zimmermann, L., Schreiber, L., … Klingberg, S. (2019). Self-assessment of negative symptoms—Critical appraisal of the motivation and pleasure—Self-report's (MAP-SR) validity and reliability. *Comprehensive Psychiatry*, *88*, 22–28. https://doi.org/10.1016/j.comppsych.2018.10.007.

Ruppin, E., Reggia, J. A., & Horn, D. (1996). Pathogenesis of schizophrenic delusions and hallucinations: A neural model. *Schizophrenia Bulletin*, *22*(1), 105–123.

Schott, B. H., Voss, M., Wagner, B., Wustenberg, T., Duzel, E., & Behr, J. (2015). Fronto-limbic novelty processing in acute psychosis: Disrupted relationship with memory performance and potential implications for delusions. *Frontiers in Behavioral Neuroscience*, *9*, 144. https://doi.org/10.3389/fnbeh.2015.00144.

Shenton, E. M., Kikinis, R., Jolesz, A. F., Pollak, D. S., LeMay, M., Wible, G., … McCarley, W. R. (1992). Abnormalities of the left temporal lobe and thought disorder in schizophrenia—A quantitative magnetic resonance imaging study. *The New England Journal of Medicine*, *327*, 604–612.

Siekmeier, P. J., & van Maanen, D. P. (2014). Dopaminergic contributions to hippocampal pathophysiology in schizophrenia: A computational study. *Neuropsychopharmacology*, *39*(7), 1713–1721. https://doi.org/10.1038/npp.2014.19.

Simeone, J. C., Ward, A. J., Rotella, P., Collins, J., & Windisch, R. (2015). An evaluation of variation in published estimates of schizophrenia prevalence from 1990-2013: A systematic literature review. *BMC Psychiatry*, *15*, 193.

Sommer, I. E., Tiihonen, J., van Mourik, A., Tanskanen, A., & Taipale, H. (2020). The clinical course of schizophrenia in women and men-a nation-wide cohort study. *NPJ Schizophrenia*, *6*(1), 12. https://doi.org/10.1038/s41537-020-0102-z.

Stake, R. E. (1995). *The art of case study research: Perspective in practice*. London: Sage.

Szeszko, P. R., Robinson, D. G., Ashtari, M., Vogel, J., Betensky, J., Sevy, S., ... Bilder, R. M. (2008). Clinical and neuropsychological correlates of white matter abnormalities in recent onset schizophrenia. *Neuropsychopharmacology*, *33*(5), 976–984. https://doi.org/10.1038/sj.npp.1301480.

Tamminga, C. A., Stan, A. D., & Wagner, A. D. (2010). The hippocampal formation in schizophrenia. *The American Journal of Psychiatry*, *167*(10), 1178–1193. doi:appi.ajp.2010.09081187 [pii] https://doi.org/10.1176/appi.ajp.2010.09081187.

Taylor, S., & Berridge, V. (2006). Medicinal plants and malaria: An historical case study of research at the London School of Hygiene and Tropical Medicine in the twentieth century. *Transactions of the Royal Society of Tropical Medicine and Hygiene*, *100*(8), 707–714.

Teixeira, B., Venancio, A., & Araujo, M. (2013). Late-onset schizophrenia: Review and case study. *European Psychiatry*, *28*(Suppl 1).

Tellis, W. (1997). Introduction to case study. *The Qualitative Report*, *3*(2).

Yin, R. K. (1984). *Case study research: Design and methods*. Beverly Hills, CA: Sage Publications.

Yin, R. K. (2017). *Case study research: Design and methods* (6th ed.). Beverly Hills, CA: Sage Publications.

Yoon, J. H., Minzenberg, M. J., Raouf, S., D'Esposito, M., & Carter, C. S. (2013). Impaired prefrontal-basal ganglia functional connectivity and substantia nigra hyperactivity in schizophrenia. *Biological Psychiatry*, *74*(2), 122–129. https://doi.org/10.1016/j.biopsych.2012.11.018.

Zaidah, Z. (2007). Case study as a research method. *Jurnal Kemanusiaan*, *9*.

Prevalence of depression in schizophrenia and related disorders

9

Pronab Ganguly[a], Ahmed A. Helal[b], Eid Abo Hamza[b,c], and Ahmed A. Moustafa[d,e]
[a]Flourish, Australia, [b]Faculty of Education, Department of Mental Health, Tanta University, Egypt, [c]College of Graduate Studies, Arabian Gulf University, Bahrain, [d]School of Psychology & Marcs Institute for Brain and Behaviour, Western Sydney University, Sydney, NSW, Australia, [e]Department of Human Anatomy and Physiology, the Faculty of Health Sciences, University of Johannesburg, South Africa

Chapter outline

Introduction

Depression occurs in different types of mental disorders (Abo Hamza, Helal, Moustafa, & Emam, 2020; Moustafa et al., 2019, 2020; Radell, Abo Hamza, & Moustafa, 2020; Sheynin et al., 2020). A major depressive episode is generally accompanied by depressed mood for 2 weeks or more. Depression is associated with a loss of interest or pleasure in daily activities, which is known as anhedonia (De Fruyt, Sabbe, & Demyttenaere, 2020; Watson, Harvey, McCabe, & Reynolds, 2020). Generally, depression goes hand in hand along with other symptoms such as feelings of emptiness, hopelessness, anxiety, worthlessness, guilt and/or irritability, changes in appetite, problems in concentrating, remembering details, or making decisions, and even thoughts of or attempts at suicide (Bosanac & Castle, 2013). These symptoms may exist along with symptoms of insomnia or hypersomnia, aches, pains, or digestive problems (Nutt, Wilson, & Paterson, 2008; Trivedi, Hollander, Nutt, & Blier, 2008).

The prevalence of major depressive disorder is approximately 7%, in the general population (Bosanac & Castle, 2013). Major depressive disorder can occur at any

Cognitive and Behavioral Dysfunction in Schizophrenia. https://doi.org/10.1016/B978-0-12-820005-6.00003-7

age, although its peak onset is in the 20s. The prevalence for 18- to 29-year-olds is generally threefold higher than that of 60-year-olds, although other studies suggest that depression is more common in older age (Beekman et al., 1995; Kramer, German, Anthony, Van Korff, & Skinner, 1985; Roberts, Kaplan, Shema, & Strawbridge, 1997). Further, the prevalence of depression in women is 1.5- to 3-fold higher than in men (Hyde & Mezulis, 2020; Kang et al., 2020), although few studies reported opposite results (Gao, Ping, & Liu, 2020). The essential feature of major depressive disorder is a period of at least 2 weeks during which there is depressed mood that represents a change in functioning as characterized by exhibiting the following: (a) depressed mood most of the day, almost every day and (b) diminished interest in nearly all activities most of the day—almost every day.

Some of the following symptoms need to be present to conclude a diagnosis of depression in schizophrenia (Siris, 2012, Mulholland & Cooper, 2000): (a) significant weight loss or gain or change in appetite (decrease or increase) almost every day; (b) sleep disturbance (insomnia or hypersomnia) almost every day; (c) restlessness or slowing down almost every day; (d) fatigue or loss of energy almost every day; (e) feelings of guilt or worthlessness almost every day; (f) decreased ability to think or concentrate or make decisions almost every day; and (g) recurrent thoughts of death, recurrent suicidal ideation, suicide attempt or specific plan for committing suicide (Hawton, Sutton, Haw, Sinclair, & Deeks, 2005). In order to meet the criteria for major depressive disorder, the symptoms must cause significant impairment in occupational, social, or other areas of functioning and the symptoms may not be attributable to another medical condition, including substance abuse.

Schizophrenia and depression

Suicide is about 13 times more likely in people with schizophrenia than in the general population and depression is the most significant mediator of suicide in people with schizophrenia (Hayes, Chang, Fernandes, et al., 2012; Saha, Chant, & McGrath, 2007). Depressive symptoms in schizophrenia is associated with deficiencies in psychosocial functioning and increase the risk of suicide (Hor & Taylor, 2010; Kasckow, Felmet, & Zisook, 2011; Palmer, Pankratz, & Bostwick, 2005; Pompili et al., 2007; Preti, Meneghelli, Pisano, Cocchi, & Programma, 2009; Ventriglio et al., 2016). Approximately 5%–6% of individuals with schizophrenia die by suicide and 20% attempt suicide, but the risk of suicidal behavior exists at all times during major depressive episodes (Hawton et al., 2005).

About 25% of people diagnosed with schizophrenia suffer from depression (Chemerinski, Bowie, Anderson, & Harvey, 2008), although different studies report different rates of prevalence (Conley, Ascher-Svanum, Zhu, Faries, & Kinon, 2007; Upthegrove et al., 2010; Upthegrove, Marwaha, & Birchwood, 2017). Depression may be prevalent throughout all phases of the illness in schizophrenia patients, including during psychotic episodes, and may be associated with themes of loss and hopelessness.

Schizophrenia patients with major depression show lower quality of life than schizophrenia patients without depressive symptoms (Karow, Wittmann, Schottle, Schafer, & Lambert, 2014). In schizophrenia patients with low quality of life, three factors are related with depression: the presence of schizophrenia symptoms, large number of medications, and lack of regular daily routine activities (Cardoso et al., 2007). Thus, there is a high prevalence of depression in schizophrenia with impact on quality of life. Risk factors for depression in schizophrenia relate to family history of depressive disorder, high levels of family and personal expectations for success in life, critical family attitudes, high levels of family expressed emotion, stigma, intelligence and insight, multiple hospitalizations, recent hospital discharge, and lack or loss of psychosocial support or support of self-esteem.

Many people with schizophrenia have a limited and solitary existence, in addition to high rates of unemployment, low income, and poor physical health (Andreu-Bernabeu et al., 2020; Knafo, 2020; Morgan, Waterreus, Jablensky, et al., 2011). Misuse of alcohol and illicit substances is common among people with schizophrenia (Cantor-Graae, Nordstrom, & McNeil, 2001; Mallard, Harden, & Fromme, 2019; Menghini-Muller et al., 2019; Moore, Mancuso, Slade, et al., 2012; Winklbaur, Ebner, Sachs, Thau, & Fischer, 2006). All these factors contribute to high rates of depression in people with schizophrenia. As mentioned above, around a quarter of people with schizophrenia meet criteria for a depressive disorder at some time in their lives (Chemerinski et al., 2008; Siris, 2000). However, many more people with schizophrenia experience subthreshold depressive symptoms, that is, patients falling below the diagnostic threshold (Morgan et al., 2011).

The difficulty of diagnosis of depression in schizophrenia

Depressive symptoms in patients with schizophrenia are often ignored by clinicians (Mulholland & Cooper, 2000). This is at least true in part because of the difficulty of distinguishing between symptoms of a concurrent mood disorder (or depressive symptoms) and those of the schizophrenia disorder itself. Further, differentiating schizophrenia from significant depressive symptoms of schizoaffective disorder and major depressive disorder with psychotic features (psychotic depression) is often difficult (APA, 2000; (Upthegrove et al., 2017). Although depressive and negative symptoms of schizophrenia may appear similar, some features can help in differentiating them. For instance, negative symptoms include blunted affect while depressive symptoms are associated with prominent low mood, hopelessness, helplessness, worthlessness, guilt, and suicidal ideation (Mulholland & Cooper, 2000). Thus, during clinical assessments, it is very useful to ask questions about patients' interest in activities to differentiate depressive symptoms from schizophrenia symptoms. For instance, a loss of interest in usual activities (anhedonia) is more common in major depressive disorder than in schizophrenia patients. On the other hand, patients with severe negative symptoms alone may describe their interests in a mild and affectively restricted manner (Bosanac & Castle, 2013).

Causes of depression in schizophrenia and related disorders

There are many factors related to the occurrence of depression in schizophrenia, including genetic and environmental factors (Park, Lee, Furnham, Jeon, & Ko, 2017). As mentioned above, the prevalence of schizophrenia is greater in men than women (Aleman, Kahn, & Selten, 2003; McGrath, Saha, Chant, & Welham, 2008). The onset of schizophrenia is generally supposed to occur earlier in men than women (Cornblatt, Lenzenweger, Dworkin, & Erlenmeyer-Kimling, 1985). It is not known if gender differences in the prevalence of schizophrenia is related to genetic or environmental factors. However, children have a 10% chance of developing schizophrenia and associated depression if one of the parents suffer from schizophrenia. In addition, stressful events might act as a trigger for the onset of schizophrenia (Nasrallah & Hwang, 2009). Sometimes anxiousness and irritability occur before the symptoms of schizophrenia becomes evident, and even act as risk factors for the development of schizophrenia symptoms.

Depression may occur in schizophrenia due to various reasons. It has been found that people with a psychotic disorder (e.g., schizophrenia) had high rates of depressed mood (79.6% at some time in their life). Depressive symptoms in schizophrenia may occur due to significant distress such as loss, grief, and hopelessness, and can occur throughout all phases of the illness, including acute psychotic episodes and the post-psychotic phase. There is an increased risk of psychotic relapse when depression persists in the chronic phase of schizophrenia. Trauma and neglect may trigger depression in schizophrenia (Upthegrove et al., 2017).

Depression in schizophrenia may be triggered by social adversity and or due to childhood maltreatment (Jauhar et al., 2014). Increasing evidence implicates that both SIRT1 (an enzyme at deacetylates proteins that contribute to cellular regulation) and BDNF (a member of the neurotrophin family of growth factors, which are related to the canonical nerve growth factor) are closely related to the development of depression. Fang, Chen, Wang, Ren, and Zhang (2019) aimed to explore the effect of BDNF and SIRT1 on the development of depressive symptoms, and also explore the risk factors for the depressive symptoms in schizophrenia patients. In this study, it was found that low BDNF and SIRT1 concentration may be responsible for the occurrence of depression in schizophrenic patients. In a recent study by Krynicki, Upthegrove, Deakin, and Barnes (2018), it was found that in schizophrenia, primary factors of low mood, suicidal ideation and pessimism are related to depressive symptoms, whereas alogia and blunted affect are related to negative symptoms in schizophrenia. Anhedonia, anergia, and avolition are common to both depressive and negative symptoms. It may be possible to further distinguish depressive features from negative symptoms in schizophrenia when detailed phenomenology is considered. However, these two domains continue to share many characteristics, highlighting their close relationship.

The treatment of depression in schizophrenia and related disorders

Below, we discuss both pharmacological and behavioral treatments (including mindfulness and cognitive behavioral therapy) for depression in schizophrenia, respectively.

Pharmacological treatment

Antidepressants prescribed along with antipsychotics have a major role in controlling depressive symptoms in schizophrenia. Hospitalization might be necessary during increased depressive episodes, to ensure safety and proper self-care (Gregory, Mallikarjun, & Upthegrove, 2017). Antidepressants along with antipsychotics can manage depressive symptoms in schizophrenia, but side effects such as constipation, urinary retention can occur (Gregory et al., 2017). Though some of the atypical antipsychotics appear to have primary antidepressant effects, the effectiveness of these drugs alone for an effective treatment of persistent depressive symptoms in schizophrenia is not well established. Siris, Van Kammen, and Docherty (1978) observed that the combination of antidepressants, such as tricyclic antidepressant (TCAs) and antipsychotics ameliorated the symptoms of depression in some patients with schizophrenia. This finding was confirmed by another clinical study (Prusoff, Williams, Weissman, & Astrachan, 1979). Siris, Bermanzohn, Mason, and Shuwall (1994) have also suggested that maintenance of supporting antidepressant therapy for schizophrenia patients with depressive symptoms could help prevent a relapse of depression and protect patients from worsening psychosis (Mao & Ming-Dao, 2015).

The side effects of tricyclic antidepressant are due to their anticholinergic properties. These side effects include constipation, urinary retention, delirium, and cognitive dysfunction. It has been observed that these side effects are more pronounced in older patients than in younger patients with schizophrenia. Sedative and anticholinergic side effects of antipsychotics are worsened by tricyclic antidepressant, although they might be helpful for extrapyramidal symptoms. If an overdose of tricyclic antidepressants is taken, it might be fatal and due to this fact it is a serious problem due to their inherent toxicity (Mao & Ming-Dao, 2015).

Serotonin antagonist and reuptake inhibitor (SARI) and selective serotonin reuptake inhibitor (SSRIs) significantly improve depressive symptoms in schizophrenia and with less adverse effects than tricyclic antidepressants. It has been observed that citalopram augmentation in schizophrenia treatment has shown a significant effect by improving depressive and negative symptoms (Zisook, Kasckow, Golshan, et al., 2009). It was also found that the use of antidepressants as an add-on therapy to antipsychotics moderately yet significantly improved the negative symptoms in chronic schizophrenia patients (Rummel, Kissling, & Leucht, 2005). Newer antidepressants, including selective serotonin reuptake inhibitors (SSRIs, including fluoxetine, fluvoxamine, citalopram), SARI (trazodone), and serotonin 5-HT_{2C} antagonist (ritanserin) exhibit more favorable results in treating depression in schizophrenia (Singh, Singh, Kar, & Chan, 2010).

Another antidepressant, bupropion, serves as a nontricyclic antidepressant and is different from SSRIs. Bupropion acts as a mild reuptake inhibitor of dopamine and norepinephrine, as well as a nicotinic acetylcholine receptor antagonist (Arias, 2009). Bupropion has been shown to be an effective antidepressant in schizophrenia and is well tolerated, even compared to selective serotonin reuptake inhibitors. One study suggested that use of bupropion in schizophrenia is favorable in alleviating depressive symptoms (Nieuwstraten & Dolovich, 2001). Noradrenergic and specific serotonergic antidepressants (NaSSAs), such as mirtazapine and mianserin, have specific antagonism of certain serotonin receptors, that reduces many side effects associated with SSRIs. Noradrenergic and specific serotonergic antidepressants can be well tolerated. Research study showed that noradrenergic and specific serotonergic antidepressants augmentation therapy in schizophrenia treatment has their beneficial effects on akathisia and extrapyramidal symptoms (Kishi & Iwata, 2014). However, there was little evidence to support any significant effect of noradrenergic and specific serotonergic antidepressants on the depressive symptoms in schizophrenia (Kishi & Iwata, 2014).

Norepinephrine reuptake inhibitors (NRIs), such as reboxetine, has been shown to be effective in alleviating depressive symptoms in schizophrenia; however, compared to other serotoninergic antidepressants, reboxetine is much less effective (Cipriani, Furukawa, Salanti, et al., 2009). From the existing clinical trials, the effectiveness of antidepressants on treating depressive symptoms is rather mixed; different studies demonstrated a significant effect of antidepressants in patients with schizophrenia, while the others did not indicate any positive results. Serotonin reuptake inhibitors, the antidepressants used in combination with antipsychotic to treat depression in schizophrenia, have less effect on cholinergic, histaminergic, and adrenergic systems. They are relatively safe even in overdose situations. Serotonin reuptake inhibitors are also associated with reductions in impulsivity, irritability, aggression, paranoia, and other behavioral disturbances (Butler, Schofield, Greenberg, et al., 2010). Common complaints of these newer antidepressants include nausea, changes in appetite, and sexual dysfunction. The combination of selective serotonin reuptake inhibitors with atypical antipsychotics is generally safer than the combination of tricyclic antidepressants with typical antipsychotics.

Side effects of both antipsychotic and antidepressant medications can be weight gain and sedation and could be potentially additive (Himelhoch et al., 2012). However, the chance of these side effects is low, in particular in patients who are at a stable chronic phase of illness. It has been found that more attention should be paid when clozapine is augmented with antidepressants (Centorrino et al., 1996). The combination of antipsychotic with antidepressant increases the risk or severity of anticholinergic side effects, such as blurred vision, dry mouth, constipation, or urinary retention. Patients with schizophrenia and depressive symptoms are recommended to be firstly treated with an optimal dose of second-generation antipsychotics and a supplemental anti-Parkinsonian agent; if significant depressive symptoms persist after optimization, antidepressants, preferably selective serotonin reuptake inhibitors, are recommended (Mao & Ming-Dao, 2015). The answer to the question of whether antidepressants could overall be beneficial in treating patients with schizophrenia is still elusive. The effectiveness of added antidepressants on treating depressive symptoms in patients with schizophrenia varies to a large extent. This variation is possibly due to divergent states of psychotic illness and depression, various psychotropic medications and substance use/abuse, different properties of antidepressants themselves, individual variance in the activity of drug metabolism enzymes, and utilization of psychosocial interventions (De Silva, Cooper, Li, Lund, & Patel, 2013). Further, there is a substantial risk of worsening psychosis and other symptoms by adding antidepressants into treatment (Mao & Ming-Dao, 2015). Appropriate use of antidepressants could improve depressive symptoms in patients with schizophrenia, but extra care should be taken in terms of adverse effects.

Mindfulness

Mindfulness can be very effective for the treatment of depressive and related symptoms in schizophrenia (Treanor, 2011), including loss of interest in daily activities, loss of appetite, among others (Boge et al., 2020; Tabak, Horan, & Green, 2015). In schizophrenia, negative thoughts might lead to negative emotions, and the development of depression. As part of mindfulness, focusing on the here and now assists individuals to be conscious of their negative thoughts and identify them without judgment and realize they are not actual reflections of reality. By using mindfulness, individuals start to see their thoughts as less overwhelming. These distorted thoughts—such as "I always make mistakes" or "I'm a horrible person"—start to become less powerful.

Mindfulness-based cognitive therapy (MBCT) is a group therapy that combines mindfulness techniques with cognitive therapy to help prevent relapse in depression in schizophrenia (Kimhy et al., 2012). Mindfulness-based cognitive therapy is based on mindfulness-based stress reduction (MBSR). Mindfulness-based cognitive therapy teaches individuals to disassociate from distorted and negative thinking patterns, which can trigger the return of depression in schizophrenia. It is suggested that MBCT is a valuable tool for intervention for depression in schizophrenia. It has been found that MBCT was highly effective in reducing relapse for major depression in schizophrenia (Tang, Holzel, & Posner, 2015).

Cognitive behavioral therapy (CBT)

Cognitive Behavioral Therapy was found to reduce depressive symptoms in schizophrenia patients (Ann, 2009; Laws, Darlington, Kondel, McKenna, & Jauhar, 2018; Sonmez et al., 2020). Cognitive Behavioral Therapy for schizophrenia involves establishing a collaborative therapeutic relationship, developing a shared understanding of the problem, setting goals, and teaching the person techniques or strategies to reduce or manage their symptoms including depression. Therapy is usually conducted in individual sessions and is time-limited (typically several months). The goal is not to "cure" depression in schizophrenia, but rather to improve the person's ability to function independently, manage their depression in schizophrenia, and to reduce the distress they experience in their daily life. Specific Cognitive Behavioral Therapy approaches used in treating depression in schizophrenia include cognitive restructuring, behavioral experiments/reality testing, self-monitoring, and coping skills training. Unique considerations in treating depression in schizophrenia include emphasis on being nonconfrontational and on normalizing psychotic experiences insomuch as they are on a continuum with nonpsychotic experiences. Cognitive Behavioral Therapy for schizophrenia can focus specifically on psychotic symptoms (i.e., hallucinations or delusional beliefs) but has also been shown to be helpful for addressing depression and/or anxiety associated with psychotic symptoms and their impact on the person's life (Rector & Beck, 2001).

Conclusion

In this article, we reviewed studies showing that depression in schizophrenia is prevalent. Depression can impact the quality of life and lead to suicidal thoughts and attempts in schizophrenia patients. We also show evidence that there are genetic and environmental factors underlying the occurrence of depression in schizophrenia. Finally, based on our review, we should that behavioral treatments, such as mindfulness and cognitive behavioral therapy, can better manage depressive symptoms than pharmacological treatments in schizophrenia patients.

References

Abo Hamza, E., Helal, A. A., Moustafa, A. A., & Emam, M. (2020). The relationship between intrusive cognition and defense mechanisms in healthy and clinical populations. *Humanities & Social Sciences Reviews*, *8*(1), 759–767.

Aleman, A., Kahn, R. S., & Selten, J. P. (2003). Sex differences in the risk of schizophrenia: Evidence from meta-analysis. *Archives of General Psychiatry*, *60*, 565–571.

American Psychiatric Association. (2000). *Diagnostic and statistical manual of mental disorders* (4th ed.). Washington, DC: American Psychiatric Publishing. text revision.

Andreu-Bernabeu, A., Diaz-Caneja, C. M., Costas, J., De Hoyos, L., Stella, C., Gurriaran, X., et al. (2020). Unraveling the relationship of loneliness and isolation in schizophrenia: Polygenic dissection and causal inference. *medRxiv*. https://doi.org/10.1101/2020.11.06.20226910.

Ann, M. K. (2009). Cognitive behavior therapy for people with schizophrenia. *Psychiatry (Edgmont)*, *6*(12), 32–39.

Arias, H. R. (2009). Is the inhibition of nicotinic acetylcholine receptors by bupropion involved in its clinical actions? *The International Journal of Biochemistry & Cell Biology*, *41*(11), 2098–2108.

Beekman, A. T. F., Deeg, D. J. H., van Tilburg, T., Smit, J. H., Hooijer, C., & van Tilburg, W. (1995). Major and minor depression in later life: A study of prevalence and risk factors. *Journal of Affective Disorders*, *36*, 65–75.

Boge, K., Karadza, A., Fuchs, L. M., Ehlen, F., Ta, T. M. T., Thomas, N., … Hahn, E. (2020). Mindfulness-based interventions for in-patients with schizophrenia spectrum disorders-a qualitative approach. *Frontiers in Psychiatry*, *11*, 600. https://doi.org/10.3389/fpsyt.2020.00600.

Bosanac, P., & Castle, D. J. (2013). Schizophrenia and depression. *The Medical Journal of Australia*, *199*, S369.

Butler, T., Schofield, P. W., Greenberg, D., et al. (2010). Reducing impulsivity in repeat violent offenders: An open label trial of a selective serotonin reuptake inhibitor. *The Australian and New Zealand Journal of Psychiatry*, *44*, 1137–1143.

Cantor-Graae, E., Nordstrom, L. G., & McNeil, T. F. (2001). Substance abuse in schizophrenia: A review of the literature and a study of correlates in Sweden. *Schizophrenia Research, 48*, 69–82.

Cardoso, C. S., Caiaffa, W. T., Bandeira, M., Siqueira, A. L., Silva, J. T., & Fonseca, J. O. (2007). Depression in schizophrenia: Prevalence and relationship to quality of life. *Cadernos de Saúde Pública, 23*(9), 2035–2048.

Centorrino, F., Baldessarini, R. J., Frankenburg, F. R., Kando, J., Volpicelli, S. A., & Flood, J. G. (1996). Serum levels of clozapine and norclozapine in patients treated with selective serotonin reuptake inhibitors. *The American Journal of Psychiatry, 153*, 820–822.

Chemerinski, E., Bowie, C., Anderson, H., & Harvey, P. (2008). Depression in schizophrenia: Methodological artifact or distinct feature of the illness. *The Journal of Neuropsychiatry and Clinical Neurosciences, 20*(4), 431–440.

Cipriani, A., Furukawa, T. A., Salanti, G., et al. (2009). Comparative efficacy and acceptability of 12 new-generation antidepressants: A multiple-treatments meta-analysis. *Lancet, 373*(9665), 746–758.

Conley, R. R., Ascher-Svanum, H., Zhu, B., Faries, D. E., & Kinon, B. J. (2007). The burden of depressive symptoms in the long-term treatment of patients with schizophrenia. *Schizophrenia Research, 90*, 186–197.

Cornblatt, A. B., Lenzenweger, M. F., Dworkin, H. R., & Erlenmeyer-Kimling, L. (1985). Positive and negative schizophrenic symptoms, attention, and information processing; Oxford journals; Medicine & Health. *Schizophrenia Bulletin, 11*(3), 397–408.

De Fruyt, J., Sabbe, B., & Demyttenaere, K. (2020). Anhedonia in depressive disorder: A narrative review. *Psychopathology*, 1–8. https://doi.org/10.1159/000508773.

De Silva, M. J., Cooper, S., Li, H. L., Lund, C., & Patel, V. (2013). Effect of psychosocial interventions on social functioning in depression and schizophrenia: Meta-analysis. *The British Journal of Psychiatry, 202*, 253–260.

Fang, X., Chen, Y., Wang, Y., Ren, J., & Zhang, C. (2019). Depressive symptoms in schizophrenia patients: A possible relationship between SIRT1 and BDNF. *Progress in Neuro-Psychopharmacology & Biological Psychiatry, 20*(95), 109673.

Gao, W., Ping, S., & Liu, X. (2020). Gender differences in depression, anxiety, and stress among college students: A longitudinal study from China. *Journal of Affective Disorders, 263*, 292–300. https://doi.org/10.1016/j.jad.2019.11.121.

Gregory, A., Mallikarjun, P., & Upthegrove, R. (2017). Treatment of depression in schizophrenia: Systematic review and meta-analysis. *The British Journal of Psychiatry, 211*(4), 198–204. https://doi.org/10.1192/bjp.bp.116.190520 (Epub 2017 Sep 7).

Hawton, K., Sutton, L., Haw, C., Sinclair, J., & Deeks, J. D. (2005). Schizophrenia and suicide: Systematic review of risk factors. *British Journal of Psychiatry, 187*, 9–20.

Hayes, R. D., Chang, C. K., Fernandes, A., et al. (2012). Associations between symptoms and all-cause mortality in individuals with serious mental illness. *Journal of Psychosomatic Research, 72*, 114–119.

Himelhoch, S., Slade, E., Kreyenbuhl, J., Medoff, D., Brown, C., & Dixon, L. (2012). Antidepressant prescribing patterns among VA patients with schizophrenia. *Schizophrenia Research, 136*, 32–35.

Hor, K., & Taylor, M. (2010). Suicide and schizophrenia: A systematic review of rates and risk factors. *Journal of Psychopharmacology, 24*(4 Suppl), 81–90. https://doi.org/10.1177/1359786810385490.

Hyde, J. S., & Mezulis, A. H. (2020). Gender differences in depression: Biological, affective, cognitive, and sociocultural factors. *Harvard Review of Psychiatry, 28*(1), 4–13. https://doi.org/10.1097/HRP.0000000000000230.

Jauhar, S., McKenna, P. J., Radua, J., Fung, E., Salvador, R., & Laws, K. R. (2014). Cognitive behavior therapy for the symptoms of schizophrenia: Systematic review and meta-analysis with examination of potential bias. *The British Journal of Psychiatry*, *204*, 20–29.

Kang, H. J., Park, Y., Yoo, K. H., Kim, K. T., Kim, E. S., Kim, J. W., … Kim, J. M. (2020). Sex differences in the genetic architecture of depression. *Scientific Reports*, *10*(1), 9927. https://doi.org/10.1038/s41598-020-66672-9.

Karow, A., Wittmann, L., Schottle, D., Schafer, I., & Lambert, M. (2014). The assessment of quality of life in clinical practice in patients with schizophrenia. *Dialogues in Clinical Neuroscience*, *16*(2), 185–195.

Kasckow, J., Felmet, K., & Zisook, S. (2011). Managing suicide risk in patients with schizophrenia. *CNS Drugs*, *25*(2), 129–143. https://doi.org/10.2165/11586450-000000000-00000.

Kimhy, D., Vakhrusheva, J., Jobson-Ahmed, L., Tarrier, N., Malaspina, D., & Gross, J. J. (2012). Emotion awareness and regulation in individuals with schizophrenia: Implications for social functioning. *Psychiatry Research*, *2012*, 193–201.

Kishi, T., & Iwata, N. (2014). Meta-analysis of noradrenergic and specific serotonergic antidepressant use in schizophrenia. *The International Journal of Neuropsychopharmacology*, *17*(2), 343–354.

Knafo, D. (2020). Alone in a crowded mind: When psychosis masks loneliness. *Psychoanalytic Psychology*, *37*(2), 108–116. https://doi.org/10.1037/pap0000257.

Kramer, M., German, P. S., Anthony, J. C., Van Korff, M., & Skinner, E. A. (1985). Patterns of mental disorders among the elderly residents of eastern Baltimore. *Journal of the American Geriatrics Society*, *33*, 236–245.

Krynicki, C. R., Upthegrove, R., Deakin, J. F. W., & Barnes, T. R. E. (2018). The relationship between negative symptoms and depression in schizophrenia: A systematic review. *Acta Psychiatrica Scandinavica*, *137*(5), 380–390.

Laws, K. R., Darlington, N., Kondel, T. K., McKenna, P. J., & Jauhar, S. (2018). Cognitive behavioural therapy for schizophrenia - outcomes for functioning, distress and quality of life: A meta-analysis. *BMC Psychology*, *6*(1), 32. https://doi.org/10.1186/s40359-018-0243-2.

Mallard, T. T., Harden, K. P., & Fromme, K. (2019). Genetic risk for schizophrenia is associated with substance use in emerging adulthood: An event-level polygenic prediction model. *Psychological Medicine*, *49*(12), 2027–2035. https://doi.org/10.1017/S0033291718002817.

Mao, Y.-M., & Ming-Dao, Z. (2015). Augmentation with antidepressants in schizophrenia treatment: benefit or risk. *Neuropsychiatric Disease and Treatment*, *11*, 701–713.

McGrath, J. L., Saha, S., Chant, D., & Welham, J. (2008). Schizophrenia: A concise overview of incidence, prevalence, and mortality. *Epidemiologic Reviews*, *30*, 67–76.

Menghini-Muller, S., Studerus, E., Ittig, S., Heitz, U., Egloff, L., Andreou, C., … van Os, J. (2019). Gender differences of patients at-risk for psychosis regarding symptomatology, drug use, comorbidity and functioning—Results from the EU-GEI study. *European Psychiatry*, *59*, 52–59. https://doi.org/10.1016/j.eurpsy.2019.04.007.

Moore, E., Mancuso, S. G., Slade, T., et al. (2012). The impact of alcohol and illicit drugs on people with psychosis: The second Australian national survey of psychosis. *The Australian and New Zealand Journal of Psychiatry*, *46*, 864–878.

Morgan, V. A., Waterreus, A., Jablensky, A., et al. (2011). *People living with psychotic illness 2010: Report on the second Australian national survey.* Canberra: Department of Health and Ageing.

Moustafa, A. A., Crouse, J. J., Herzallah, M. M., Salama, M., Mohamed, W., Misiak, B., … Mattock, K. (2019). Depression following major life transitions in women: A review and theory. *Psychological Reports*.

Moustafa, A. A., Tindle, R., Cashel, S., Parkes, D., Mohamed, E., & Abo Hamza, E. (2020). Bidirectional relationship between heroin addiction and depression: Behavioural and neural studies. *Current Psychology*.

Mulholland, C., & Cooper, S. (2000). The symptom of depression in schizophrenia and its management. *Advances in Psychiatric Treatment*, *6*, 169–177.

Nasrallah, H., & Hwang, M. (2009). Psychiatric and physical comorbidity in schizophrenia. *A Psychiatric Clinic*, *32*(4), 719–914.

Nieuwstraten, C. E., & Dolovich, L. R. (2001). Bupropion versus selective serotonin-reuptake inhibitors for treatment of depression. *The Annals of Pharmacotherapy*, *35*(12), 1608–1613.

Nutt, D., Wilson, S., & Paterson, L. (2008). Sleep disorders as core symptoms of depression. *Dialogues in Clinical Neuroscience*, *10*(3), 329–336.

Palmer, B. A., Pankratz, V. S., & Bostwick, J. M. (2005). The lifetime risk of suicide in schizophrenia: A reexamination. *Archives of General Psychiatry*, *62*(3), 247–253. https://doi.org/10.1001/archpsyc.62.3.247.

Park, S., Lee, M., Furnham, A., Jeon, M., & Ko, Y. M. (2017). Lay beliefs about the causes and cures of schizophrenia. *The International Journal of Social Psychiatry*. 20764017717283 Y.

Pompili, M., Amador, X. F., Girardi, P., Harkavy-Friedman, J., Harrow, M., Kaplan, K., … Tatarelli, R. (2007). Suicide risk in schizophrenia: Learning from the past to change the future. *Annals of General Psychiatry*, *6*, 10. https://doi.org/10.1186/1744-859X-6-10.

Preti, A., Meneghelli, A., Pisano, A., Cocchi, A., & Programma, T. (2009). Risk of suicide and suicidal ideation in psychosis: Results from an Italian multi-modal pilot program on early intervention in psychosis. *Schizophrenia Research*, *113*(2–3), 145–150. https://doi.org/10.1016/j.schres.2009.06.007.

Prusoff, B. A., Williams, D. H., Weissman, M. M., & Astrachan, B. M. (1979). Treatment of secondary depression in schizophrenia: A double-blind, placebo-controlled trial of amitriptyline added to perphenazine. *Archives of General Psychiatry*, *36*, 569.

Radell, M., Abo Hamza, E., & Moustafa, A. A. (2020). Depression in posttraumatic stress disorder. *Reviews in the Neurosciences*.

Rector, N. A., & Beck, A. T. (2001). Cognitive behavioral therapy for schizophrenia: An empirical review. *The Journal of Nervous and Mental Disease*, *189*(5), 278–287.

Roberts, R. E., Kaplan, G. A., Shema, S. J., & Strawbridge, W. J. (1997). Does growing old increase the risk for depression? *The American Journal of Psychiatry*, *154*, 1384–1390.

Rummel, C., Kissling, W., & Leucht, S. (2005). Antidepressants as add-on treatment to antipsychotics for people with schizophrenia and pronounced negative symptoms: A systematic review of randomized trials. *Schizophrenia Research*, *80*, 85–97.

Saha, S., Chant, D., & McGrath, J. (2007). A systematic review of mortality in schizophrenia: Is the differential mortality gap worsening over time? *Archives of General Psychiatry*, *64*, 1123–1131.

Sheynin, J., Baetu, I., Collins-Praino, L. E., Myers, C. E., Winwood-Smith, R., & Moustafa, A. A. (2020). Maladaptive avoidance patterns in Parkinson's disease are exacerbated by symptoms of depression. *Behavioural Brain Research*.

Singh, S. P., Singh, V., Kar, N., & Chan, K. (2010). Efficacy of antidepressants in treating the negative symptoms of chronic schizophrenia: Meta-analysis. *The British Journal of Psychiatry*, *197*, 174–179.

Siris, S. G. (2000). Depression in schizophrenia: Perspective in the era of "atypical" antipsychotic agents. *The American Journal of Psychiatry*, *157*, 1379–1389.

Siris, S. (2012). Treating "depression" in patients with schizophrenia. *Current Psychiatry*, *11*(8), 35–39.

Siris, S. G., Bermanzohn, P. C., Mason, S. E., & Shuwall, M. A. (1994). Maintenance imipramine therapy for secondary depression in schizophrenia: A controlled trial. *Archives of General Psychiatry*, *51*, 109.

Siris, S. G., Van Kammen, D. P., & Docherty, J. P. (1978). Use of antidepressant drugs in schizophrenia. *Archives of General Psychiatry*, *35*, 1368.

Sonmez, N., Romm, K. L., Ostefjells, T., Grande, M., Jensen, L. H., Hummelen, B., … Rossberg, J. I. (2020). Cognitive behavior therapy in early psychosis with a focus on depression and low self-esteem: A randomized controlled trial. *Comprehensive Psychiatry*, *97*, 152157. https://doi.org/10.1016/j.comppsych.2019.152157.

Tabak, N. T., Horan, W. P., & Green, M. F. (2015). Mindfulness in schizophrenia: Associations with self-reported motivation, emotion regulation, dysfunctional attitudes, and negative symptoms. *Schizophrenia Research*, *168*(1–2), 537–542. https://doi.org/10.1016/j.schres.2015.07.030.

Tang, Y.-Y., Holzel, B. K., & Posner, M. I. (2015). The neuroscience of mindfulness meditation. *Nature Reviews. Neuroscience*, *16*, 213–225.

Treanor, M. (2011). The potential impact of mindfulness on exposure and extinction learning in anxiety disorders. *Clinical Psychology Review*, *31*, 617–625.

Trivedi, M. H., Hollander, E., Nutt, D., & Blier, P. (2008). Clinical evidence and potential neurobiological underpinnings of unresolved symptoms of depression. *The Journal of Clinical Psychiatry*, *69*(2), 246–258. https://doi.org/10.4088/jcp.v69n0211.

Upthegrove, R., Birchwood, M., Ross, K., Brunett, K., McCollum, R., & Jones, L. (2010). The evolution of depression and suicidality in first episode psychosis. *Acta Psychiatrica Scandinavica*, *122*, 211–218.

Upthegrove, R., Marwaha, S., & Birchwood, M. (2017). Depression and schizophrenia: Cause, consequence, or trans-diagnostic issue? *Schizophrenia Bulletin*, *43*(2), 240–244. https://doi.org/10.1093/schbul/sbw097.

Ventriglio, A., Gentile, A., Bonfitto, I., Stella, E., Mari, M., Steardo, L., & Bellomo, A. (2016). Suicide in the early stage of schizophrenia. *Frontiers in Psychiatry*, *7*, 116. https://doi.org/10.3389/fpsyt.2016.00116.

Watson, R., Harvey, K., McCabe, C., & Reynolds, S. (2020). Understanding anhedonia: A qualitative study exploring loss of interest and pleasure in adolescent depression. *European Child & Adolescent Psychiatry*, *29*(4), 489–499. https://doi.org/10.1007/s00787-019-01364-y.

Winklbaur, B., Ebner, N., Sachs, G., Thau, K., & Fischer, G. (2006). Substance abuse in patients with schizophrenia. *Dialogues in Clinical Neuroscience*, *8*(1), 37–43.

Zisook, S., Kasckow, J. W., Golshan, S., et al. (2009). Citalopram augmentation for subsyndromal symptoms of depression in middle-aged and older outpatients with schizophrenia and schizoaffective disorder: A randomized controlled trial. *The Journal of Clinical Psychiatry*, *70*, 562.

Sleep and psychosis

10

Noémi Báthori[a], *Ahmed A. Moustafa*[b,c], *and Bertalan Polner*[a]
[a]Budapest University of Technology and Economics, Budapest, Hungary, [b]School of Psychology & Marcs Institute for Brain and Behaviour, Western Sydney University, Sydney, NSW, Australia, [c]Department of Human Anatomy and Physiology, the Faculty of Health Sciences, University of Johannesburg, South Africa

Chapter outline

Introduction

We spend about one-third of our lives asleep, and sleep is essential for our daily optimal functioning and well-being. Sufficient and satisfactory sleep is necessary to protect our physical and mental health. Inadequate sleep is linked to different health problems including obesity, cardiovascular diseases, and type 2 diabetes. Moreover, insufficient sleep is associated with lower performance at school and work and also increases the risk of traffic, work, and household accidents. Therefore, sleep improvement is crucial in healthcare and equally important at the individual, family, and social levels. In this article, we discuss the relationship between sleep and psychosis and how improving sleep can decrease psychotic episodes and help manage schizophrenia symptoms.

Sleep disorders are often linked to different psychopathologies, and for some several mental disorders, variable sleep duration and quality are listed as diagnostic criteria. The alteration of sleep is also linked to schizophrenia, although it is not included in DSM-5 as a diagnostic criterion. Nonetheless, most patients with schizophrenia reported different sleep disturbances before the illness onset or the aggravation of

Cognitive and Behavioral Dysfunction in Schizophrenia. https://doi.org/10.1016/B978-0-12-820005-6.00010-4

psychosis. Additionally, human physiological and clinical studies have shown that schizophrenia patients demonstrate altered sleep quality using both subjective- and objective measures. Furthermore, there is evidence suggesting that treating sleep disturbances in patients with schizophrenia is important for preventing and/or reducing psychotic experiences (Benson, 2006, 2015; Kaskie, Graziano, & Ferrarelli, 2017; Waters, 2012).

Nowadays, psychosis and sleep research are both dynamically and interactively developing. Accordingly, in the past decade, the study of the link between psychosis and sleep has also been extensively exploded (Benson, 2006, 2015; Kaskie et al., 2017; Waters, 2012). Inconsistencies and conflicting results in the literature leave countless unanswered questions that should be investigated using neural, behavioral, and clinical studies. Before we discuss the relationship between psychosis and sleep, we will first discuss sleep basics.

Sleep basics

Sleep is essential not only for humans but for most animals and appears to have evolutionary roots. Although it could seem maladaptive in terms of foraging, mating and defence against predators, sleep is preserved across evolution (Joiner, 2016). This suggests that sleep is crucial for humans and animals, and its absence has physiological, health, and functional consequences. In humans, sleep is essential for the maintenance and restoration of physiological functions (Fultz et al., 2019) and different mental processes such as cognitive processing, memory consolidation, and emotional brain processes (Walker, 2009). In spite of that, our understanding of the function of sleep is far from complete.

Sleep is not just the mere absence of wakefulness. From a behavioral point of view, sleep is marked by specific attributes such as an increased sensory threshold, a typical sleeping posture, decreased movement and by its approximately 24-hour cycle. Comparing sleep and wakefulness from phenomenological and physiological perspectives, sleep can be described as a transiently altered state of consciousness with decreased sensory activity and specific brainwave patterns, muscle atony, and rapid eye movements. In addition, we can divide sleep into two general types: rapid-eye-movement (REM) and nonrapid-eye-movement (NREM) sleep. NREM sleep is further subdivided into four different stages (N1, N2, N3-N4) according to the stage-specific patterns of the electrical activity of the brain that can be measured with electroencephalography (EEG) (Hori et al., 2001; Moser et al., 2009).

Measurement of sleep states

Qualifying and quantifying sleep is the key role of a sleep study. Objective measurement of specific sleep parameters can help detect nocturnal abnormalities (i.e., difficulty in falling or staying asleep, nocturnal awakenings, sleep-related movement, and breathing disorders) (Littner et al., 2003; Montplaisir et al., 2010; Uhlig et al., 2019).

Polysomnography (PSG) is the gold standard method to collect physiological parameters during sleep and investigate wakefulness and different sleep states and diagnose sleep disorders in the laboratory. PSG is a multi-parametric test to collect, monitor and record data in a sleep study and it usually includes (but is not limited to) EEG for neural electroencephalographic activity, electrooculography (EOG) for eye movements, electromyography (EMG) for movements of the skeletal muscles, electrocardiography (ECG) for the electrical activity of the heart, pulse oximeter (SaO2) for monitoring oxygen saturation, piezoelectric belts for respiratory effort on chest-wall and abdominal movement (Chesson et al., 1997; Krystal & Edinger, 2008). Together, these measures provide a more accurate and better understanding of sleep and helps distinguish normal and pathological sleep patterns and architectures.

In addition, several self-report instruments have been developed to measure the subjective quality of sleep; these questionnaires can measure not only quantitative aspects such as insufficient and disturbed sleep but also the individual's perceived experience of poor sleep quality and daytime sleepiness (Ji & Liu, 2016). The subjective perception of sleep quality is as crucial as the objective measures (e.g., PSG) and they complement each other because there is a high discrepancy of variability and uncertainty in subjective evaluations and the objective measures of sleep (PSG). Nonetheless, variables such as total sleep time (TST) and sleep onset latency (SOL) correlate adequately with each other and suggest an explicit relationship between these subjective and objective sleep parameters (Zhang & Zhao, 2007). Nonrestorative sleep (NRS) is an important concept referring to the subjective impression that sleep was rather poor than refreshing, despite physiologically normal sleep, and it may co-occur with cognitive and affective complaints (Wilkinson & Shapiro, 2013).

Sleep states and architecture

Sleep architecture refers to the basic structural organization, the cyclic patterns, and the shifts between the distinct sleep stages (REM, NREM 1, 2, 3–4) and awakenings that can be assessed using PSG data and summarized in a graph named hypnogram (sleep histogram) (Colten et al., 2006; Swihart, Caffo, Bandeen-Roche, & Punjabi, 2008). It represents the transitions between sleep stages, awakenings, and abnormal events during the recording as a function of time (Fig. 1). Different sleep stages are characterized by specific brainwave patterns supplemented by specific behavioral patterns. The brain waves in wakefulness typically show a high frequency and low amplitude cortical neuronal activity; wakefulness is typically characterized by beta (13-32 Hz) and gamma (32-100 Hz) waves. NREM sleep N1 (stage I sleep) is a very relaxed state, associated with experiencing drowsiness, which leads to a transition from wakefulness into a light sleep. The most typical changes in the EEG activity pattern are that brain waves begin to slow down. First the alpha waves (8-13 Hz) appear, followed by an increase in theta waves (4–7 Hz). Eye-rolling or slow eye movements (SEM) are also typical in this state. NREM sleep N2 (stage II sleep) is the step before deeper sleep. The skeletal muscles are more relaxed, the heartbeat and breathing slow further and SEM stops. Sleep spindles (12–16 Hz), vertex waves and K-complex waveforms are hallmarks of this stage. NREM sleep N3-N4 (stage 3 and 4 sleep) are also called slow-wave sleep (SWS)

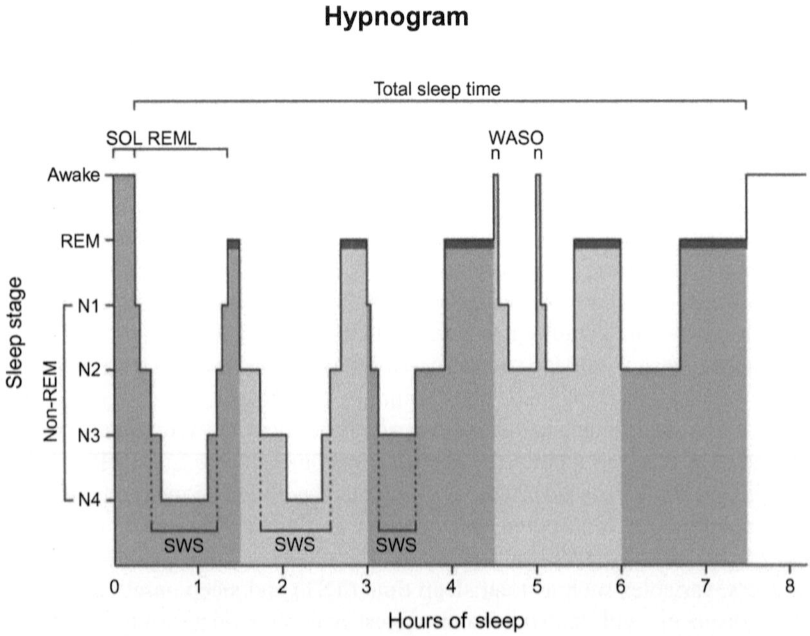

Fig. 1 A hypnogram of a typical night of sleep representing changes between wakefulness and sleep stages as a function of time. The hypnogram is informative about the sleep cycles, the sequence of sleep stages and continuity of sleep. The darker and lighter shades show the approximately 90-min-long cycles of REM and NREM sleep. We note that previously NREM was divided into four different phases, whereas recent theories acknowledge only N1, N2, and N3 (with N3 comprising N3 and N4 from the former model); in recent theories, N3 is also called slow wave sleep (SWS) or deep sleep. NREM sleep is more dominant in the first half of the night, while REM sleep is more prevalent during the second half of the night. *SOL*, sleep onset latency; *REML*, REM latency; *WASO*, wake after sleep onset.

or deep sleep where the dominant activities are delta waves (0.5–4 Hz) oscillations. As we shall see, these aspects of sleep show specific alterations in psychosis. The heartbeat and breathing are in their slowest state. This is the most restorative phase, and awareness of external sensory stimuli is the lowest in this stage, so waking up is the most difficult during this period. REM phase is also known as paradoxical sleep because its brain activity is similar to waking states as it is characterized by a high-frequency and low-amplitude activity, plus rapid side-to-side eye movements. Normally, REM sleep first occurs about 80-100 minutes after falling asleep. Blood pressure and heart rate are elevated during REM sleep, and the skeletal muscles become paralyzed in this stage, which prevents acting out dreams. Most dreams occur during this period, while dreams in NREM stages are less typical (Colten et al., 2006; Hori et al., 2001; Moser et al., 2009; Roehrs, 2000; Silber et al., 2007).

According to according to Academy of Sleep Medicine (AASM), sleep stage scoring, and spectral analysis are the most common analyses for sleep EEG recordings (Campbell, 2009). After scoring of sleep based on PSG data, the hypnogram shows one's sleep architecture, where normally a cyclic sleep stage iteration can be observed in the following order: N1-N2-N3-4-REM. After the end of the REM sleep the cycle starts again with stage N1-2. A whole NREM-REM sleep cycle is approximately 90–110min long. NREM sleep is more prevalent in the first half of the night, while REM sleep more pronounced during the second half of the night. Hypnogram is an acceptable tool to detect and report altered sleep architecture, abnormal cycle order, disrupted and fragmented sleep and prolonged or shortened duration at different stages. These abnormal phenomena are frequently linked to different sleep and mental dysfunctions. A normal sleep stage distribution is approximately 5% of N1, 50% of N2, 20% of N3-4, 20-25% of REM (Shrivastava, Jung, Saadat, Sirohi, & Crewson, 2014) and a few arousals, with significant variability between individuals and with age. The hypnogram represents the sleep macrostructure that visualizes the cyclic changes of sleep stages (Barcaro et al., 1998; Muzet, 2005), while microstructure refers to the characteristics of the sleep EEG features and phasic phenomena that are the basics of categorizing sleep stages (Muzet, 2005). For example, both macro- and microstructure provide important information about sleep quality and could help distinguish normal and pathological sleep. Indeed, abnormal macro- and microstructure changes are found in psychotic patients (Baran et al., 2019; Kaskie, Gill, & Ferrarelli, 2019; Keshavan, Montrose, Miewald, & Jindal, 2011; Muzet, 2005; Sharma & Mazmanian, 2003; Wilson & Argyropoulos, 2012; Zanini et al., 2013).

A PSG assessment in a laboratory also reveals quantitative information about sleep which is important in order to identify insomnia. Total recording time (TRT) or time in bed (TIB) is the total amount of time when the subject is in bed with the activated PSG equipment, including nonsleep-related activity as watching television, reading, or using smart devices. Lights out time are when the lights and devices are turned off and it is assumed that this is the moment when the participant decided to try to fall asleep. The time of falling asleep is called sleep onset time (ST) which is defined as the time when the first epoch of sleep was scored. The overall quantity of sleep is indicated by total sleep time (TST) which is the amount of sleep time is the sum of time spent in N1, N2, N3–4, REM stages in minutes without wake times. Furthermore, these parameters provide the opportunity to derive important sleep indicators such as sleep efficiency (SE) which is the percentage of total time in bed divided by total time spent in sleep which is a hallmark of insomnia. Difficulties with falling asleep may be reflected in prolonged sleep latency or sleep onset latency (SOL) which is the duration from lights out till the first sleep onset epoch. REM onset is the time between the first sleep onset epoch and the first REM onset epoch. Fragmented sleep can be mirrored by altered wake after sleep onset (WASO) which refers to the frequency and duration of nocturnal awakenings. (Shrivastava et al., 2014). These parameters could be crucial diagnostic signs of different sleep disorders such as insomnia or narcolepsy and also of various mental disorders (e.g., major depressive disorder, anxiety disorders, schizophrenia-spectrum disorders, or post-traumatic stress disorder) (Chouinard, Poulin, Stip, & Godbout, 2004; Gupta, Dahiya, & Bhatia, 2009; Kobayashi, Boarts, & Delahanty, 2007).

Aging is associated with changes in the sleep pattern and the sleep cycle across the human lifespan. The recommended sleep duration varies across different stages of life in healthy individuals and sleep duration may be different from person to person as well. The ideal amount of sleep for a newborn is between 14 and 17 h, for a school-aged child between 9 and 11 h, adolescents between 8 and 10 h, young adults 7–9 h, and older adults 7–8 h (Hirshkowitz et al., 2015). PSG studies of sleep architecture frequently described that TST, SE, SWS, REM, and REM latency decrease with age, while WASO increases (Ohayon, Carskadon, Guilleminault, & Vitiello, 2004).

Transitions between wakefulness and sleep

The sleep-wake cycle in humans is typically monophasic (e.g., nocturnal sleep) or biphasic (e.g., napping during afternoon) (Tobler, 1995). The rhythm of sleep and wakefulness is regulated by the interaction of two opposing systems: the sleep-dependent process S that represents homeostatic sleep pressure which constantly increases during wakefulness and decreases during sleep (i.e., the greater the sleep debt, the greater sleep pressure), and the circadian process C which promotes wakefulness and oscillates with a period of circa 24 hours (Blatter & Cajochen, 2007; Borbély, 1982). Process S can be inferred from slow-wave activity in the EEG (Borbély, 1982): increasing sleep pressure correlates with increasing power in low frequency EEG, especially above frontal areas (Cajochen, Foy, & Dijk, 1999; Cajochen, Knoblauch, Kräuchi, Renz, & Wirz-Justice, 2001; Tinguely, Finelli, Landolt, Borbély, & Achermann, 2006). Circadian rhythms are organized by the master circadian pacemaker located in the suprachiasmatic nucleus (SCN) of the hypothalamus which receives input from the retina in order to synchronize with cycles of the environment and sends signals to peripheral clocks located in other brain areas and also in various other organs of the body (Kondratova & Kondratov, 2012). Indeed, circadian rhythms are apparent in gene expression, secretion of hormones such as melatonin or cortisol, and in physiological functions such as body temperature or heart rate (Blatter & Cajochen, 2007; Kondratova & Kondratov, 2012). Moreover, diurnal rhythms in cognitive functions such as vigilance, attention, cognitive control, and memory are correlated with circadian processes (see Blatter & Cajochen, 2007; Schmidt, Collette, Cajochen, & Peigneux, 2007 for reviews).

Sleep-wake cycles are regulated through neuronal mechanisms. Different wake- and sleep-promoting areas were first predicted by von Economo (Economo, 1930) who hypothesized that the posterior hypothalamus promotes wakefulness, and the preoptic area and the basal forebrain contain sleep-promoting neurons; recent studies mostly confirmed his predictions. In the case of a stable sleep-wake cycle sleep- and wake-promoting neurons inhibit each other; the damage of these pathways generates impaired daily cycle (Saper, Chou, & Scammell, 2001) which is related to different sleep-wake disorders such as narcolepsy or hypersomnolence. Sleep-wake control mechanisms regulate the alteration between wakefulness, NREM, and REM sleep. The ascending arousal system promotes wakefulness; it sends projections to the forebrain from the brainstem and the posterior hypothalamus. Several brainstem regions, producing different neurotransmitters, are involved in increasing arousal. Cholinergic (acetylcholine, Ach) fibers that arise from the laterodorsal tegmental nuclei (LDT) and the pedunculopontine tegmental nuclei (PPT) project to the thalamus and indirectly regulate cortical activity. On the other hand, aminergic nuclei and their neurotransmitters directly regulate cortical activity: these are the locus coeruleus (LC, a nucleus that produces norepinephrine), the raphe nuclei (RN, produces serotonin), the ventral tegmental area (VTA, a nucleus that produces dopamine) and the tuberomammillary nucleus (TMN a nucleus that produces histamine). The ventrolateral preoptic nucleus (VLPO, produces gamma-aminobutyric acid (GABA) and galanin) in the anterior thalamus is involved in sleep promotion and projects to TMN and the brainstem to inhibit the arousal system (Saper et al., 2001).

How do dreams arise and why do we dream? Most dreams occur during REM periods, which are mostly bizarre, vivid, and hallucination-like complex stories (Hobson, 2009), which contrasts with dreaming in NREM sleep stage that has a lower dream recall frequency, with more thought-like and less coherent and complex perceptual experiences (Hobson, 2009; Noreika, Valli, Lahtela, & Revonsuo, 2009). The role of dreaming in cognitive functioning, memory and learning is a riddle yet several researchers tried to prove or confine hypotheses about it (Nielsen & Stenstrom, 2005; Stickgold, 2001; Wamsley, Tucker, Payne, Benavides, & Stickgold, 2010). Numerous findings show evidence that dreaming supports memory consolidation, brain plasticity (Frank & Benington, 2006), and emotional-memory processing (Walker, 2009; Walker & van der Helm, 2009) yet a mechanistic understanding of how sleep and dreaming accomplish these functions is still to be investigated.

Wakefulness, REM sleep, and NREM sleep are distinct conscious states that vary during the wake-sleep cycle and can be described by different mentation content and behavioral and physiological parameters (Hobson, 2009; Kahn, Pace-Schott, & Hobson, 1997). These three conscious states are characterized by diverse arousal levels and content; however, it is still debated whether these states are distinct phenomena or rather lie on a continuum (Blume, del Giudice, Wislowska, Lechinger, & Schabus, 2015; Hobson, 2009). From a neural point of view, these conscious states are not homogenous global brain phenomena with distinct physiological event markers, but also a local phenomenon where these state marker physiological events may overlap with each other (Mahowald, Cramer Bornemann, & Schenck, 2011), where these different states could be present in various combinations. These may be associated with hybrid states and unusual sleep-related experiences (e.g., narcoleptic symptoms, lucid dreaming, night terror, sleepwalking, etc.) and also with clinical disorders or symptoms or associated traits (e.g., autism, schizotypy, schizophrenia and psychotic-like experiences) (Koffel & Watson, 2009; Mahowald et al., 2011). Accordingly, it has been proposed that unusual sleep experiences could be described as involuntary wake-like intrusions during sleep, while unusual daytime experiences may be explained as intrusions of sleep-like states into wakefulness (Koffel & Watson, 2009; Watson, 2001). Furthermore, some have argued that dreaming could be seen as a model of psychosis (Dresler et al., 2015; Scarone et al., 2008; Waters et al., 2016) as it shows physiological, neurochemical and functional similarities with hallucinations and delusions. The human brain creates a fictious world during sleep based on conscious experiences collected during the day. The most vivid and intense dreams appear during REM sleep, where mental experiences are typically independent of external stimuli, thinking can be bizarre, or even delusional, and the judgment of facts are inadequate. These characteristics resemble features of psychosis (Castro-Zaballa et al., 2019; Dresler et al., 2015; Mota, Resende, Mota-Rolim, Copelli, & Ribeiro, 2016), and behind this overlap there might be shared electrophysiological and neurochemical features as well.

Sleep disorders and psychosis

As we discuss below, research convincingly suggests a link between poor sleep and psychosis. Nevertheless, it is still to be determined to what extent is there bidirectional or one-directional causality between these domains (i.e., poor sleep predicts unusual daytime experiences and/or vice versa) and to what extent are sleep disturbances associated with psychotic symptoms because of a common cause. To identify poor sleep is important to consider both its qualitative and quantitative features. At present, there are different diagnostic procedures and tools for the assessment of sleep disorders such as (1) the Diagnostic and Statistical Manual of Mental Disorders, fifth edition (DSM-5), published by the American Psychiatric Association (American Psychiatric Association & American Psychiatric Association, 2013), (2) International Statistical Classification of Diseases and Related Health Problems, tenth edition (ICD-10), published by the World Health Organization (ICD-10, 2011), and (3) the International Classification of Sleep Disorders (ICSD-3) that was published by the American Academy of Sleep Medicine (American Academy of Sleep Medicine, 2014). The main difference between these tools is that the former two (DSM-5, ICD-10) are medical classification lists used by mental health and general medical clinicians, while the latter classification system (ISCD-3) is mostly used by sleep experts (Bassetti, 2014). Here, we followed the Third Edition of the International Classification of Sleep Disorders (ICSD-3) to structure our review of the common sleep disorders that are mostly linked to psychosis and psychotic disorders. ICSD-3 describes seven major categories of sleep disorders: (1) insomnia, (2) sleep-related breathing disorders, (3) central disorder of hypersomnolence, (4) circadian rhythm sleep-wake disorders, (5) parasomnias, (6) sleep-related movement disorders and (7) other sleep disorders (Sateia, 2014). We only consider those of these that are usually linked to psychosis or psychotic symptoms.

Insomnia disorder

Insomnia is the most common sleep disorder in the general population (American Psychiatric Association & American Psychiatric Association, 2013; Miyagawa & Tokunaga, 2019). Its symptoms are subjective perception of (1) difficulty initiating or (2) maintaining sleep, (3) early morning awakening, (4) nonrestorative sleep with daytime consequences; at least one of the symptoms occur even if the opportunity is given and environmental conditions are suitable for sleep (i.e., dark, quiet place and ideal temperature) (Billiard & Bentley, 2004; Schutte-Rodin, 2008). This definition includes different subtypes of insomnia, such as nonorganic insomnia and insomnia comorbid with different somatic and mental disorders (Riemann et al., 2017). Presently, in all three diagnostic classification systems (DSM-5, ICD-10, ICSD-3), insomnia disorder is rather an umbrella category that includes different insomnia subtypes (Riemann et al., 2017; Sateia, 2014).

Insomnia can be verified by objective measures obtained with PSG such as increased sleep latency, decreased total sleep time and frequent awakenings during the night (PSG can also facilitate detection of other, comorbid sleep disorders such as sleep-related breathing disorders (i.e., sleep apnea) or restless-leg syndrome or circadian rhythm disorder (Sutton, 2014)). Yet, there is an objective/subjective dichotomy in insomnia subtypes (Edinger & Krystal, 2003): in some cases, insomnia manifests as a subjective impression of sleep loss and sleep complains without objective (PSG) evidence. This sleep state misperception (Salin-Pascual, Roehrs, Merlotti, Zorick, & Roth, 1992) can be confirmed by subjective instruments such as sleep diaries and validated questionnaires which could also tap into the daytime consequences of sleep disturbances. Objectively and subjectively assessed alterations may capture different aspects of sleep disturbances that may not covary (Werner, Griffin, & Galovski, 2016); nevertheless, both could predict diminished next-day functioning, and increased psychotic symptoms in a recent experience sampling study (Mulligan, Haddock, Emsley, Neil, & Kyle, 2016). In this study, 22 outpatient patients participated who have been diagnosed with various psychotic disorders but have not had any past or present sleep disorder other than insomnia. Their sleep-wake pattern was measured by a wrist actigraphy and subjective sleep quality was measured by sleep diary. Participants' psychotic symptoms, functioning and positive and negative affect were assessed five times per day for a week. However, psychotic symptoms were assessed with simplistic questions which may not capture the multidimensional complexity of delusions and hallucinations. Furthermore, the participants were taking antipsychotic medication which may have confounded the results; thus, further research is needed with antipsychotic naïve patients (Mulligan et al., 2016). Nevertheless, objective and subjective sleep measures should be considered in clinical investigations (Zhang & Zhao, 2007).

As mentioned above, insomnia is the most common sleep disorder in both the general and the medical population (Roth & Roehrs, 2003). One-third of the adult population report insomnia symptoms, and 6%–10% fulfil the criteria for insomnia disorder (American Psychiatric Association & American Psychiatric Association, 2013). Female sex, older age (> 60 years), medication side effects, shift work (i.e., work that does not follow the standard 9 AM-5 PM schedule), pregnancy, and substance use are known risk factors (Zhou, Gardiner, & Bertisch, 2017). Comorbid insomnia-related symptoms among patients with schizophrenia are around 80% and the prevalence of clinical insomnia is estimated to be between 30% and 40% (Robertson, Cheung, & Fan, 2019). Yet, comorbid insomnia in schizophrenia is frequently neglected, and as disrupted sleep is linked to more severe schizophrenia symptoms and poorer clinical outcomes, insomnia could be an important target of the therapy (Robertson et al., 2019).

Association of insomnia with psychosis

Insomnia seems to correlate with and temporally precede the appearance of psychotic experiences during the day not only in clinically diagnosed groups and also in the general population (Hennig, Schlier, & Lincoln, 2019; Reeve, Emsley, Sheaves, &

Freeman, 2017; Simor, Báthori, Nagy, & Polner, 2019). Several recent cross-sectional, longitudinal and experience sampling studies using both clinical and nonclinical samples investigated this issue. In an experimental study involving healthy participants, sleep loss and poor sleep were associated with increases in negative affect and daytime psychotic-like experiences (i.e., sub-clinical hallucinations, paranoia, and cognitive disorganization), and negative affect appeared to mediate the effect of poor sleep on psychotic experiences (Reeve et al., 2017). Another study has found that insomnia symptoms were linked to elevated persecutory ideation in healthy adults, and this association was mediated by anxiety and depression; furthermore, insomnia was present in more than half of the individuals diagnosed with persecutory delusions (Freeman, Pugh, Vorontsova, & Southgate, 2009). A study investigating the link between subjectively and objectively monitored insomnia, negative affect, and paranoid thinking found that self-reported delayed sleep onset was associated with paranoia and the effect was mediated by negative affect (Scott, Rowse, & Webb, 2017). However, self-reported problems with sleep maintenance or objective measures of difficulties with initiating and maintaining sleep were not significantly associated with paranoid thinking.

Sleep problems could influence attenuated psychotic and prodromal symptoms (e.g., suspiciousness, perceptual abnormalities) in those having Clinical High Risk (CHR) for psychosis, where depression appears to be the mediator of the cross-sectional link between sleep problems and paranoid symptoms (Goines et al., 2019). The conjecture that insomnia contributes to the development of psychotic experiences through negative affect gained additional support from a clinical longitudinal study where insomnia was a significant predictor of both paranoia and hallucinations over time, and again, the effect was mediated by negative affect (Reeve, Emsley, Sheaves, & Freeman, 2018). Moreover, paranoia was a significant predictor of insomnia, while hallucinations were not.

Treatment of insomnia

Adequate sleep hygiene (appropriate sleep habits and practice) is a necessary but not a sufficient condition of treating chronic insomnia. If insomnia is causally related to psychotic experiences, then improving sleep should decrease psychotic experiences and improve mental health (Freeman et al., 2017). A randomized controlled trial study that applied a psychological intervention for insomnia in a large sample of university students found that a 10-week long digital cognitive behavioral therapy for insomnia (CBT-I) effectively reduced insomnia, paranoia, and hallucinations (Freeman et al., 2017). CBT-I is considered to be the most effective, first-line treatment of insomnia (Bollu & Kaur, 2019; Riemann et al., 2017). In a pilot study, Freeman and colleagues tested the effectiveness of CBT-I in schizophrenia patients with current psychotic symptoms (e.g., distressing delusions and hallucinations) and insomnia diagnosis in an assessor-blind, randomized controlled, progressive study (Freeman et al., 2015). The results showed that CBT-I had a significant effect on insomnia severity but there was no significant decline in hallucinations and delusions. In addition, there are several highly specific medications for insomnia which provide varying clinical effect through regulating the molecular factors of sleep- and wake-promoting brain areas. Patient-specifically selected drugs—taking comorbid psychiatric disorders and patient-specific sleep difficulty into account—could help effectively improving sleep quality (Krystal, 2015).

Further complicating the issue, a qualitative study in patients with showed that the patients not only had insomnia, but several additional symptoms and comorbid sleep problems of insomnia such as sleep/wake circadian dysfunctions and different parasomnias (nightmare, night terrors, sleepwalking), and REM sleep-related disturbances (acting out dreams) and sleep-disordered breathing (sleep apnoea) schizophrenia (Chiu, Ree, Janca, & Waters, 2016). Additionally, they found that patients believed that sleep disturbances were an unchangeable and uncontrollable part of schizophrenia, therefore psychoeducation should be considered when planning CBT-I interventions in patients with psychosis (Chiu et al., 2016). It is important to consider that the constructs of insomnia and schizophrenia both cover a broad range of symptoms and experiences (Cosgrave, Wulff, & Gehrman, 2018), therefore, studies should examine associations at the level of symptoms of schizophrenia and insomnia. For instance, reduction of N3-4 slow wave sleep seems to be linked to negative symptoms in patients with schizophrenia (see Monti & Monti, 2004 for a review). We recommend that future studies consider associations between different dimensions of schizophrenia schizophrenia-spectrum and the subtypes of insomnia and comorbid sleep disorders.

Nightmare disorder

Nightmares are vivid, well-remembered, story-like scenes of dreams that seem realistic and stimulate fear, anxiety, and dysphoric emotions and usually terminate with awakening and full alertness (American Psychiatric Association & American Psychiatric Association, 2013; Thorpy, 2017). Frequent nightmares could interfere with adequate sleep especially if they lead to awakening or cause fear of falling asleep. The diagnostic criteria for nightmare disorder in DSM-5, ICD-10 and ICDS-3 are highly similar and follow the above definition. Nightmares typically arise during REM sleep therefore they are more likely to occur in the second half of the sleep episode when REM sleep is longer and more intense. Polysomnographic markers are abrupt awakenings from REM sleep with elevated autonomic activation where heart, respiratory and eye-movement rate may be elevated before awakening (American Psychiatric Association & American Psychiatric Association, 2013). Nightmares could cause significant subjective distress and sleep avoidance, and the frequent awakenings associated with nightmares may result in excessive daytime sleepiness and poor executive functioning and emotion regulation. Nightmare disorder is defined by repeated episodes of nightmares that threaten the individuals (Thorpy, 2017). The severity is rated by the frequency of nightmare occurrence: it is mild if on average someone has less than one nightmare per week, moderate if one or more, and severe if one has nightmares every night (American Psychiatric Association & American Psychiatric Association, 2013). The prevalence in childhood lies between 1.3 and 3.9% (American Psychiatric Association & American Psychiatric Association, 2013), and among adults, the prevalence of at least monthly occurring nightmares is 6%, while the prevalence of frequent nightmares is

1%–2% and it can be twice as high for females than for males. Nightmares are comorbid with various medical conditions such as coronary heart disease, parkinsonism, pain, substance abuse, whereas nightmare disorder is frequently comorbid with mental disorders such as PTSD, insomnia disorder, schizophrenia, psychosis, mood, anxiety, and personality disorders (American Psychiatric Association & American Psychiatric Association, 2013).

Several studies have reported that frequent nightmares are associated with elevated suicide risk and more severe psychotic symptoms (Lemyre, Bastien, & Vallières, 2019). Patients with schizophrenia experienced more nightmares than healthy controls, although the contents of the dreams reported by the two groups did not differ in terms of negative emotionality (Lemyre et al., 2019). In another study, four-fifth of patients with early nonaffective psychosis (primary affective disorder was exclusion criteria) reported chronic, frequent, and distressing sleep problems (Reeve, Sheaves, & Freeman, 2019), and patients with comorbid sleep disorders had more severe psychotic symptoms (paranoia, hallucinations, cognitive disorganization, depression, and anxiety). Importantly, nightmare disorder was the second most prevalent disorder after insomnia (Reeve et al., 2019). In a retrospective study of patients with psychotic symptoms, 55% reported at least weekly nightmares, and more distressing nightmares were associated with greater delusional severity (Sheaves, Onwumere, Keen, Stahl, & Kuipers, 2015). An 8-year longitudinal study (Li et al., 2016) investigated the link between sleep disturbances and suicide risk in a schizophrenia-spectrum disorder group. The most common sleep disorder was insomnia with prevalence of 19%, followed by frequent nightmares having a prevalence of 9%. They found that insomnia and insomnia comorbid nightmare predicted elevated risk of a subsequent suicide attempt. Although nightmare seems to be a key predictor of suicide risk in both inpatient and community samples, how it exactly contributes to suicide is currently unclear (Titus et al., 2018). In light of that, it is not negligible that nightmares and nightmares comorbid with insomnia were associated with an increased risk of suicide risk in a schizophrenia-spectrum disorder group (Li et al., 2016). It is worth paying attention to nightmares in the detection and treatment of suicide risk.

Circadian rhythm sleep-wake disorder

Circadian rhythm disruption (SCRD) (e.g., advanced or delayed sleep phase, bidian (48 h) or non-24h periods and different irregular and fragmented sleep patterns) could also be a hallmark of schizophrenia, as the prevalence of CRD is 80% among patients with schizophrenia (Cosgrave et al., 2018). DSM-5, ICD-10, and ICDS-3 all include the same diagnostic category of circadian rhythm sleep-wake disorder (CRSWD) with the same subcategories (e.g., delayed-, advanced-, irregular sleep phase, non-24h-, shift work, and jet lag disorder) (Thorpy, 2017). Circadian rhythm disorder is a considerable and persistent misalignment between the internal circadian rhythm and the optimal sleep-wake schedule of the external physical environment (American Academy of Sleep Medicine, 2014; Thorpy, 2017). It could lead to excessive sleepiness and/or insomnia, and causes significant distress, impaired social and occupational functioning (American Psychiatric Association & American Psychiatric Association, 2013).

In a high-risk for psychosis group, a study has reported disturbed sleep-wake patterns and desynchronization of sleep-wake rhythm from the light-darkness cycle of the environment. Furthermore, decreased daily activity was associated with more severe psychotic symptoms (Cosgrave et al., 2018). In another study, adolescents with clinical high-risk psychotic syndromes showed more fragmented circadian rhythm and later onset of nocturnal sleep, and fragmented circadian rhythm and lower daily activity were linked to elevated psychotic symptoms (Lunsford-Avery et al., 2017). Another study examined circadian misalignment in 66 patients with schizophrenia (Chung, Poon, Ng, & Kan, 2018). For 1 week, the patients completed a sleep diary and wore actigraphy. Higher sleep and actigraphy square successive difference (SSD) scores were associated with positive and depressive symptoms, poor sleep quality, evening chronotype and delayed sleep-wake phase disorder.

Although dopamine dysregulation is typically linked to aberrant salience in psychosis (for a review see Howes & Kapur, 2009), it seems to be relevant to sleep-wake regulation as well. Disrupted sleep could elevate dopamine release and sensitivity and increased dopamine levels may disturb sleep and circadian rhythms, which suggests that treating circadian disturbances could be a useful target in patients with schizophrenia (Yates, 2016). Sleep and wake-promoting brain regions could be affected by hyperactivity of the dopaminergic system and the dysfunction of the GABAergic system, which could partly relate to circadian disruption (Monti et al., 2013). Further, stress vulnerability could also contribute to altered circadian patterns in schizophrenia (Coulon, Brailly-Tabard, Walter, & Tordjman, 2016). Cortisol is a hormone key to the stress response, and it has a circadian rhythm. High cortisol level was supported as an endophenotype in schizophrenia and studying cortisol circadian pattern alteration by measuring salivary cortisol could open a new possibility to identify CHR individuals for schizophrenia.

Furthermore, circadian clock gene expression could be altered in patients with schizophrenia (Johansson, Owe-Larsson, Hetta, & Lundkvist, 2016). A study compared mononuclear blood cells and fibroblast cells of skin from patients with chronic schizophrenia and healthy controls. They found an altered expression of clock genes in the group of patients with schizophrenia, as compared to healthy controls. Seney and colleagues investigated the diurnal rhythms in gene expression in the human dorsolateral prefrontal cortex (dlPFC) (Seney et al., 2019), the results show 24h transcript rhythmicity in healthy subjects but not in subjects of schizophrenia.

Light therapy could be a promising way to improve intrinsic circadian rhythm in neuro-psychiatric illnesses (Faulkner, Bee, Meyer, Dijk, & Drake, 2019). A meta-analysis indicated that light schedule interventions could improve sleep and avoidance of light during the evening was associated with a greater increase in total sleep time. Surprisingly, at the moment, the application of bright light therapy (BLT) to improve sleep in patients with psychosis and schizophrenia is understudied, while its efficacy for treating patients with seasonal affective disorder, major depression, and bipolar depression is well established (see Pail et al., 2011). Therefore, more research is needed to investigate the possibility and efficacy of BLT in patients diagnosed with psychotic disorders.

Narcolepsy

The DSM-5, the ICD-10 and the ICSD-3 identify narcolepsy as a sleep disorder. Narcolepsy is a chronic neurological sleep disorder described as recurrent periods of irrepressible need to sleep, lapses into sleep or repeated napping during the same day along with one of the additional symptoms, such as cataplexy, hypocretin deficiency, or different polysomnographic markers as sleep-onset REM period (SOREMP) and fragmented sleep. (American Psychiatric Association & American Psychiatric Association, 2013; Miyagawa & Tokunaga, 2019 ; Thorpy, 2017). Narcolepsy could cause insomnia symptoms—because of the difficulties with sustaining wakefulness and sleeping for normal periods; however, it differs from insomnia disorder in that its dominant symptoms are excessive daytime sleepiness, cataplexy, sleep paralysis, and sleep-related hallucinations (hypnagogic/hypnopompic hallucinations) (American Psychiatric Association & American Psychiatric Association, 2013; Miyagawa & Tokunaga, 2019). Narcolepsy often produces cataplexy (bilateral loss of muscle tone, sometimes the whole body is affected and could end with complete falls) usually triggered by intense emotions. In addition, approximately 20%–60% of individuals with narcolepsy reported vivid hypnagogic hallucinations during falling asleep, or hypnopompic hallucinations right after awakening. ICDS-3 define two different types of narcolepsy, type 1 (NT1) and type 2 (NT2) (Thorpy, 2017). NT1 is characterized by cataplexy, hypnagogic/hypnopompic hallucinations, excessive daytime sleepiness, and sleep paralysis (Miyagawa & Tokunaga, 2019) and low hypocretin-1 (orexin) level—due to hypothalamic deficiency in hypcretin-1 (orexin) production neurons—that could be measured in cerebrospinal fluid (Cavalier & Kothare, 2018; Thorpy, 2017). NT2 shows most of NT1's symptoms except for cataplexy (Miyagawa & Tokunaga, 2019; Thorpy, 2017). NT1 patients carry the specific human leukocyte antigen (HLA) allele HLA-DQB1*06:02 which is strictly related to hypocretin deficiency (Miyagawa & Tokunaga, 2019; Sansa et al., 2016).

Narcolepsy is not a frequent sleep disorder but its symptoms such as unusual experiences (hybrid-like states of body and mind) and hallucination-like events during sleep and wakefulness makes it relevant in the context of psychosis. In the light of these symptoms, narcolepsy could be misdiagnosed (Cavalier & Kothare, 2018). Furthermore, NT1 is not uncommon in adults with schizophrenia (Sansa et al., 2016). If we consider the reduced dopaminergic tone of narcolepsy, than it could suggest a reverse association between narcolepsy and psychotic illnesses where dopaminergic transmission is increased (Sansa et al., 2016; Walterfang, Upjohn, & Velakoulis, 2005). In psychotic disorders comorbid with narcolepsy, narcolepsy appears first in childhood or adolescence (Canellas et al., 2014; Walterfang et al., 2005), later followed by psychotic symptoms (auditory hallucinations, fixed delusional beliefs, persecutory delusional thoughts, psychosocial decline). Narcolepsy medication may be a trigger for psychotic symptoms which does not seem to reverse after changing the therapy (Canellas et al., 2014; Walterfang et al., 2005).

What are the differences and similarities between hypnagogic/hypnopompic and psychotic hallucinations at the phenomenological level? Hypnagogic or hypnopompic hallucinations usually occur during the sleep-wake transition phase while psychotic hallucinations occur in full wake state (Fortuyn et al., 2009; Waters et al., 2016). Narcoleptic hallucinations are usually multimodal (visual, auditory, and tactile) "holistic" hallucinatory experiences largely distinct from reality without concurrent delusions, while hallucinations of schizophrenia patients are generally present in verbal-auditory sensory mode overlaid on veridical perception and occur simultaneously with other psychotic symptoms (Fortuyn et al., 2009; Sarkanen, Niemel, Landtblom, & Partinen, 2014; Waters et al., 2016).

Sleep EEG patterns in schizophrenia

There are common sleep architecture disturbances associated with schizophrenia. PSG studies reported (see review: (Manoach, Pan, Purcell, & Stickgold, 2016)) different abnormalities of sleep architecture in schizophrenia patients such as decreased N3 (SWS) sleep and REM sleep latency, and increased REM density, but the findings are inconsistent. The spectral characteristics of sleep EEG show reduced sleep spindle oscillation during N2 sleep and reduced delta power in N3 sleep.

Finding biomarkers for schizophrenia in sleep EEG abnormalities is a major research area but the findings are yet inconsistent and confounding by medication complicates research. The investigated characteristic features of sleep polysomnography studies in schizophrenia concentrated mostly on (1) difficulties in sleep initiation and maintenance, and sleep efficiency (i.e., insomnia), (2) SWS sleep, (3) REM sleep, (4) sleep spindle, and (5) delta activity alterations.

A meta-analysis study showed that polysomnographic abnormalities are common in schizophrenia; however, there is a heterogeneity between studies due to medication status and duration, and the duration of the illness (Chan, Chung, Yung, & Yeung, 2017). They found consistent results in sleep macrostructure such as significantly shorter total sleep time, longer sleep onset latency and more awakenings after sleep onset, which together result in lower sleep efficiency, as compared to healthy controls. In sleep macrostructure reduced slow-wave sleep and decreased duration and latency of REM sleep were consistently reported, as compared to healthy controls; however, in case of drug-naïve patients, no significant sleep architecture alterations were found. In sleep microstructure, the alterations of delta waves and sleep spindles were inconsistent (Chan et al., 2017). A qualitative sleep EEG study (Oh, Lee, Kim, Choi, & Jeong, 2017) compared the activity in bilateral frontal, central and occipital areas with EEG spectral analysis in nine patients with schizophrenia and matched healthy controls. Patients showed elevated sleep latency, and in N2 sleep they had significantly lower 0.5-1 Hz power, higher theta power in the left prefrontal region, and a higher beta power in the left occipital region, relative to the control group. Patients showed a significantly higher alpha power in the left occipital region during N3 sleep than controls. It is worth noting that this study did not find significant differences between patients and controls in terms of total sleep time, total wake time after sleep onset, sleep efficiency, and SWS and REM sleep latency (Oh et al., 2017). It should be mentioned that this study is limited by the low sample size and potential effects of antipsychotic medications. Another study investigated the relationship between EEG parameters and the severity of clinical symptoms (Yang & Winkelman, 2006) in 15 drug-free inpatients with schizophrenia and matched controls. Besides poor sleep quality, an SWS deficit and an increased REM density were seen in the patients. They also found an inverse correlation between SWS and cognitive symptoms while REM density inversely correlated with emotional and cognitive discomfort as well as with overall symptom severity (as reflected by the PANSS total score).

In sleep microstructure, schizophrenia patients show a specific sleep spindle deficit which may be a possible biomarker for psychotic disorders and serve as an endophenotype for schizophrenia (Ferrarelli & Tononi, 2016). Sleep spindles are characteristic bursts of 11–15 Hz activities with a duration between 0.5 and 2s that occur during NREM N2 sleep. They are generated in the thalamic reticular nucleus and they are involved in sleep regulation and in cognitive functioning such as memory and learning (Purcell et al., 2017) and sleep spindles are also involved in protecting sleep and preventing awakening (Sasidharan et al., 2017). Sigma power in EEG is a stable fingerprint-like feature across the night within individuals, but there is a qualitative and quantitative variability between individuals that is related to age, sex, and genetic factors. There may be two types of sleep spindles with different topological associations: slow spindles (below ~13 Hz) occurring usually over the frontal derivation while fast spindles occurring mostly over the centroparietal derivations (Purcell et al., 2017). fMRI studies also suggest that both spindles type have different cortical sources. A review showed (Manoach et al., 2016) that spindle activity is heritable and schizophrenia risk genes may be associated with spindle deficit. Patients with schizophrenia and their first-degree relatives have reduced sleep spindle activity, which are associated with impaired memory consolidation and positive symptoms. Importantly, some studies suggest that sleep spindles can be enhanced. A randomized placebo-controlled study (Wamsley et al., 2013) investigated the effect of Eszopiclone (a non-benzodiazepine hypnotic, that acts on GABA neurons in the thalamic reticular nucleus where sleep spindles originate) on sleep spindle activity. Their question was whether eszopiclone could improve memory consolidation through increasing sleep spindle activity. The results showed that eszopiclone ($n = 10$) significantly increased the number and density of sleep spindles compared to placebo group ($n = 11$) and this increase correlated with improvement on a motor sequence task, while the study did not show a significant effect on memory (potentially due to low statistical power) (Wamsley et al., 2013). To conclude, the role of sleep spindles in psychotic disorders is little understood, not to mention the controversies surrounding the functional relevance of sleep spindles in general. Nonetheless, the results suggested that schizophrenia patients show sleep spindle deficit, that may serve as a hallmark of sleep in schizophrenia (Ferrarelli & Tononi, 2016).

Individual differences in sleep EEG patterns seem to be temporally stable traits (Buckelmüller, Landolt, Stassen, & Achermann, 2006), but can we consider sleep EEG patterns endophenotypes of schizophrenia? A study investigated the main brain oscillations during NREM sleep with high density EEG in first degree relatives of patients with schizophrenia (D'Agostino et al., 2018). They found that the relatives did not have reduced sleep spindle density, so sleep spindle density may be specific to the disease. They investigated slow-wave slope parameters—because the slope of evoked wakes is usually defined as an electrophysiological measure of cortical synchronization—and they showed significant differences in slow-wave amplitude and slope parameters (average down-slope, maximal down-slope, average up-slope, maximal up-slope) this finding suggest a possible cortical synchronization impairment rather than a slow-waves generation deficit. They suggested that spindle activity could represent an endophenotype for schizophrenia nevertheless slow-wave deficits—that are associated with disrupted cortical synchronization—in relatives are associated with increased risk for schizophrenia, but the thalamic dysfunction is the key factor for developing the disorder (Scarone et al., 2008). Relatedly, Kaskie and colleagues investigated slow-wave abnormalities in patients with first-episode psychosis (FEP) and found a significant reduction in slow-wave density over frontal areas, and slow-wave density inversely correlated with positive symptoms severity (Kaskie et al., 2019). They drew further questions to determine the direction of these associations if the clinical symptoms or the SW deficits were presented first. A study (Sasidharan et al., 2017) investigated sleep macro- and micro-structure and sleep-cycle abnormalities in patients with schizophrenia (n = 45) and healthy controls (n = 39). They replicated former findings of sleep-architecture abnormalities and sleep spindle deficit in schizophrenia, furthermore, they showed abnormalities in sleep-cycles that may lead to inefficient sleep-stabilizing mechanisms. The patients showed significant alterations in sleep dynamics during the first three sleep cycles that were analyzed. As compared to healthy controls, patients showed spindle density deficits but no delta density deficits during the first three cycles. Increased sleep instability was present between sleep-cycles in association with sleep arousability and stage transitions during NREM and REM periods—which affect sleep continuity with wake intrusions. Put more broadly, these findings supported the thalamocortical dysfunction hypothesis of schizophrenia (Sasidharan et al., 2017).

Cognitive alterations mediating the association between sleep and psychosis

Why are various sleep disturbances and anomalous sleep experiences associated with psychotic-like experiences and psychotic symptoms, ranging from perceptual anomalies, suspiciousness, and difficulties with concentrating to hallucinations, paranoid delusions and disorganisztion of thought? Notwithstanding that the above subjective phenomena are likely to emerge from complex interactions between various cognitive alterations and interpersonal dynamics (see the excellent reviews by Bentall & Fernyhough, 2008; Freeman, 2007, 2016), and also keeping in mind that any mechanistic explanation of psychosis is likely to be reductionist, we outline empirically testable hypotheses about a selected set of cognitive alterations that may mediate the association between disturbed sleep and psychosis. Although we are not discussing emotion regulation here, it is important to note that sleep disturbances have an impact on it and there is evidence consistent with its mediating role (Simon, Rossi, Harvey, & Walker, 2019; Simor et al., 2019; Simor, Krietsch, Köteles, & McCrae, 2015).

Reduced prepulse inhibition

One potential mediator is impaired sensorimotor gating which can be indexed by the prepulse inhibition (PPI) of the acoustic startle reflex. Prepulse inhibition is the reduction of the startle reflex to an intense stimulus—the pulse—when a weak stimulus—the prepulse—shortly precedes it (Petrovsky et al., 2014). There is evidence showing that PPI has good test-retest reliability in healthy participants and also in patients with schizophrenia (Ludewig, Geyer, Etzensberger, & Vollenweider, 2002). The validity of the PPI construct as a correlate of vulnerability to psychosis is underscored by the fact that reduction of PPI is robustly documented in patients with schizophrenia (Braff, Swerdlow, & Geyer, 1999; Swerdlow et al., 2014) and it has also been reported in patients with schizotypal personality disorder (Cadenhead, Geyer, & Braff, 1993). Moreover, reduced PPI has been found in unaffected siblings of patients with schizophrenia (Kumari, Das, Zachariah, Ettinger, & Sharma, 2005), suggesting that it could indicate familial liability for schizophrenia. However, it remains an open question whether PPI maps to a specific symptom domain of the schizophrenia-spectrum. In some studies, PPI deficit significantly correlated with positive (Braff et al., 1999; Weike, Bauer, & Hamm, 2000) and negative symptoms (Braff et al., 1999) of schizophrenia, while in a larger sample, no significant association was found neither with positive nor with negative symptoms (Swerdlow et al., 2014).

Crucially for the purpose of the present article, it has been shown in healthy volunteers that one night of full sleep deprivation impairs PPI and induces perceptual alterations, cognitive disorganization, and anhedonia (Petrovsky et al., 2014). Thus, sleep deprivation is likely to have a causal effect on psychosis and the reduction of PPI. This argument is further strengthened by data from an animal experiment: in the rat, sleep deprivation reduced PPI, and this deficit could be prevented by the administration of antipsychotic drugs (Frau et al., 2008). However, experimentally induced sleep deprivation and insufficient sleep occurring in daily life probably differ in many aspects; therefore, data on sleep impairment in natural environments is informative. In a sample of women two months postpartum, partial sleep deprivation (sleeping less than four hours during the preceding night), and postpartum depression were independent predictors of reduced PPI (Comasco et al., 2016). It still remains to be examined whether the emergence of psychotic-like experiences or psychotic symptoms in postpartum women is predicted by the reduction of PPI. Furthermore, its correlation with depression implicates that diminished PPI might not be specific to schizophrenia but may indicate a general vulnerability to psychopathology (see (Kohl, Heekeren, Klosterkötter, & Kuhn, 2013) for a review), which might be closer to the disorganized aspect of the psychosis-spectrum (Caspi & Moffitt, 2018). Mapping PPI impairment to disorganization seems plausible given that not only PPI (Braff et al., 1999; Weike et al., 2000) but also self-reported cognitive disorganization correlates with the positive and negative aspects of psychosis (Polner et al., 2019). In the following sections, we turn our attention to higher-level cognitive processes and functions whose theorized connection with specific aspects of psychosis has received rich empirical support.

Impaired reasoning, analytical thinking, and cognitive rigidity

Several reasoning biases—such as jumping to conclusions, confirmation bias, or bias against disconfirmatory evidence—have been suggested to be involved in the formation and the maintenance of delusions (see Bronstein, Pennycook, Joormann, Corlett, & Cannon, 2019; Ward & Garety, 2019 for recent reviews). Belief flexibility is a higher-level construct that involves the ability to override strongly held (delusional) beliefs in light of potentially contradicting information, to make decisions under uncertainty, and to consider alternative interpretations. Critically, lack of belief flexibility is commonly found in people with delusions. Moreover, some studies have shown that impoverished belief flexibility can contribute to variation in subclinical delusional ideation as well (Ward & Garety, 2019); for instance, analytic thinking had a weak negative correlation with odd beliefs, magical thinking, and ideas of reference in an online community sample (Barron et al., 2018). It has recently been proposed that dual-process theories of reasoning can be particularly useful to understand reasoning biases associated with delusions; these theories distinguish between two main types of reasoning: a fast, intuitive, nonreflective system/process that does not depend on working memory (Type 1), and a slow, analytical, reflective system/process that relies on working memory (Type 2). According to cognitive models of psychosis, reduced engagement in analytical reasoning and deficits of working memory can impair critical reappraisal, leading to belief inflexibility and also allowing jumping to conclusions on the basis of fast, intuitive judgements (Ward & Garety, 2019).

Can sleep disturbances cause impairments in analytical thinking? Although meta-analytic evidence from healthy adults shows that total sleep deprivation impairs attention, processing speed, working memory, and short-term memory, no significant effect was reported for performance on reasoning tasks (Lim & Dinges, 2010). On the other hand, it seems that sleep deprivation is detrimental to cognitive flexibility, which is arguably crucial to reasoning and analytical thinking, as impaired cognitive control (Buonocore et al., 2015) and working memory (Garety et al., 2013) have been found to correlate with reasoning biases. For instance, sleep deprived healthy subjects were impaired at shifting between response categories on a divergent thinking task and showed reduced performance improvement on the trail making task that demands set shifting (Wimmer, Hoffmann, Bonato, & Moffitt, 1992). Moreover, in a game simulating marketing decision making in a dynamically changing environment, sleep-deprived participants achieved less profit and made more production errors (Harrison & Horne, 1999). Importantly, sleep deprivation made participants more prone to make perseverative errors and to continue using the same strategies in the decision-making game despite changed circumstances (although it did not significantly impair their performance on a simple test of critical reasoning). Further studies applying computerised experimental assessment of cognitive flexibility has yielded convergent findings. One night of sleep deprivation impaired task-switching ability (alternating between deciding whether a number is odd or even vs. smaller or larger than 5), while performance on nonswitch trials was intact (Couyoumdjian et al., 2010). In another study, two nights of sleep deprivation negatively affected maintenance in working memory and sustained attention, and also impaired learning stimulus-response mapping and reversal of such contingencies (Whitney, Hinson, Jackson, & Van Dongen, 2015). Paralleling the above findings, a sleep fragmentation manipulation impaired set-shifting in rats (McCoy et al., 2007). Furthermore, modelling of decision making suggested that sleep deprived participants reduce weighing of novel information during inference (Dickinson & Drummond, 2008), which is especially interesting in light of studies showing a stronger influence of previous knowledge on inference in psychosis (Sterzer et al., 2018). To conclude, because cognitive flexibility as assessed in the above studies resembles the construct of belief flexibility as defined in the delusion literature (Ward & Garety, 2019), we suggest that impaired analytical reasoning may mediate the association between disturbed sleep and delusional ideation.

Source monitoring errors and false memories

Source monitoring theories of psychosis propose that errors of attributing self-generated or imagined representations to external sources and an overall proneness for false memories are key mechanisms setting the stage for hallucinations and delusions (Bentall & Fernyhough, 2008; Ditman & Kuperberg, 2005; Griffin & Fletcher, 2017). Accordingly, a study has found that relative to healthy controls, patients with schizophrenia were more prone to false recognition errors in a visual memory task if the distractors only weakly resembled the target stimuli, and patients were more confident in the erroneous recognitions and a larger proportion of their high confidence responses were mistaken (Moritz, Woodward, Jelinek, & Klinge, 2008). However, performance on the task did not correlate significantly with positive symptomatology (which could be due to insufficient statistical power). Another study using a word recognition memory task found an impairment of source monitoring in patients with schizophrenia: relative to healthy controls, they attributed self-generated and also new words to an external source, suggesting two independent deficits behind source monitoring difficulties (Vinogradov et al., 1997). Source monitoring errors were associated with hostility and lower IQ. A later study found impaired source monitoring in patients with schizophrenia who were more likely to remember an imagined action as having been performed, relative to healthy controls (Mammarella et al., 2010). In this study, source monitoring impairment correlated with conceptual disorganization and context processing on a sustained attention task. Corroborating the conjecture that false memories and impaired reality monitoring are specifically associated with positive symptoms, patients with schizophrenia currently experiencing delusions were especially prone to false memories, as compared to controls and patients with schizophrenia without an acute delusion (Bhatt, Laws, & McKenna, 2010), while other studies have shown that patients with schizophrenia who had auditory hallucinations were more prone to attribute self-generated items to an external source, relative to patients with schizophrenia without auditory hallucinations (Brunelin et al., 2006; Woodward, Menon, & Whitman, 2007). Furthermore, source monitoring impairment is associated with psychosis-spectrum traits in the general population. In an early study, overall schizotypal traits were associated with poor source monitoring (Peters, Smeets, Giesbrecht, Jelicic, & Merckelbach, 2007), while a later study revealed that positive and disorganized schizotypy predicted impaired source monitoring (confusing imagined and performed actions) and reality monitoring (confusing whether the target was imagined or generated by the self or an external source) (Humpston, Linden, & Evans, 2017). Other studies have used the Deese-Roediger-McDermott (DRM; Roediger & McDermott, 1995) paradigm to assess false memories: in the DRM participants are shown lists of semantically related words (e.g., *bed, pillow, dream*) and at a subsequent test participants may have false memory for items that were not presented but are semantically connected to the studied items (e.g., *sleep*). Such false recall was associated with anomalous experiences, magical thinking (Corlett et al., 2009) and delusion-proneness (Bhatt et al., 2010; Laws & Bhatt, 2005).

Several studies have used the DRM paradigm to examine the impact of sleep on false memories and source monitoring. Sleep deprivation before retrieval produced false memories in the DRM paradigm with recognition testing (Diekelmann, Landolt, Lahl, Born, & Wagner, 2008), while sleep between study and retrieval has been shown to reduce false memories, relative to an equally long wake retention interval (Fenn, Gallo, Margoliash, Roediger, & Nusbaum, 2009). Moreover, it has been shown that women during pregnancy and after childbirth had more fragmented sleep and were more prone to false recognition in the DRM (Berndt, Diekelmann, Alexander, Pustal, & Kirschbaum, 2014). However, in another study, where participants were either partially or fully sleep deprived before studying the lists, it was found that both manipulations reduced veridical and false memory in the DRM paradigm (Chatburn, Kohler, Payne, & Drummond, 2017), suggesting that timing of sleep deprivation relative to study and test could be critical in predicting its effect on false memories. Relatedly, false recall in the DRM was enhanced by nocturnal sleep following learning and by sleep deprivation as well, relative to a daytime retention condition (Diekelmann, Born, & Wagner, 2010). The authors suggest two different mechanisms behind these effects: post-encoding sleep may enhance consolidation of false memories whereas sleep deprivation could impair control processes that support source monitoring at retrieval. In line with this speculation, sleep deprivation reduced word fluency and also self-reported motivation, activation, and concentration at retrieval. Other studies have used a misinformation paradigm where participants are first shown photographs of events, and then read a narrative of the events that contains information contradicting the photographs—at test, participants' memory for details where the narrative conflicts the photographs is critical in assessing susceptibility for false memories (Frenda, Patihis, Loftus, Lewis, & Fenn, 2014). When sleep deprivation preceded encoding, participants produced more false memories (reported seeing a detail in the photos that was actually mentioned only in the misinformation narrative), but if sleep deprivation occurred between misinformation and encoding it did not have a significant effect on false memories, suggesting that in the misinformation paradigm sleep deprivation may lead to false memories by impairing encoding. On the other hand, partially sleep deprived participants were more prone to have false memories about news events occurring years before test, implicating sleep deprivation can also impair source monitoring at retrieval (Frenda et al., 2014). Another study that applied either partial or full sleep deprivation before encoding found that both manipulations made participants respond more consistently with the misinformation presented in the narrative (Lo, Chong, Ganesan, Leong, & Chee, 2016). To sum up, it appears that source monitoring is specifically associated with the positive aspects of the psychosis spectrum, particularly hallucinations, and most studies indicate that source monitoring is impaired by sleep deprivation; thus, we hypothesize that source monitoring mediates the association between disturbed sleep and hallucinations.

Outstanding questions on the links between sleep and psychosis

What is the nature of the relationship between disturbed sleep and psychosis? Although the former is likely to have a causal effect on psychotic symptoms and experiences, one may also argue that disturbed sleep and psychosis correlate because they have a common cause. According to the review by Lunsford-Avery and Mittal (2013), various sleep disturbances (including nonspecific sleep problems, reduced sleep time, sleep fragmentation) appear to be core features of psychosis that are present before the onset of acute psychosis, suggesting that they are not merely secondary effects of disease processes and disease burden (Lunsford-Avery & Mittal, 2013). This conclusion was well supported by numerous retrospective studies of patients with schizophrenia, while scarce data available from genetic high-risk and prodromal ultra high-risk studies seemed inconclusive, making the authors suggest that further research was warranted in these populations. Differences in sleep macrostructure (i.e., characteristics of NREM and REM sleep) are well documented yet somewhat variable in patients with schizophrenia, while data on alterations of sleep macrostructure in at-risk states is rather scarce. Lunsford-Avery and Mittal (2013) has outlined multiple pathways between distal and proximal risk factors of schizophrenia, sleep disturbances and psychosis: they argue that distal risk factors (such as genetic risk and early environmental insults) predict disturbed brain maturation during adolescence and cognitive dysfunction, and that the latter is further amplified by abnormal brain maturation, which also increases vulnerability to stressors. Crucially, in light of abnormalities in brain structures involved in sleep and aberrant memory consolidation during sleep in schizophrenia, Lunsford-Avery and Mittal (2013) hypothesized that distal risk factors and neural maldevelopment during adolescence can also contribute to sleep disturbances, which in turn can cause cognitive impairment and reciprocally interact with distress.

Summary and conclusions

As we have seen, sleep problems are often comorbid with psychotic symptoms and schizophrenia. As yet, the evidence about the direction of causality between sleep and psychotic symptoms has not been consistent. Sleep and sleep disorders are as complex as psychosis which makes understanding their connection difficult.

We started with discussing that wakefulness, NREM sleep, and REM sleep are different states with distinct behavioral and physiological features, arousal levels and phenomenology. Even so, the transitions between these states can be fuzzy which may explain hybrid states of sleep and wakefulness that could share features with psychosis. The involuntary intrusion of wakefulness and sleep states into each other may create unusual experiences during such as lucid dreaming, narcoleptic symptoms and sleepwalking during sleep and psychotic-like symptoms during wakefulness. Additionally, others have argued that considering their shared features, dreaming can be considered as a model for psychosis.

Insomnia disorder, nightmare disorder, and circadian rhythm sleep-wake disorder are the most prevalent sleep problems associated with psychosis and schizophrenia which could be a significant additional burden impacting the wellbeing of these patients and could also worsen the symptoms of the disorder. Investigating sleep EEG patterns in patients with schizophrenia and psychosis is another important research field: it is a key question in this topic whether sleep EEG abnormalities can be used as biomarkers of schizophrenia and psychotic symptoms.

Restorative and sufficient sleep is necessary for optimal cognitive and emotional functioning during the day. Alteration of cognitive functioning could mediate the association between sleep and psychosis. We summarized evidence showing that disruption of sleep reduces prepulse inhibition, impairs reasoning, analytical thinking, and cognitive flexibility, induces source monitoring errors and increases susceptibility for false memories. Importantly, we have also cited studies showing that such cognitive alterations are associated with psychosis; therefore, we have concluded that they are likely to mediate the association between disturbed sleep and psychosis.

The literature clearly suggests that sleep disturbances and psychotic symptoms are related to each other, but our knowledge about the direction of the effect (i.e., sleep quality affects psychotic symptoms, vice versa, and they have a common cause) is yet inconsistent and insufficient. We suggest that further research is needed to clarify the fine details of this association and to uncover the contributing factors. It could be argued that several studies in this research area use constructs that are rather umbrella terms (e.g., insomnia, psychotic symptoms) that may include multiple subdimensions, symptoms or subtypes. Identifying associations at the levels of symptom dimensions and of subtypes would be fruitful for patients and clinicians as well.

Funding

Bertalan Polner was supported by the BME-Biotechnology FIKP grant of EMMI (BME FIKP-BIO), and by the National Research, Development and Innovation Office (NKFI/OTKA K 128599).

References

American Academy of Sleep Medicine. (2014). *International classification of sleep disorders*. American Academy of Sleep Medicine.

American Psychiatric Association, & American Psychiatric Association. (2013). *Diagnostic and statistical manual of mental disorders: DSM-5* (5th ed.). American Psychiatric Association.

Baran, B., Karahanoğlu, F. I., Mylonas, D., Demanuele, C., Vangel, M., Stickgold, R., … Manoach, D. S. (2019). Increased thalamocortical connectivity in schizophrenia correlates with sleep spindle deficits: Evidence for a common pathophysiology. *Biological Psychiatry: Cognitive Neuroscience and Neuroimaging*, *4*(8), 706–714. https://doi.org/10.1016/j.bpsc.2019.04.012.

Barcaro, U., Navona, C., Belloli, S., Bonanni, E., Gneri, C., & Murri, L. (1998). A simple method for the quantitative description of sleep microstructure. *Electroencephalography and Clinical Neurophysiology*, *106*(5), 429–432. https://doi.org/10.1016/S0013-4694(98)00008-X.

Barron, D., Furnham, A., Weis, L., Morgan, K. D., Towell, T., & Swami, V. (2018). The relationship between schizotypal facets and conspiracist beliefs via cognitive processes. *Psychiatry Research*, *259*, 15–20. https://doi.org/10.1016/j.psychres.2017.10.001.

Bassetti, C. L. (2014). *ESRS-sleep medicine textbook*. European Sleep Research Society.

Benson, K. L. (2006). Sleep in schizophrenia: Impairments, correlates, and treatment. *Psychiatric Clinics of North America*, *29*(4), 1033–1045. https://doi.org/10.1016/j.psc.2006.08.002.

Benson, K. L. (2015). Sleep in schizophrenia: Pathology and treatment. *Sleep Medicine Clinics*, *10*(1), 49–55. https://doi.org/10.1016/j.jsmc.2014.11.001.

Bentall, R. P., & Fernyhough, C. (2008). Social predictors of psychotic experiences: Specificity and psychological mechanisms. *Schizophrenia Bulletin*, *34*(6), 1012–1020. https://doi.org/10.1093/schbul/sbn103.

Berndt, C., Diekelmann, S., Alexander, N., Pustal, A., & Kirschbaum, C. (2014). Sleep fragmentation and false memories during pregnancy and motherhood. *Behavioural Brain Research*, *266*, 52–57. https://doi.org/10.1016/j.bbr.2014.02.030.

Bhatt, R., Laws, K. R., & McKenna, P. J. (2010). False memory in schizophrenia patients with and without delusions. *Psychiatry Research*, *178*(2), 260–265. https://doi.org/10.1016/j.psychres.2009.02.006.

Billiard, M., & Bentley, A. (2004). Is insomnia best categorized as a symptom or a disease? *Sleep Medicine*, *5*, S35–S40. https://doi.org/10.1016/S1389-9457(04)90006-8.

Blatter, K., & Cajochen, C. (2007). Circadian rhythms in cognitive performance: Methodological constraints, protocols, theoretical underpinnings. *Physiology & Behavior*, *90*(2), 196–208. https://doi.org/10.1016/j.physbeh.2006.09.009.

Blume, C., del Giudice, R., Wislowska, M., Lechinger, J., & Schabus, M. (2015). Across the consciousness continuum—From unresponsive wakefulness to sleep. *Frontiers in Human Neuroscience*, *9*. https://doi.org/10.3389/fnhum.2015.00105.

Bollu, P. C., & Kaur, H. (2019). Sleep medicine: Insomnia and sleep. *Missouri Medicine*, *116*(1), 68–75.

Borbély, A. A. (1982). A two process model of sleep regulation. *Human Neurobiology*, *1*(3), 195–204.

Braff, D. L., Swerdlow, N. R., & Geyer, M. A. (1999). Symptom correlates of prepulse inhibition deficits in male schizophrenic patients. *American Journal of Psychiatry*, *156*(4), 596–602. https://doi.org/10.1176/ajp.156.4.596.

Bronstein, M. V., Pennycook, G., Joormann, J., Corlett, P. R., & Cannon, T. D. (2019). Dual-process theory, conflict processing, and delusional belief. *Clinical Psychology Review*, *72*, 101748. https://doi.org/10.1016/j.cpr.2019.101748.

Brunelin, J., Combris, M., Poulet, E., Kallel, L., D'Amato, T., Dalery, J., & Saoud, M. (2006). Source monitoring deficits in hallucinating compared to non-hallucinating patients with schizophrenia. *European Psychiatry: The Journal of the Association of European Psychiatrists*, *21*(4), 259–261. https://doi.org/10.1016/j.eurpsy.2006.01.015.

Buckelmüller, J., Landolt, H.-P., Stassen, H. H., & Achermann, P. (2006). Trait-like individual differences in the human sleep electroencephalogram. *Neuroscience*, *138*(1), 351–356. https://doi.org/10.1016/j.neuroscience.2005.11.005.

Buonocore, M., Bosia, M., Riccaboni, R., Bechi, M., Spangaro, M., Piantanida, M., … Cavallaro, R. (2015). Combined neurocognitive and metacognitive rehabilitation in schizophrenia: Effects on bias against disconfirmatory evidence. *European Psychiatry*, *30*(5), 615–621. https://doi.org/10.1016/j.eurpsy.2015.02.006.

Cadenhead, K. S., Geyer, M. A., & Braff, D. L. (1993). Impaired startle prepulse inhibition and habituation in patients with schizotypal personality disorder. *The American Journal of Psychiatry*, *150*(12), 1862–1867. https://doi.org/10.1176/ajp.150.12.1862.

Cajochen, C., Foy, R., & Dijk, D. J. (1999). Frontal predominance of a relative increase in sleep delta and theta EEG activity after sleep loss in humans. *Sleep Research Online*, *2*(3), 65–69.

Cajochen, C., Knoblauch, V., Kräuchi, K., Renz, C., & Wirz-Justice, A. (2001). Dynamics of frontal EEG activity, sleepiness and body temperature under high and low sleep pressure. *Neuroreport*, *12*(10), 2277–2281. https://doi.org/10.1097/00001756-200107200-00046.

Campbell, I. G. (2009). EEG recording and analysis for sleep research. *Current Protocols in Neuroscience/Editorial Board*. https://doi.org/10.1002/0471142301.ns1002s49. Jacqueline N. Crawley … [et al.], CHAPTER, Unit10.2.

Canellas, F., Lin, L., Julià, M. R., Clemente, A., Vives-Bauza, C., Ollila, H. M., … Mignot, E. (2014). Dual cases of type 1 narcolepsy with schizophrenia and other psychotic disorders. *Journal of Clinical Sleep Medicine*, *10*(9), 1011–1018. https://doi.org/10.5664/jcsm.4040.

Caspi, A., & Moffitt, T. E. (2018). All for one and one for all: Mental disorders in one dimension. *American Journal of Psychiatry*, *175*(9), 831–844. https://doi.org/10.1176/appi.ajp.2018.17121383.

Castro-Zaballa, S., Cavelli, M. L., Gonzalez, J., Nardi, A. E., Machado, S., Scorza, C., & Torterolo, P. (2019). EEG 40 Hz coherence decreases in REM sleep and ketamine model of psychosis. *Frontiers in Psychiatry*, *9*. https://doi.org/10.3389/fpsyt.2018.00766.

Cavalier, Y., & Kothare, S. V. (2018). The association of schizophrenia and narcolepsy in adolescents. *Pediatric Neurology*, *83*, 56–57. https://doi.org/10.1016/j.pediatrneurol.2018.01.001.

Chan, M.-S., Chung, K.-F., Yung, K.-P., & Yeung, W.-F. (2017). Sleep in schizophrenia: A systematic review and meta-analysis of polysomnographic findings in case-control studies. *Sleep Medicine Reviews*, *32*, 69–84. https://doi.org/10.1016/j.smrv.2016.03.001.

Chatburn, A., Kohler, M. J., Payne, J. D., & Drummond, S. P. A. (2017). The effects of sleep restriction and sleep deprivation in producing false memories. *Neurobiology of Learning and Memory*, *137*, 107–113. https://doi.org/10.1016/j.nlm.2016.11.017.

Chesson, A. L., Ferber, R. A., Fry, J. M., Grigg-Damberger, M., Hartse, K. M., Hurwitz, T. D., … Sher, A. (1997). The indications for polysomnography and related procedures. *Sleep*, *20*(6), 423–487. https://doi.org/10.1093/sleep/20.6.423.

Chiu, V. W., Ree, M., Janca, A., & Waters, F. (2016). Sleep in schizophrenia: Exploring subjective experiences of sleep problems, and implications for treatment. *Psychiatric Quarterly*, *87*(4), 633–648. https://doi.org/10.1007/s11126-015-9415-x.

Chouinard, S., Poulin, J., Stip, E., & Godbout, R. (2004). Sleep in untreated patients with schizophrenia: A meta-analysis. *Schizophrenia Bulletin*, *30*(4), 957–967. https://doi.org/10.1093/oxfordjournals.schbul.a007145.

Chung, K.-F., Poon, Y. P. Y.-P., Ng, T.-K., & Kan, C.-K. (2018). Correlates of sleep irregularity in schizophrenia. *Psychiatry Research*, *270*, 705–714. https://doi.org/10.1016/j.psychres.2018.10.064.

Colten, H. R., Altevogt, B. M., & Institute of Medicine (US) Committee on Sleep Medicine and Research. (2006). *Sleep physiology*. National Academies Press (US). https://www.ncbi.nlm.nih.gov/books/NBK19956/.

Comasco, E., Gulinello, M., Hellgren, C., Skalkidou, A., Sylven, S., & Sundström-Poromaa, I. (2016). Sleep duration, depression, and oxytocinergic genotype influence prepulse inhibition of the startle reflex in postpartum women. *European Neuropsychopharmacology*, *26*(4), 767–776. https://doi.org/10.1016/j.euroneuro.2016.01.002.

Corlett, P. R., Simons, J. S., Pigott, J., Gardner, J. M., Murray, G. K., Krystal, J. H., & Fletcher, P. C. (2009). Illusions and delusions: Relating experimentally-induced false memories to anomalous experiences and ideas. *Frontiers in Behavioral Neuroscience*, *3*. https://doi.org/10.3389/neuro.08.053.2009.

Cosgrave, J., Wulff, K., & Gehrman, P. (2018). Sleep, circadian rhythms, and schizophrenia: Where we are and where we need to go. *Current Opinion in Psychiatry*, *31*(3), 176–182. https://doi.org/10.1097/YCO.0000000000000419.

Coulon, N., Brailly-Tabard, S., Walter, M., & Tordjman, S. (2016). Altered circadian patterns of salivary cortisol in individuals with schizophrenia: A critical literature review. *Journal of Physiology, Paris*, *110*(4, Part B), 439–447. https://doi.org/10.1016/j.jphysparis.2017.05.002.

Couyoumdjian, A., Sdoia, S., Tempesta, D., Curcio, G., Rastellini, E., Gennaro, L. D., & Ferrara, M. (2010). The effects of sleep and sleep deprivation on task-switching performance. *Journal of Sleep Research*, *19*(1-Part-I), 64–70. https://doi.org/10.1111/j.1365-2869.2009.00774.x.

D'Agostino, A., Castelnovo, A., Cavallotti, S., Casetta, C., Marcatili, M., Gambini, O., … Sarasso, S. (2018). Sleep endophenotypes of schizophrenia: Slow waves and sleep spindles in unaffected first-degree relatives. *NPJ Schizophrenia*, *4*(1). https://doi.org/10.1038/s41537-018-0045-9.

Dickinson, D. L., & Drummond, S. P. A. (2008). The effects of total sleep deprivation on Bayesian updating. *Judgment and Decision making*, *3*(2), 10.

Diekelmann, S., Born, J., & Wagner, U. (2010). Sleep enhances false memories depending on general memory performance. *Behavioural Brain Research*, *208*(2), 425–429. https://doi.org/10.1016/j.bbr.2009.12.021.

Diekelmann, S., Landolt, H.-P., Lahl, O., Born, J., & Wagner, U. (2008). Sleep loss produces false memories. *PLoS One*, *3*(10). https://doi.org/10.1371/journal.pone.0003512, e3512.

Ditman, T., & Kuperberg, G. R. (2005). A source-monitoring account of auditory verbal hallucinations in patients with schizophrenia. *Harvard Review of Psychiatry*, *13*(5), 280–299. https://doi.org/10.1080/10673220500326391.

Dresler, M., Wehrle, R., Spoormaker, V. I., Steiger, A., Holsboer, F., Czisch, M., & Hobson, J. A. (2015). Neural correlates of insight in dreaming and psychosis. *Sleep Medicine Reviews*, *20*, 92–99. https://doi.org/10.1016/j.smrv.2014.06.004.

Economo, C. V. (1930). Sleep as a problem of localization. *The Journal of Nervous and Mental Disease*, *71*(3), 249–259. https://doi.org/10.1097/00005053-193003000-00001.

Edinger, J. D., & Krystal, A. D. (2003). Subtyping primary insomnia: Is sleep state misperception a distinct clinical entity? *Sleep Medicine Reviews*, *7*(3), 203–214. https://doi.org/10.1053/smrv.2002.0253.

Faulkner, S. M., Bee, P. E., Meyer, N., Dijk, D.-J., & Drake, R. J. (2019). Light therapies to improve sleep in intrinsic circadian rhythm sleep disorders and neuro-psychiatric illness: A systematic review and meta-analysis. *Sleep Medicine Reviews*, *46*, 108–123. https://doi.org/10.1016/j.smrv.2019.04.012.

Fenn, K. M., Gallo, D. A., Margoliash, D., Roediger, H. L., & Nusbaum, H. C. (2009). Reduced false memory after sleep. *Learning & Memory*, *16*(9), 509–513. https://doi.org/10.1101/lm.1500808.

Ferrarelli, F., & Tononi, G. (2016). What are sleep spindle deficits telling us about schizophrenia? *Biological Psychiatry*, *80*(8), 577–578. https://doi.org/10.1016/j.biopsych.2016.08.012.

Fortuyn, H. A. D., Lappenschaar, G. A., Nienhuis, F. J., Furer, J. W., Hodiamont, P. P., Rijnders, C. A., … Overeem, S. (2009). Psychotic symptoms in narcolepsy: Phenomenology and a comparison with schizophrenia. *General Hospital Psychiatry*, *31*(2), 146–154. https://doi.org/10.1016/j.genhosppsych.2008.12.002.

Frank, M. G., & Benington, J. H. (2006). The role of sleep in memory consolidation and brain plasticity: Dream or reality? *The Neuroscientist*, *12*(6), 477–488. https://doi.org/10.1177/1073858406293552.

Frau, R., Orrù, M., Puligheddu, M., Gessa, G. L., Mereu, G., Marrosu, F., & Bortolato, M. (2008). Sleep deprivation disrupts prepulse inhibition of the startle reflex: Reversal by antipsychotic drugs. *International Journal of Neuropsychopharmacology*, *11*(7), 947–955. https://doi.org/10.1017/S1461145708008900.

Freeman, D. (2007). Suspicious minds: The psychology of persecutory delusions. *Clinical Psychology Review*, *27*(4), 425–457. https://doi.org/10.1016/j.cpr.2006.10.004.

Freeman, D. (2016). Persecutory delusions: A cognitive perspective on understanding and treatment. *The Lancet Psychiatry*, *3*(7), 685–692. https://doi.org/10.1016/S2215-0366(16)00066-3.

Freeman, D., Pugh, K., Vorontsova, N., & Southgate, L. (2009). Insomnia and paranoia. *Schizophrenia Research*, *108*(1), 280–284. https://doi.org/10.1016/j.schres.2008.12.001.

Freeman, D., Sheaves, B., Goodwin, G. M., Yu, L.-M., Nickless, A., Harrison, P. J., … Espie, C.A. (2017). The effects of improving sleep on mental health (OASIS): A randomised controlled trial with mediation analysis. *The Lancet Psychiatry*, *4*(10), 749–758. https://doi.org/10.1016/S2215-0366(17)30328-0.

Freeman, D., Waite, F., Startup, H., Myers, E., Lister, R., McInerney, J., … Yu, L.-M. (2015). Efficacy of cognitive behavioural therapy for sleep improvement in patients with persistent delusions and hallucinations (BEST): A prospective, assessor-blind, randomised controlled pilot trial. *The Lancet Psychiatry*, *2*(11), 975–983. https://doi.org/10.1016/S2215-0366(15)00314-4.

Frenda, S. J., Patihis, L., Loftus, E. F., Lewis, H. C., & Fenn, K. M. (2014). Sleep deprivation and false memories. *Psychological Science*, *25*(9), 1674–1681. https://doi.org/10.1177/0956797614534694.

Fultz, N. E., Bonmassar, G., Setsompop, K., Stickgold, R. A., Rosen, B. R., Polimeni, J. R., & Lewis, L. D. (2019). Coupled electrophysiological, hemodynamic, and cerebrospinal fluid oscillations in human sleep. *Science*, *366*(6465), 628–631. https://doi.org/10.1126/science.aax5440.

Garety, P., Joyce, E., Jolley, S., Emsley, R., Waller, H., Kuipers, E., … Freeman, D. (2013). Neuropsychological functioning and jumping to conclusions in delusions. *Schizophrenia Research*, *150*(2), 570–574. https://doi.org/10.1016/j.schres.2013.08.035.

Goines, K. B., LoPilato, A. M., Addington, J., Bearden, C. E., Cadenhead, K. S., Cannon, T. D., … Walker, E. F. (2019). Sleep problems and attenuated psychotic symptoms in youth at clinical high-risk for psychosis. *Psychiatry Research*, *282*, 112492. https://doi.org/10.1016/j.psychres.2019.112492.

Griffin, J. D., & Fletcher, P. C. (2017). Predictive processing, source monitoring, and psychosis. *Annual Review of Clinical Psychology*, *13*, 265–289. https://doi.org/10.1146/annurev-clinpsy-032816-045145.

Gupta, R., Dahiya, S., & Bhatia, M. S. (2009). Effect of depression on sleep: Qualitative or quantitative? *Indian Journal of Psychiatry*, *51*(2), 117–121. https://doi.org/10.4103/0019-5545.49451.

Harrison, Y., & Horne, J. A. (1999). One night of sleep loss impairs innovative thinking and flexible decision making. *Organizational Behavior and Human Decision Processes*, *78*(2), 128–145. https://doi.org/10.1006/obhd.1999.2827.

Hennig, T., Schlier, B., & Lincoln, T. M. (2019). Sleep and psychotic symptoms: An actigraphy and diary study with young adults with low and elevated psychosis proneness. *Schizophrenia Research*. https://doi.org/10.1016/j.schres.2019.09.012.

Hirshkowitz, M., Whiton, K., Albert, S. M., Alessi, C., Bruni, O., DonCarlos, L., … Adams Hillard, P. J. (2015). National Sleep Foundation's sleep time duration recommendations: Methodology and results summary. *Sleep Health*, *1*(1), 40–43. https://doi.org/10.1016/j.sleh.2014.12.010.

Hobson, J. A. (2009). REM sleep and dreaming: Towards a theory of protoconsciousness. *Nature Reviews Neuroscience*, *10*(11), 803–813. https://doi.org/10.1038/nrn2716.

Hori, T., Sugita, Y., Koga, E., Shirakawa, S., Inoue, K., Uchida, S., … Fukuda, N. (2001). Proposed supplements and amendments to 'A Manual of Standardized Terminology, Techniques and Scoring System for Sleep Stages of Human Subjects', the Rechtschaffen & Kales (1968) standard. *Psychiatry and Clinical Neurosciences*, *55*(3), 305–310. https://doi.org/10.1046/j.1440-1819.2001.00810.x.

Howes, O. D., & Kapur, S. (2009). The dopamine hypothesis of schizophrenia: version III—The final common pathway. *Schizophrenia Bulletin*, *35*(3), 549–562. https://doi.org/10.1093/schbul/sbp006.

Humpston, C. S., Linden, D. E. J., & Evans, L. H. (2017). Deficits in reality and internal source monitoring of actions are associated with the positive dimension of schizotypy. *Psychiatry Research*, *250*, 44–49. https://doi.org/10.1016/j.psychres.2017.01.063.

ICD-10. (2011). *International statistical classification of diseases and related health problems*. World Health Organization.

Ji, X., & Liu, J. (2016). Subjective sleep measures for adolescents: A systematic review. *Child: Care, Health and Development*, *42*(6), 825–839. https://doi.org/10.1111/cch.12376.

Johansson, A.-S., Owe-Larsson, B., Hetta, J., & Lundkvist, G. B. (2016). Altered circadian clock gene expression in patients with schizophrenia. *Schizophrenia Research*, *174*(1), 17–23. https://doi.org/10.1016/j.schres.2016.04.029.

Joiner, W. J. (2016). Unraveling the evolutionary determinants of sleep. *Current Biology*, *26*(20), R1073–R1087. https://doi.org/10.1016/j.cub.2016.08.068.

Kahn, D., Pace-Schott, E. F., & Hobson, J. A. (1997). Consciousness in waking and dreaming: The roles of neuronal oscillation and neuromodulation in determining similarities and differences. *Neuroscience*, *78*, 13–38.

Kaskie, R. E., Gill, K. M., & Ferrarelli, F. (2019). Reduced frontal slow wave density during sleep in first-episode psychosis. *Schizophrenia Research*, *206*, 318–324. https://doi.org/10.1016/j.schres.2018.10.024.

Kaskie, R., Graziano, B., & Ferrarelli, F. (2017). Schizophrenia and sleep disorders: Links, risks, and management challenges. *Nature and Science of Sleep*, *9*, 227–239. https://doi.org/10.2147/NSS.S121076.

Keshavan, M. S., Montrose, D. M., Miewald, J. M., & Jindal, R. D. (2011). Sleep correlates of cognition in early course psychotic disorders. *Schizophrenia Research*, *131*(1), 231–234. https://doi.org/10.1016/j.schres.2011.05.027.

Kobayashi, I., Boarts, J. M., & Delahanty, D. L. (2007). Polysomnographically measured sleep abnormalities in PTSD: A meta-analytic review. *Psychophysiology*, *44*(4), 660–669. https://doi.org/10.1111/j.1469-8986.2007.537.x.

Koffel, E., & Watson, D. (2009). Unusual sleep experiences, dissociation, and schizotypy: Evidence for a common domain. *Clinical Psychology Review*, *29*(6), 548–559. https://doi.org/10.1016/j.cpr.2009.06.004.

Kohl, S., Heekeren, K., Klosterkötter, J., & Kuhn, J. (2013). Prepulse inhibition in psychiatric disorders—Apart from schizophrenia. *Journal of Psychiatric Research*, *47*(4), 445–452. https://doi.org/10.1016/j.jpsychires.2012.11.018.

Kondratova, A. A., & Kondratov, R. V. (2012). The circadian clock and pathology of the ageing brain. *Nature Reviews Neuroscience*, *13*(5), 325–335. https://doi.org/10.1038/nrn3208.

Krystal, A. D. (2015). New developments in insomnia medications of relevance to mental health disorders. *The Psychiatric Clinics of North America*, *38*(4), 843–860. https://doi.org/10.1016/j.psc.2015.08.001.

Krystal, A. D., & Edinger, J. D. (2008). Measuring sleep quality. *Sleep Medicine*, *9*, S10–S17. https://doi.org/10.1016/S1389-9457(08)70011-X.

Kumari, V., Das, M., Zachariah, E., Ettinger, U., & Sharma, T. (2005). Reduced prepulse inhibition in unaffected siblings of schizophrenia patients. *Psychophysiology*, *42*(5), 588–594. https://doi.org/10.1111/j.1469-8986.2005.00346.x.

Laws, K. R., & Bhatt, R. (2005). False memories and delusional ideation in normal healthy subjects. *Personality and Individual Differences*, *39*(4), 775–781. https://doi.org/10.1016/j.paid.2005.03.005.

Lemyre, A., Bastien, C., & Vallières, A. (2019). Nightmares in mental disorders: A review. *Dreaming*, *29*(2), 144–166. https://doi.org/10.1037/drm0000103.

Li, S. X., Lam, S. P., Zhang, J., Yu, M. W. M., Chan, J. W. Y., Chan, C. S. Y., … Wing, Y.-K. (2016). Sleep disturbances and suicide risk in an 8-year longitudinal study of schizophrenia-spectrum disorders. *Sleep*, *39*(6), 1275–1282. https://doi.org/10.5665/sleep.5852.

Lim, J., & Dinges, D. F. (2010). A meta-analysis of the impact of short-term sleep deprivation on cognitive variables. *Psychological Bulletin*, *136*(3), 375–389. https://doi.org/10.1037/a0018883.

Littner, M., Hirshkowitz, M., Kramer, M., Kapen, S., Anderson, W. M., Bailey, D., … Woodson, B. T. (2003). Practice parameters for using polysomnography to evaluate insomnia: An update. *Sleep*, *26*(6), 754–760. https://doi.org/10.1093/sleep/26.6.754.

Lo, J. C., Chong, P. L. H., Ganesan, S., Leong, R. L. F., & Chee, M. W. L. (2016). Sleep deprivation increases formation of false memory. *Journal of Sleep Research*, *25*(6), 673–682. https://doi.org/10.1111/jsr.12436.

Ludewig, K., Geyer, M. A., Etzensberger, M., & Vollenweider, F. X. (2002). Stability of the acoustic startle reflex, prepulse inhibition, and habituation in schizophrenia. *Schizophrenia Research*, *55*(1), 129–137. https://doi.org/10.1016/S0920-9964(01)00198-0.

Lunsford-Avery, J. R., da Silva Brandão Gonçalves, B., Brietzke, E., Bressan, R. A., Gadelha, A., Auerbach, R. P., & Mittal, V. A. (2017). Adolescents at clinical-high risk for psychosis: Circadian rhythm disturbances predict worsened prognosis at 1-year follow-up. *Schizophrenia Research*, *189*, 37–42. https://doi.org/10.1016/j.schres.2017.01.051.

Lunsford-Avery, J. R., & Mittal, V. A. (2013). Sleep dysfunction prior to the onset of schizophrenia: A review and neurodevelopmental diathesis–stress conceptualization. *Clinical Psychology: Science and Practice*, *20*(3), 291–320. https://doi.org/10.1111/cpsp.12041.

Mahowald, M., Cramer Bornemann, M., & Schenck, C. (2011). State dissociation, human behavior, and consciousness. *Current Topics in Medicinal Chemistry*, *11*, 2392–2402. https://doi.org/10.2174/156802611797470277.

Mammarella, N., Altamura, M., Padalino, F. A., Petito, A., Fairfield, B., & Bellomo, A. (2010). False memories in schizophrenia? An imagination inflation study. *Psychiatry Research*, *179*(3), 267–273. https://doi.org/10.1016/j.psychres.2009.05.005.

Manoach, D. S., Pan, J. Q., Purcell, S. M., & Stickgold, R. (2016). Reduced sleep spindles in schizophrenia: A treatable endophenotype that links risk genes to impaired cognition? *Biological Psychiatry*, *80*(8), 599–608. https://doi.org/10.1016/j.biopsych.2015.10.003.

McCoy, J. G., Tartar, J. L., Bebis, A. C., Ward, C. P., McKenna, J. T., Baxter, M. G., … Strecker, R. E. (2007). Experimental sleep fragmentation impairs attentional set-shifting in rats. *Sleep*, *30*(1), 52–60. https://doi.org/10.1093/sleep/30.1.52.

Miyagawa, T., & Tokunaga, K. (2019). Genetics of narcolepsy. *Human Genome Variation*, *6*. https://doi.org/10.1038/s41439-018-0033-7.

Monti, J. M., BaHammam, A. S., Pandi-Perumal, S. R., Bromundt, V., Spence, D. W., Cardinali, D. P., & Brown, G. M. (2013). Sleep and circadian rhythm dysregulation in schizophrenia. *Progress in Neuro-Psychopharmacology and Biological Psychiatry*, *43*, 209–216. https://doi.org/10.1016/j.pnpbp.2012.12.021.

Monti, J. M., & Monti, D. (2004). Sleep in schizophrenia patients and the effects of antipsychotic drugs. *Sleep Medicine Reviews*, *8*(2), 133–148. https://doi.org/10.1016/S1087-0792(02)00158-2.

Montplaisir, J., Gagnon, J.-F., Fantini, M. L., Postuma, R. B., Dauvilliers, Y., Desautels, A., … Paquet, J. (2010). Polysomnographic diagnosis of idiopathic REM sleep behavior disorder. *Movement Disorders*, *25*(13), 2044–2051. https://doi.org/10.1002/mds.23257.

Moritz, S., Woodward, T. S., Jelinek, L., & Klinge, R. (2008). Memory and metamemory in schizophrenia: A liberal acceptance account of psychosis. *Psychological Medicine*, *38*(6), 825–832. https://doi.org/10.1017/S0033291707002553.

Moser, D., Anderer, P., Gruber, G., Parapatics, S., Loretz, E., Boeck, M., … Dorffner, G. (2009). Sleep classification according to AASM and Rechtschaffen & Kales: Effects on sleep scoring parameters. *Sleep*, *32*(2), 139–149.

Mota, N. B., Resende, A., Mota-Rolim, S. A., Copelli, M., & Ribeiro, S. (2016). Psychosis and the control of lucid dreaming. *Frontiers in Psychology*, *7*. https://doi.org/10.3389/fpsyg.2016.00294.

Mulligan, L. D., Haddock, G., Emsley, R., Neil, S. T., & Kyle, S. D. (2016). High resolution examination of the role of sleep disturbance in predicting functioning and psychotic symptoms in schizophrenia: A novel experience sampling study. *Journal of Abnormal Psychology*, *125*(6), 788–797. https://doi.org/10.1037/abn0000180.

Muzet, A. (2005). Alteration of sleep microstructure in psychiatric disorders. *Dialogues in Clinical Neuroscience*, *7*(4), 315–321.

Nielsen, T. A., & Stenstrom, P. (2005). What are the memory sources of dreaming? *Nature*, *437*(7063), 1286–1289. https://doi.org/10.1038/nature04288.

Noreika, V., Valli, K., Lahtela, H., & Revonsuo, A. (2009). Early-night serial awakenings as a new paradigm for studies on NREM dreaming. *International Journal of Psychophysiology*, *74*(1), 14–18. https://doi.org/10.1016/j.ijpsycho.2009.06.002.

Oh, S. M., Lee, Y. J., Kim, J. W., Choi, J. W., & Jeong, D.-U. (2017). Preliminary study on quantitative sleep EEG characteristics in patients with schizophrenia. *Psychiatry Investigation*, *14*(2), 219–225. https://doi.org/10.4306/pi.2017.14.2.219.

Ohayon, M. M., Carskadon, M. A., Guilleminault, C., & Vitiello, M. V. (2004). Meta-analysis of quantitative sleep parameters from childhood to old age in healthy individuals: Developing normative sleep values across the human lifespan. *Sleep*, *27*(7), 1255–1273. https://doi.org/10.1093/sleep/27.7.1255.

Pail, G., Huf, W., Pjrek, E., Winkler, D., Willeit, M., Praschak-Rieder, N., & Kasper, S. (2011). Bright-light therapy in the treatment of mood disorders. *Neuropsychobiology*, *64*(3), 152–162. https://doi.org/10.1159/000328950.

Peters, M. J. V., Smeets, T., Giesbrecht, T., Jelicic, M., & Merckelbach, H. (2007). Confusing action and imagination: Action source monitoring in individuals with schizotypal traits. *The Journal of Nervous and Mental Disease*, *195*(9), 752–757. https://doi.org/10.1097/NMD.0b013e318142cc02.

Petrovsky, N., Ettinger, U., Hill, A., Frenzel, L., Meyhöfer, I., Wagner, M., ... Kumari, V. (2014). Sleep deprivation disrupts prepulse inhibition and induces psychosis-like symptoms in healthy humans. *Journal of Neuroscience*, *34*(27), 9134–9140. https://doi.org/10.1523/JNEUROSCI.0904-14.2014.

Polner, B., Faiola, E., Urquijo, M. F., Meyhöfer, I., Steffens, M., Rónai, L., ... Ettinger, U. (2019). The network structure of schizotypy in the general population. *European Archives of Psychiatry and Clinical Neuroscience*. https://doi.org/10.1007/s00406-019-01078-x.

Purcell, S. M., Manoach, D. S., Demanuele, C., Cade, B. E., Mariani, S., Cox, R., ... Stickgold, R. (2017). Characterizing sleep spindles in 11,630 individuals from the National Sleep Research Resource. *Nature Communications*, *8*(1), 1–16. https://doi.org/10.1038/ncomms15930.

Reeve, S., Emsley, R., Sheaves, B., & Freeman, D. (2017). Disrupting sleep: The effects of sleep loss on psychotic experiences tested in an experimental study with mediation analysis. *Schizophrenia Bulletin*. https://doi.org/10.1093/schbul/sbx103.

Reeve, S., Emsley, R., Sheaves, B., & Freeman, D. (2018). Disrupting sleep: The effects of sleep loss on psychotic experiences tested in an experimental study with mediation analysis. *Schizophrenia Bulletin*, *44*(3), 662–671. https://doi.org/10.1093/schbul/sbx103.

Reeve, S., Sheaves, B., & Freeman, D. (2019). Sleep disorders in early psychosis: Incidence, severity, and association with clinical symptoms. *Schizophrenia Bulletin*, *45*(2), 287–295. https://doi.org/10.1093/schbul/sby129.

Riemann, D., Baglioni, C., Bassetti, C., Bjorvatn, B., Dolenc Groselj, L., Ellis, J. G., ... Spiegelhalder, K. (2017). European guideline for the diagnosis and treatment of insomnia. *Journal of Sleep Research*, *26*(6), 675–700. https://doi.org/10.1111/jsr.12594.

Robertson, I., Cheung, A., & Fan, X. (2019). Insomnia in patients with schizophrenia: Current understanding and treatment options. *Progress in Neuro-Psychopharmacology and Biological Psychiatry*, *92*, 235–242. https://doi.org/10.1016/j.pnpbp.2019.01.016.

Roediger, H. L., & McDermott, K. B. (1995). Creating false memories: Remembering words not presented in lists. *Journal of Experimental Psychology: Learning, Memory, and Cognition*, *21*(4), 803–814. https://doi.org/10.1037/0278-7393.21.4.803.

Roehrs, T. (2000). Sleep physiology and pathophysiology. *Clinical Cornerstone*, *2*(5), 1–12. https://doi.org/10.1016/S1098-3597(00)90036-X.

Roth, T., & Roehrs, T. (2003). Insomnia: Epidemiology, characteristics, and consequences. *Clinical Cornerstone*, *5*(3), 5–15. https://doi.org/10.1016/S1098-3597(03)90031-7.

Salin-Pascual, R. J., Roehrs, T. A., Merlotti, L. A., Zorick, F., & Roth, T. (1992). Long-term study of the sleep of insomnia patients with sleep state misperception and other insomnia patients. *The American Journal of Psychiatry*, *149*(7), 904–908. https://doi.org/10.1176/ajp.149.7.904.

Sansa, G., Gavaldà, A., Gaig, C., Monreal, J., Ercilla, G., Casamitjana, R., ... Santamaria, J. (2016). Exploring the presence of narcolepsy in patients with schizophrenia. *BMC Psychiatry*, *16*. https://doi.org/10.1186/s12888-016-0859-9.

Saper, C. B., Chou, T. C., & Scammell, T. E. (2001). The sleep switch: Hypothalamic control of sleep and wakefulness. *Trends in Neurosciences*, *24*(12), 726–731. https://doi.org/10.1016/S0166-2236(00)02002-6.

Sarkanen, T., Niemel, Ã. V., Landtblom, A.-M., & Partinen, M. (2014). Psychosis in patients with narcolepsy as an adverse effect of sodium oxybate. *Frontiers in Neurology*, *5*. https://doi.org/10.3389/fneur.2014.00136.

Sasidharan, A., Kumar, S., Nair, A. K., Lukose, A., Marigowda, V., John, J. P., & Kutty, B. M. (2017). Further evidences for sleep instability and impaired spindle-delta dynamics in schizophrenia: A whole-night polysomnography study with neuroloop-gain and sleep-cycle analysis. *Sleep Medicine*, *38*, 1–13. https://doi.org/10.1016/j.sleep.2017.02.009.

Sateia, M. J. (2014). International classification of sleep disorders-third edition. *Chest*, *146*(5), 1387–1394. https://doi.org/10.1378/chest.14-0970.

Scarone, S., Manzone, M. L., Gambini, O., Kantzas, I., Limosani, I., D'Agostino, A., & Hobson, J. A. (2008). The dream as a model for psychosis: An experimental approach using bizarreness as a cognitive marker. *Schizophrenia Bulletin*, *34*(3), 515–522. https://doi.org/10.1093/schbul/sbm116.

Schmidt, C., Collette, F., Cajochen, C., & Peigneux, P. (2007). A time to think: Circadian rhythms in human cognition. *Cognitive Neuropsychology*, *24*(7), 755–789. https://doi.org/10.1080/02643290701754158.

Schutte-Rodin, S. (2008). Clinical guideline for the evaluation and management of chronic insomnia in adults. *Journal of Clinical Sleep Medicine*, *4*(5), 19.

Scott, A. J., Rowse, G., & Webb, T. L. (2017). A structural equation model of the relationship between insomnia, negative affect, and paranoid thinking. *PLoS One*, *12*(10). https://doi.org/10.1371/journal.pone.0186233.

Seney, M. L., Cahill, K., Enwright, J. F., Logan, R. W., Huo, Z., Zong, W., … McClung, C. A. (2019). Diurnal rhythms in gene expression in the prefrontal cortex in schizophrenia. *Nature Communications*, *10*(1), 1–11. https://doi.org/10.1038/s41467-019-11335-1.

Sharma, V., & Mazmanian, D. (2003). Sleep loss and postpartum psychosis. *Bipolar Disorders*, *5*(2), 98–105. https://doi.org/10.1034/j.1399-5618.2003.00015.x.

Sheaves, B., Onwumere, J., Keen, N., Stahl, D., & Kuipers, E. (2015). Nightmares in patients with psychosis: The relation with sleep, psychotic, affective, and cognitive symptoms. *The Canadian Journal of Psychiatry*, *60*(8), 354–361. https://doi.org/10.1177/070674371506000804.

Shrivastava, D., Jung, S., Saadat, M., Sirohi, R., & Crewson, K. (2014). How to interpret the results of a sleep study. *Journal of Community Hospital Internal Medicine Perspectives*, *4*(5), 24983. https://doi.org/10.3402/jchimp.v4.24983.

Silber, M. H., Ancoli-Israel, S., Bonnet, M. H., Chokroverty, S., Grigg-Damberger, M. M., Hirshkowitz, M., … Iber, C. (2007). The visual scoring of sleep in adults. *Journal of Clinical Sleep Medicine*, *3*(2), 121–131.

Simon, E. B., Rossi, A., Harvey, A. G., & Walker, M. P. (2019). Overanxious and underslept. *Nature Human Behaviour*, 1–11. https://doi.org/10.1038/s41562-019-0754-8.

Simor, P., Báthori, N., Nagy, T., & Polner, B. (2019). Poor sleep quality predicts psychotic-like symptoms: An experience sampling study in young adults with schizotypal traits. *Acta Psychiatrica Scandinavica*, *140*(2), 135–146. https://doi.org/10.1111/acps.13064.

Simor, P., Krietsch, K. N., Köteles, F., & McCrae, C. S. (2015). Day-to-day variation of subjective sleep quality and emotional states among healthy university students—A 1-week prospective study. *International Journal of Behavioral Medicine*, *22*(5), 625–634. https://doi.org/10.1007/s12529-015-9464-4.

Sterzer, P., Adams, R. A., Fletcher, P., Frith, C., Lawrie, S. M., Muckli, L., … Corlett, P. R. (2018). The predictive coding account of psychosis. *Biological Psychiatry*, *84*(9), 634–643. https://doi.org/10.1016/j.biopsych.2018.05.015.

Stickgold, R. (2001). Sleep, learning, and dreams: Off-line memory reprocessing. *Science*, *294*(5544), 1052–1057. https://doi.org/10.1126/science.1063530.

Sutton, E. L. (2014). Insomnia. *Medical Clinics of North America*, *98*(3), 565–581. https://doi.org/10.1016/j.mcna.2014.01.008.

Swerdlow, N. R., Light, G. A., Sprock, J., Calkins, M. E., Green, M. F., Greenwood, T. A., ... Braff, D.L. (2014). Deficient prepulse inhibition in schizophrenia detected by the multi-site COGS. *Schizophrenia Research, 152*(2), 503–512. https://doi.org/10.1016/j.schres.2013.12.004.

Swihart, B. J., Caffo, B., Bandeen-Roche, K., & Punjabi, N. M. (2008). Characterizing sleep structure using the hypnogram. *Journal of Clinical Sleep Medicine, 4*(4), 349–355.

Thorpy, M. (2017). International classification of sleep disorders. In S. Chokroverty (Ed.), *Sleep disorders medicine* (pp. 475–484). New York: Springer. https://doi.org/10.1007/978-1-4939-6578-6_27.

Tinguely, G., Finelli, L. A., Landolt, H.-P., Borbély, A. A., & Achermann, P. (2006). Functional EEG topography in sleep and waking: State-dependent and state-independent features. *NeuroImage, 32*(1), 283–292. https://doi.org/10.1016/j.neuroimage.2006.03.017.

Titus, C. E., Speed, K. J., Cartwright, P. M., Drapeau, C. W., Heo, Y., & Nadorff, M. R. (2018). What role do nightmares play in suicide? A brief exploration. *Current Opinion in Psychology, 22*, 59–62. https://doi.org/10.1016/j.copsyc.2017.08.022.

Tobler, I. (1995). Is sleep fundamentally different between mammalian species? *Behavioural Brain Research, 69*(1), 35–41. https://doi.org/10.1016/0166-4328(95)00025-O.

Uhlig, B. L., Hagen, K., Engstrøm, M., Stjern, M., Gravdahl, G. B., & Sand, T. (2019). The relationship between obstructive sleep apnea and insomnia: A population-based cross-sectional polysomnographic study. *Sleep Medicine, 54*, 126–133. https://doi.org/10.1016/j.sleep.2018.10.026.

Vinogradov, S., Willis-Shore, J., Poole, J. H., Marten, E., Ober, B. A., & Shenaut, G. K. (1997). Clinical and neurocognitive aspects of source monitoring errors in schizophrenia. *American Journal of Psychiatry, 154*(11), 1530–1537. https://doi.org/10.1176/ajp.154.11.1530.

Walker, M. P. (2009). The role of sleep in cognition and emotion. *Annals of the New York Academy of Sciences, 1156*(1), 168–197. https://doi.org/10.1111/j.1749-6632.2009.04416.x.

Walker, M. P., & van der Helm, E. (2009). Overnight therapy? The role of sleep in emotional brain processing. *Psychological Bulletin, 135*(5), 731–748. https://doi.org/10.1037/a0016570.

Walterfang, M., Upjohn, E., & Velakoulis, D. (2005). Is schizophrenia associated with narcolepsy? *Cognitive and Behavioral Neurology, 18*(2), 113–118. https://doi.org/10.1097/01.wnn.0000160822.53577.2c.

Wamsley, E. J., Shinn, A. K., Tucker, M. A., Ono, K. E., McKinley, S. K., Ely, A. V., ... Manoach, D. S. (2013). The effects of eszopiclone on sleep spindles and memory consolidation in schizophrenia: A randomized placebo-controlled trial. *Sleep, 36*(9), 1369–1376. https://doi.org/10.5665/sleep.2968.

Wamsley, E. J., Tucker, M., Payne, J. D., Benavides, J. A., & Stickgold, R. (2010). Dreaming of a learning task is associated with enhanced sleep-dependent memory consolidation. *Current Biology, 20*(9), 850–855. https://doi.org/10.1016/j.cub.2010.03.027.

Ward, T., & Garety, P. A. (2019). Fast and slow thinking in distressing delusions: A review of the literature and implications for targeted therapy. *Schizophrenia Research, 203*, 80–87. https://doi.org/10.1016/j.schres.2017.08.045.

Waters, F. (2012). Sleep dysfunctions in schizophrenia: A practical review. *Open Journal of Psychiatry, 02*, 384–392. https://doi.org/10.4236/ojpsych.2012.224054.

Waters, F., Blom, J. D., Dang-Vu, T. T., Cheyne, A. J., Alderson-Day, B., Woodruff, P., & Collerton, D. (2016). What is the link between hallucinations, dreams, and hypnagogic–hypnopompic experiences? *Schizophrenia Bulletin, 42*(5), 1098–1109. https://doi.org/10.1093/schbul/sbw076.

Watson, D. (2001). Dissociations of the night: Individual differences in sleep-related experiences and their relation to dissociation and schizotypy. *Journal of Abnormal Psychology, 110*(4), 526–535. https://doi.org/10.1037/0021-843X.110.4.526.

Weike, A. I., Bauer, U., & Hamm, A. O. (2000). Effective neuroleptic medication removes prepulse inhibition deficits in schizophrenia patients. *Biological Psychiatry*, *47*(1), 61–70. https://doi.org/10.1016/S0006-3223(99)00229-2.

Werner, K. B., Griffin, M. G., & Galovski, T. E. (2016). Objective and subjective measurement of sleep disturbance in female trauma survivors with posttraumatic stress disorder. *Psychiatry Research*, *240*, 234–240. https://doi.org/10.1016/j.psychres.2016.04.039.

Whitney, P., Hinson, J. M., Jackson, M. L., & Van Dongen, H. P. A. (2015). Feedback blunting: Total sleep deprivation impairs decision making that requires updating based on feedback. *Sleep*, *38*(5), 745–754. https://doi.org/10.5665/sleep.4668.

Wilkinson, K., & Shapiro, C. (2013). Development and validation of the nonrestorative sleep scale (NRSS). *Journal of Clinical Sleep Medicine*, *9*(9), 929–937. https://doi.org/10.5664/jcsm.2996.

Wilson, S., & Argyropoulos, S. (2012). Sleep in schizophrenia: Time for closer attention. *The British Journal of Psychiatry*, *200*(4), 273–274. https://doi.org/10.1192/bjp.bp.111.104091.

Wimmer, F., Hoffmann, R. F., Bonato, R. A., & Moffitt, A. R. (1992). The effects of sleep deprivation on divergent thinking and attention processes. *Journal of Sleep Research*, *1*(4), 223–230. https://doi.org/10.1111/j.1365-2869.1992.tb00043.x.

Woodward, T. S., Menon, M., & Whitman, J. C. (2007). Source monitoring biases and auditory hallucinations. *Cognitive Neuropsychiatry*, *12*(6), 477–494. https://doi.org/10.1080/13546800701307198.

Yang, C., & Winkelman, J. W. (2006). Clinical significance of sleep EEG abnormalities in chronic schizophrenia. *Schizophrenia Research*, *82*(2–3), 251–260. https://doi.org/10.1016/j.schres.2005.10.021.

Yates, N. J. (2016). Schizophrenia: The role of sleep and circadian rhythms in regulating dopamine and psychosis. *Reviews in the Neurosciences*, *27*(7). https://doi.org/10.1515/revneuro-2016-0030.

Zanini, M., Castro, J., Coelho, F. M., Bittencourt, L., Bressan, R. A., Tufik, S., & Brietzke, E. (2013). Do sleep abnormalities and misaligned sleep/circadian rhythm patterns represent early clinical characteristics for developing psychosis in high risk populations? *Neuroscience & Biobehavioral Reviews*, *37*(10, Part 2), 2631–2637. https://doi.org/10.1016/j.neubiorev.2013.08.012.

Zhang, L., & Zhao, Z.-X. (2007). Objective and subjective measures for sleep disorders. *Neuroscience Bulletin*, *23*(4), 236–240. https://doi.org/10.1007/s12264-007-0035-9.

Zhou, E. S., Gardiner, P., & Bertisch, S. M. (2017). Integrative medicine for insomnia. *The Medical Clinics of North America*, *101*(5), 865–879. https://doi.org/10.1016/j.mcna.2017.04.005.

Index

Note: Page numbers followed by *f* indicate figures and *t* indicate tables.

D

E

F

G

H

FSC
www.fsc.org
MIX
Papier | Fördert
gute Waldnutzung
FSC® C083411

Kolibri 360 GmbH
Ferdinand-Jühlke-Straße 7
99095 Erfurt, Deutschland
produktsicherheit@kolibri360.de